# Practical
# Diabetes Mellitus

# Practical Diabetes Mellitus

**Seventh Edition**

### Pradeep G Talwalkar
Senior Consultant Diabetologist
SL Raheja Hospital
All India Institute of Diabetes
Mumbai, Maharashtra, India
Formerly Honorary Professor of Medicine
Grant Medical College
Mumbai, Maharashtra, India

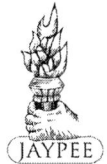

JAYPEE BROTHERS MEDICAL PUBLISHERS
*The Health Sciences Publisher*
New Delhi | London

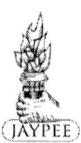 **Jaypee Brothers Medical Publishers (P) Ltd**

**Headquarters**
EMCA House
23/23-B, Ansari Road, Daryaganj
New Delhi 110 002, India
Landline: +91-11-23272143, +91-11-23272703
+91-11-23282021, +91-11-23245672
E-mail: jaypee@jaypeebrothers.com

**Corporate Office**
Jaypee Brothers Medical Publishers (P) Ltd.
4838/24, Ansari Road, Daryaganj
New Delhi 110 002, India
Phone: +91-11-43574357
Fax: +91-11-43574314
E-mail: jaypee@jaypeebrothers.com

**Overseas Office**
JP Medical Ltd.
83, Victoria Street, London
SW1H 0HW (UK)
Phone: +44-20 3170 8910
Fax: +44(0)20 3008 6180
E-mail: info@jpmedpub.com

Website: www.jaypeebrothers.com
Website: www.jaypeedigital.com

© 2023, Jaypee Brothers Medical Publishers

The views and opinions expressed in this book are solely those of the original contributor(s)/author(s) and do not necessarily represent those of editor(s) or publisher of the book.

All rights reserved. No part of this publication may be reproduced, stored or transmitted in any form or by any means, electronic, mechanical, photocopying, recording or otherwise, without the prior permission in writing of the publishers.

All brand names and product names used in this book are trade names, service marks, trademarks or registered trademarks of their respective owners. The publisher is not associated with any product or vendor mentioned in this book.

Medical knowledge and practice change constantly. This book is designed to provide accurate, authoritative information about the subject matter in question. However, readers are advised to check the most current information available on procedures included and check information from the manufacturer of each product to be administered, to verify the recommended dose, formula, method and duration of administration, adverse effects and contraindications. It is the responsibility of the practitioner to take all appropriate safety precautions. Neither the publisher nor the author(s)/editor(s) assume any liability for any injury and/or damage to persons or property arising from or related to use of material in this book.

This book is sold on the understanding that the publisher is not engaged in providing professional medical services. If such advice or services are required, the services of a competent medical professional should be sought.

Every effort has been made where necessary to contact holders of copyright to obtain permission to reproduce copyright material. If any have been inadvertently overlooked, the publisher will be pleased to make the necessary arrangements at the first opportunity.

**Inquiries for bulk sales may be solicited at:** jaypee@jaypeebrothers.com

*Practical Diabetes Mellitus / Pradeep G Talwalkar*

*Third Edition:* 2006
*Reprint,* 2006
*Fourth Edition:* 2012
*Fifth Enlarged Edition:* 2014
*Sixth Edition:* 2015
*Seventh Edition:* **2023**

ISBN: 978-93-5696-119-7

*Printed in India:*

**Dedicated to**

*My late parents
Dr Gopal Vasudeo Talvalkar* (MD)
*and
Mrs Indumati Gopal Talwalkar* (MA)

# Preface to the Seventh Edition

More than 7 years have elapsed after publishing sixth edition of *Practical Diabetes Mellitus*. During this period, prevalence of diabetes has not shown any signs of abetting, particularly in rapidly industrializing, urbanizing, and westernizing developing counties such as India. Diabesity, the duel epidemic of obesity and type 2 diabetes mellitus (T2DM) has struck the globe in the form of tsunami and has fuelled downstream epidemics of atherosclerotic cardiovascular diseases and hypertension.

However on the brighter side, significant strides have been made in understanding the pathophysiology of the disease and also in the prevention and treatment of the disease. Remission has been successfully induced in obese patients with T2DM. There has been a paradigm shift in the principles of management of diabetes from glucocentric approach to patient-centric approach with emphasis on protection of target organs such as heart and kidneys and prevention of drug-induced hypoglycemia as well as prevention and treatment of weight gain. Sodium-glucose cotransporter-2 (SGLT-2) inhibitors and glucagon-like peptide 1 receptor agonists (GLP-1 RAs) have followed dipeptidyl peptidase 4 (DPP-4) inhibitors to occupy center stage in the management of diabetes. Pharmaceutical science has translated our better understanding of pathophysiology to introduce abovementioned new classes of agents and continued further progress to give us more and more patient-friendly, safe, and effective products. About a decade ago, GLP-1 RAs were introduced in the form of twice daily subcutaneous injection, now we have two well established once a week injections as well as oral GLP-1 RA. Rapid strides have been made in surgical techniques of bariatric surgery and there has been a significant increase in number of surgeries performed at various specialized centers across the globe, including in India.

Around the end of first decade of 20th century, when cardiovascular outcome studies to prove safety of new antidiabetic agents were made mandatory by Food and Drug Administration (FDA), the drug regulatory authority of the United States of America, some pessimists forecasted end of new drug introductions in the field of diabetology. On the contrary, the medical world was pleasantly surprised to find out that not only all SGLT-2 inhibitors and GLP-1 RAs were safe but many actually offered very significant cardiorenal protection, thus turning management algorithms upside down.

The primary care physicians, the postgraduates, and internists need latest and ready information in simplified manner on these exiting recent developments in the field of diabetology for the benefit of their patients. The frequency of telephonic inquiries from clinicians from every nook and corner of our vast country regarding availability of the book and the new edition was constantly rising. Thus, I decided, it was high time I should embark on the project of seventh edition of *Practical Diabetes Mellitus*; it is never too late to start a meaningful project. The seventh edition contains additional chapters such as "COVID-19 and Diabetes" and "Travel and Diabetes" and a comprehensive information on nonalcoholic fatty liver disease (NAFLD) in chapter on Chronic Complications of Diabetes. In addition, many chapters, particularly those on antidiabetic medications have been thoroughly updated and new color photographs have been added. It is hoped that the book will meet the expectations of the readers.

**Pradeep G Talwalkar**

# Preface to the First Edition

Prevalence of diabetes mellitus, particularly, type 2 diabetes mellitus, is increasing by leaps and bounds, in India. We reached a dubious distinction of having highest number of diabetics in the year 1995 and we have still maintained the "leading position", only the gap between India and China, a country having second highest number of diabetics, has increased significantly. Diabetes is not merely a metabolic disease but very much a vascular disease. Various macrovascular complications of diabetes are responsible for 75% of deaths in diabetics, 66% among these, are due to coronary artery disease. Microvascular complications account for significant morbidity in diabetics. In the last decade, two major trials, namely the Diabetes Control and Complications Trial (DCCT) and the UK Prospective Diabetes Study (UKPDS), addressing the role of persistent tight blood glucose control in preventing or postponing microvascular complications of diabetes were completed. It was clearly proved in both the trials that persistent tight blood glucose control definitely helps in prevention of microvascular complications. Nonspecialists manage about 80% of diabetic patients. Thus, it has become vitally important for a family physician or a general duty medical officer to have a thorough working knowledge of pathophysiology, diagnosis, and management of diabetes.

Even though there are many excellent books on diabetes, a paucity of concise book on practical aspects of diabetes, written in simple, easy-to-understand language was felt by family physicians and expressed by them during my interactions with them at innumerable symposia and CMEs in which I regularly participate as a faculty. Thus, this effort from my side, I have tried to give many practical *Take Home Messages*, which can be applied in day-to-day practice. I hope that the book will serve its purpose. I dedicate the book to all my patients who gave me an opportunity to treat them and thus provided me with a large data pool and rich experience, which I would like to share with others for the benefit of diabetic patients.

**Pradeep G Talwalkar**

# Acknowledgments

I thank innumerable family physicians and general duty medical officers who have expressed their appreciations of my style of medical writing, and thus encouraged me to keep on writing for them. My thanks are due to my wife, Dr Vandana, whose support, encouragement, help and sacrifice led to successful culmination of my efforts. My thanks are also due to my friend and surgical colleague, Dr Sunil R Vaze, who has expertly looked after surgical conditions of my patients, particularly, diabetic foot. He has provided some of the colored photographs printed in the book.

Last but not the least; I thank Shri Jitender P Vij (Group Chairman), Mr Ankit Vij (Managing Director), Mr MS Mani (Group President), Ms Chetna Malhotra (Senior Director – Professional Publishing, Marketing, and Business Development), Ms Pooja Bhandari (Production Head), Mr Ramesh Krishnamachari (Commissioning Editor) and Mr Anand Kumar (Development Editor), M/s Jaypee Brothers Medical Publishers (P) Ltd, New Delhi, India, for constant encouragement.

# Contents

1. **Introduction**   1

2. **Classification and Clinical Manifestations**   4
   Type 1 Diabetes Mellitus: Previously Known as Insulin-dependent Diabetes Mellitus or Juvenile Diabetes  4; Type 2 Diabetes Mellitus: Previously Known as Noninsulin-Dependent Diabetes Mellitus or Maturity Onset Diabetes Mellitus  7; Type 2 Diabetes Mellitus in Children and Adolescents  9; Maturity-onset Diabetes of the Young  10; Other Specific Types of Diabetes  11; A Note on Older Classification of Diabetes  12; Peculiarities of Diabetics in India  14; A New Way of Classifying Diabetes in Clusters  14

3. **Type 2 Diabetes Mellitus in Children and Adolescents**   17
   Clinical Features  18; Management of T2DM in Children  19

4. **Epidemiology of Diabetes**   21
   Epidemiology of Type 1 Diabetes Mellitus  23; Epidemiology of Type 2 Diabetes Mellitus  24; Epidemiology of Gestational Diabetes Mellitus  27

5. **Diabesity**   29
   Central Obesity  33; How do we Become Fat?  34; Disorders Associated with Obesity  35; Management of Diabesity  36

6. **Metabolic Syndrome**   45
   Prevalence of Metabolic Syndrome  46; The Importance of Metabolic Syndrome  47; Management of Metabolic Syndrome  48; The Controversy on Metabolic Syndrome  48

7. **Diagnosis and Laboratory Investigations**   49
   Criteria for Diagnosis of Diabetes  50; Diagnosis of Gestational Diabetes Mellitus  51; Investigations in Diabetics and Suspected Diabetics  55; Glycosylated Hemoglobin Estimation  56; Recommendations and Conclusions of International Committee  59

## 8. Use of Glucometer in Family Practice — 62
Equipment Required for Home Blood Glucose Monitoring *63*; Reliability of Glucometer *64*; Training the Patients Using Glucometers *65*

## 9. Metabolic Memory (Legacy Effect) — 70
Pathogenesis of Metabolic Memory *73*; Therapeutic Implications and Future Prospects *74*

## 10. Management of Diabetes — 78
Why Control Diabetes? *78*; Difference Between Onset and Progression of Microvascular and Macrovascular Complications *80*; Accord Trial *81*; Advance Trial *81*; VADT Trial *82*; Take Home Message *82*; Management of Diabetes *82*

## 11. Role of Exercise in the Management of Diabetes Mellitus — 85
Benefits of Exercise *86*; Other Benefits *86*; What are the Precautions to be Observed before Starting Exercise? *87*; Which Type of Exercise? *88*; How Long? *89*; How Often? *90*; Some Walking Tips *90*; Cross Training *91*; Resistance Exercise *92*; Stretching or Flexibility Exercise *93*

## 12. Meal Planning in Diabetes — 94
What is a Balanced Food? *95*; The Food Exchange *101*; General Guideline *104*; Some Tools Used in Meal Planning *107*

## 13. Oral Antidiabetic Agents and Injectable $GLP_1 RAs$ — 113
History of Development of OADs *113*; Pharmacology *115*; Sulfonylureas and Other Insulin Secretagogues *116*; Progressive β-cell Failure in T2DM *117*; Biguanides *125*; Thiazolidinediones *130*; Alpha-glucosidase Inhibitors *138*; Incretin-based Therapy *140*; Sodium-glucose Cotransporter-2 Inhibitors *152*; Criteria for Control *162*; Failure of Control *164*; Drug Interactions *165*

## 14. Role of Insulin in Management of Diabetes — 170
Insulin Physiology and Pathophysiology in Diabetes *171*; Insulin Pharmacology *172*; Tricks of the Trade in Difficult Situations *186*; Mistakes While Taking/Prescribing Insulin *187*

## 15. Combination Therapy in Diabetes — 196
Combinations of Oral Antidiabetic Medications *196*; Combinations of Insulin with Oral Antidiabetic Drugs *203*; GLP$_1$RAs Combinations with Insulin/Metformin/Pioglitazone/Sulfonylurea *205*

## 16. Management of Diabetes in Elderly — 207
Prevention of Diabetes in the Elderly *208*; Management of Diabetes *209*

## 17. Prescribing Antidiabetic Medications in Renal Impairment — 214
Metformin *215*; Sulfonylureas *215*; Nonsulfonylurea Insulin Secretagogues *216*; Pioglitazone *216*; Alpha-glucosidase Inhibitors *216*; Insulin *216*; DPP$_4$I'S and GLP$_1$RA'S *216*

## 18. Acute Metabolic Complications of Diabetes — 219
Acute Metabolic Complications *220*; Hypoglycemia *220*; Diabetic Ketoacidosis and Coma *226*; Nonketotic Hyperosmolar Hyperglycemic State *228*; Lactic Acidosis *230*

## 19. Chronic Complications of Diabetes — 233
Microvascular Complications *233*; Macrovascular Complications of Diabetes *237*; Nonalcoholic Fatty Liver Disease *239*; Infections in Diabetes *241*; Musculoskeletal and Rheumatologic Complications of Diabetes *245*

## 20. The Diabetic Foot — 248
Etiopathogenesis *249*; Prevention *249*; Management *251*

## 21. Hypertension in Diabetes — 254
Definition *254*; Blood Pressure Measurement *255*; Note on 8th Joint National Committee Guidelines *255*; Epidemiology *256*; Types of Hypertension in Diabetes Mellitus *256*; Management of Hypertension in Diabetics *258*; Stepwise Management of Hypertension in Diabetics *264*

## 22. Management of Dyslipidemia and Cardiovascular Risk in Diabetes Mellitus — 268
Investigations *272*; Management of Dyslipidemia and CV Risk *272*; Hypertriglyceridemia *277*

### 23. Surgery in a Diabetic Patient 280
Metabolic Effects of Surgery and Anesthesia *281*; Anesthetic Agents and Anesthesia *281*; Preoperative Evaluation *282*; Insulin Therapy *282*; On the Day of Surgery *283*; Alternative Insulin Regimens *284*; Minor Surgical Procedures *285*; Postoperative Care *286*; Special Situations *287*

### 24. COVID-19 and Diabetes 288
Antidiabetic Medications and COVID-19 *290*; Effect of COVID-19 on Glycemic Control *292*; COVID-19 Vaccination for Patients with Diabetes *293*

### 25. Travel and Diabetes 294
Before Going *295*; While Traveling *299*; At the Destination *300*

### 26. Some of the Advances in the Management of Diabetes 301
Continuous Glucose Monitoring Systems *301*; Insulin Delivery *305*; Future of Artificial Pancreas *309*; Embryonic Stem Cell Research *311*; Gene Therapy *311*; Newer Insulin *311*; Routes of Administration of Insulin *313*; Immunosuppression in the Management of Type 1 Diabetes Mellitus *315*; Emerging Antidiabetic Agents (Other than Insulin) *315*; Diabetes in the 21st Century *319*

### 27. Prevention of Diabetes 320
Important Diabetes Primary Prevention Studies *321*; Summary *325*; Other Measures to Prevent Type 2 Diabetes Mellitus *326*; Prevention of Type 1 Diabetes Mellitus *326*

### 28. Instructions on Selfcare 328
Foot Care in Diabetes *328*; Mixing Insulin *329*; Correct Technique for Self-injection *335*; Stepwise Procedure for Using Reusable Insulin Pen *337*; Tips for Painless Insulin Injection *342*; What are the Best Parts of the Body for Injection? *342*

**Index** 345

# PLATE 1

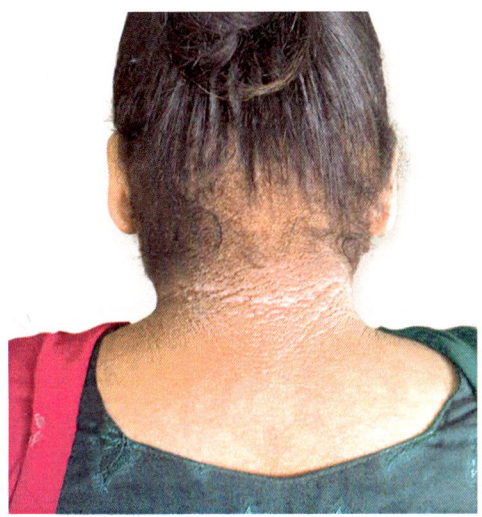

**FIG. 1:** The picture above depicts classical acanthosis nigricans. *(Chapter 3)*

*Note*: The hypertrophic dark brownish gray skin at the back of neck. Acanthosis nigricans is a sign of insulin resistance. Other manifestations of insulin resistance include hypertension, hypertriglyceridemia, and obesity. The patient depicted above had all these manifestations.

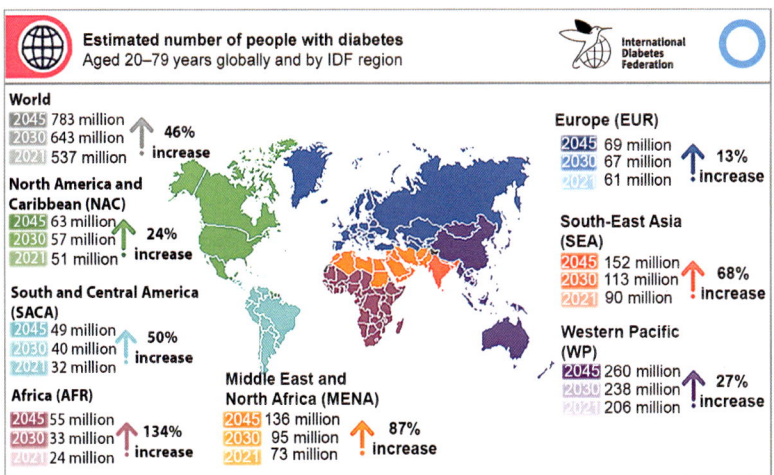

**FIG. 1:** Number of adults with diabetes in 2021, region wise distribution International Diabetes Federation (IDF) 2011. *(Chapter 4)*

*Source*: IDF Diabetes Atlas 2021, 10th edition. www.idf.org. @IntDiabetesFed.

# PLATE 2

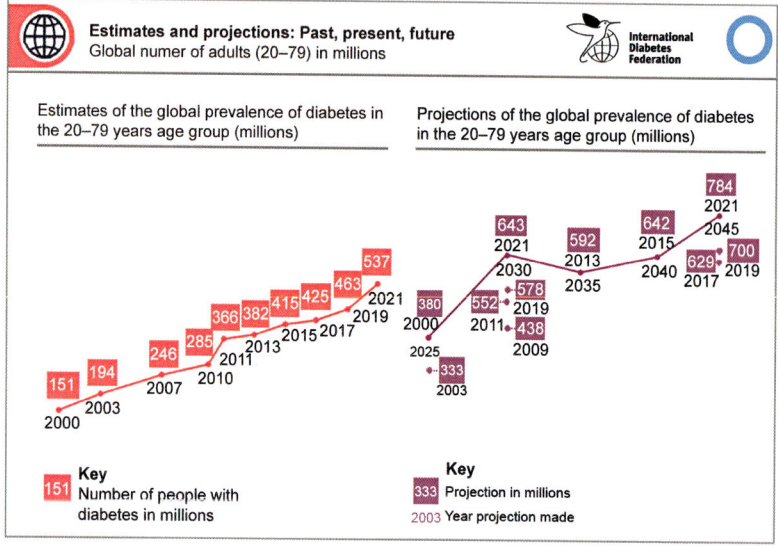

**FIG. 2:** Number of adults with diabetes in 2021 and projections for 2045-IDF (International Diabetes Federation) data. *(Chapter 4)*

*Source*: IDF Diabetes Atlas 2021, 10th edition. www.idf.org. @IntDiabetesFed.

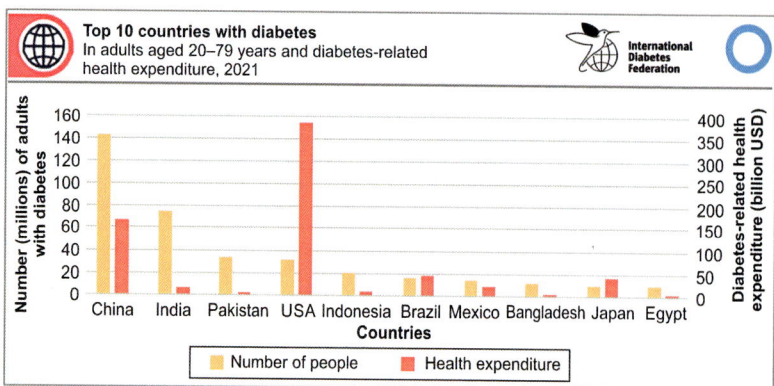

**FIG. 5:** Top 10 countries with adult diabetes and diabetes-related health expenditure as per International Diabetes Federation (IDF) 2021 data. *(Chapter 4)*

*Source*: IDF Diabetes Atlas 2021, 10th edition. www.idf.org. @IntDiabetesFed.

# PLATE 3

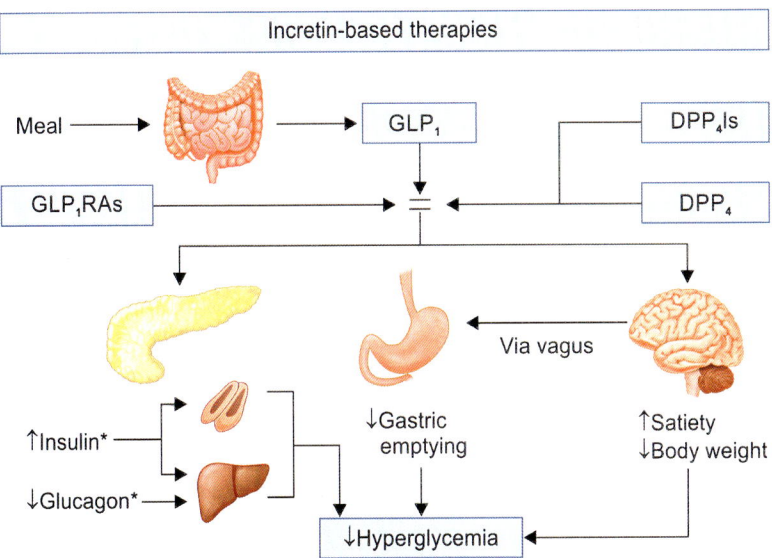

*Glucose-dependent effects.

**FIG. 3:** Mechanism of action of $DPP_4I$'s and $GLP_1RAs$. *(Chapter 13)*

($DPP_4$: dipeptidyl peptidase 4; $GLP_1$: glucagon-like peptide 1)

*Source*: Drucker DJ, Nauck MA. The incretin system: glucagon-like peptide-1 receptor agonists and dipeptidyl peptidase-4 inhibitors in type 2 diabetes. Lancet. 2006;368(9548):1696-705; Tahrani AA, Bailey CJ, Del Prato S, Barnett AH. Management of type 2 diabetes: new and future developments in treatment. Lancet. 2011;378(9786):182-97.

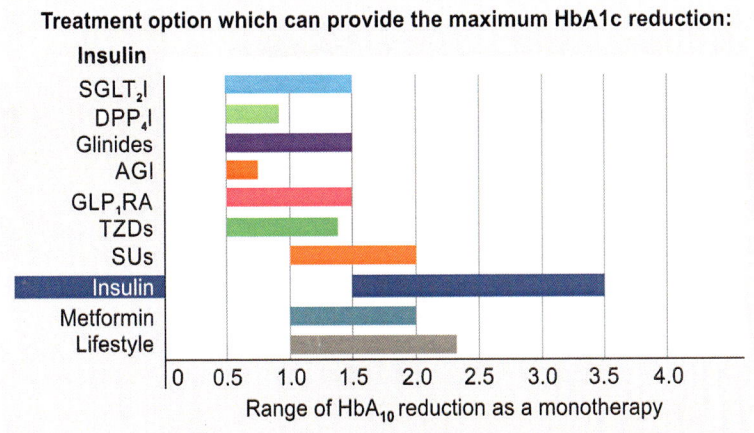

**FIG. 4:** Comparative glycemic efficacies of antidiabetic agents. *(Chapter 13)*

# PLATE 4

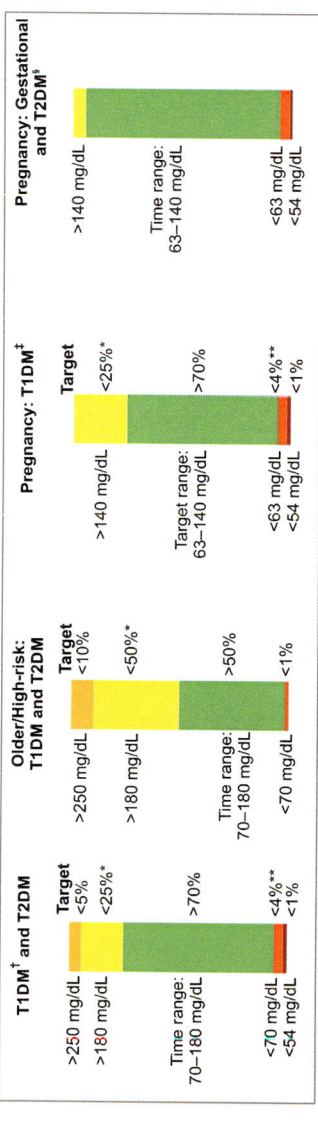

⁰ For age <25 year, if the A1c goal is 7.5, then set TIR target to approximately 60%.
† Percentages of time-in-ranges are based on limited evidence. More research is needed.
§ Percentages of time-in-ranges have not been included because there is very limited evidence in this area. More research is needed.
\* Includes percentage of values >250 mg/dL (13.9).
\*\* Includes percentage of values <54 mg/dL (3.0).

**FIG. 5:** CGM-based targets for different diabetes populations. *(Chapter 13)*

(CGM: continuous glucose monitoring; TIR: time-in-range; T1DM: type 1 diabetes mellitus; T2DM: type 2 diabetes mellitus)

*Source:* Battelino T, Danne T, Bergenstal R, et al. Clinical Targets for Continous glucose monitoring data interpretation: Recommendations from the international consensus on time in range. Diabetes Care. 2019;42(8): 593-1603.

# PLATE 5

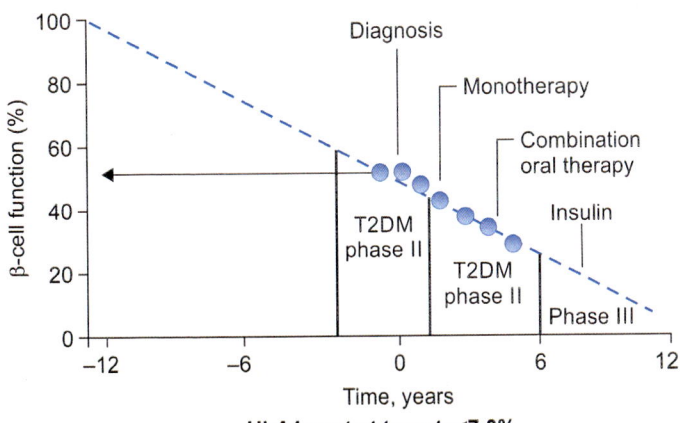

**FIG. 6:** Progressive β-cell failure. *(Chapter 13)*

(HbA1c: glycated hemoglobin; T2DM: type 2 diabetes mellitus)

*Source*: Based on data from U.K. prospective diabetes study 16. Overview of 6 years' therapy of type 2 diabetes: a progressive disease. U.K. Prospective Diabetes Study Group. Diabetes. 1995;44(11):1249-58; Kendall DM, Cuddihy RM, Bergenstal RM. Clinical application of incretin-based therapy: therapeutic potential, patient selection and clinical use. Am J Med. 2009;122 (6 Suppl): S37-50; Kendall DM, Bergenstal RM. Comprehensive management of patients with type 2 diabetes: establishing priorities of care. Am J Manag Care. 2001;7(10 Suppl):S327-43; quiz S344-8.

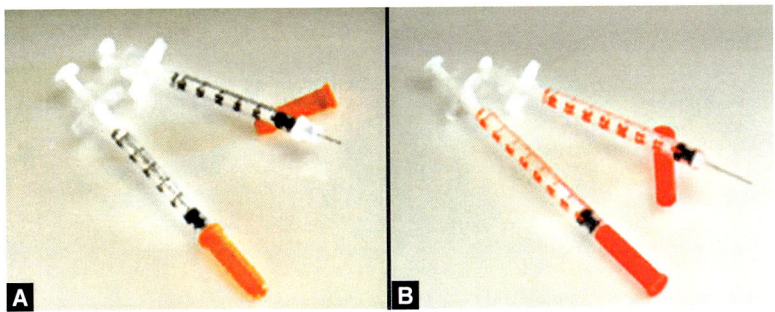

**FIGS. 1A AND B:** (A) U/100 syringe and (B) U/40 syringe. *(Chapter 18)*

# PLATE 6

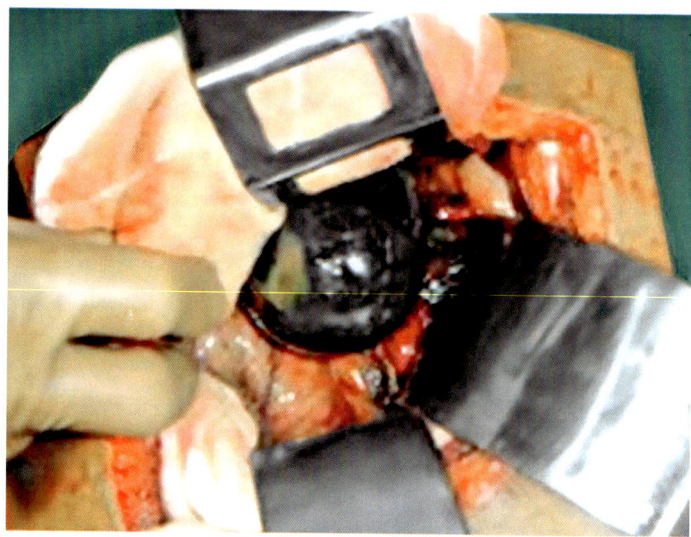

**FIG. 2:** Fulminant, gangrenous cholecystitis. *(Chapter 19)*

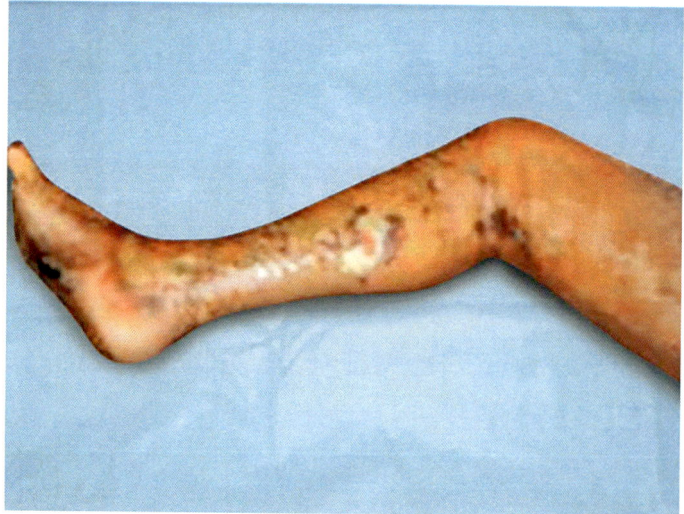

**FIG. 3:** Necrotizing fasciitis of right leg. *(Chapter 19)*

# PLATE 7

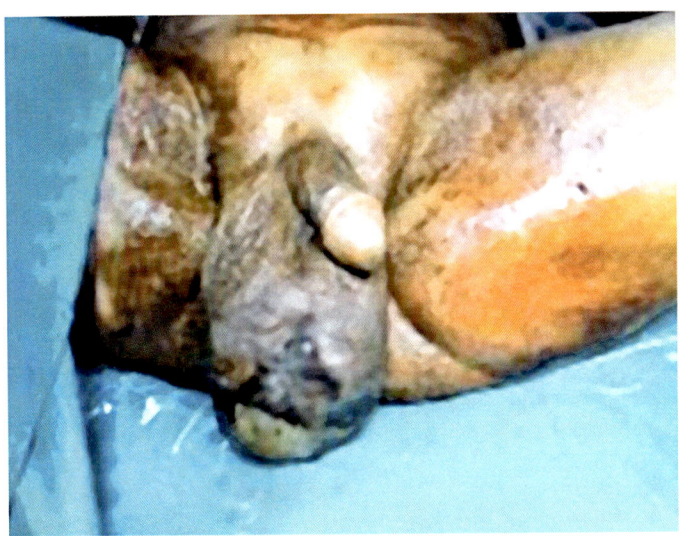

**FIG. 4:** Fournier's gangrene of scrotum. *(Chapter 19)*

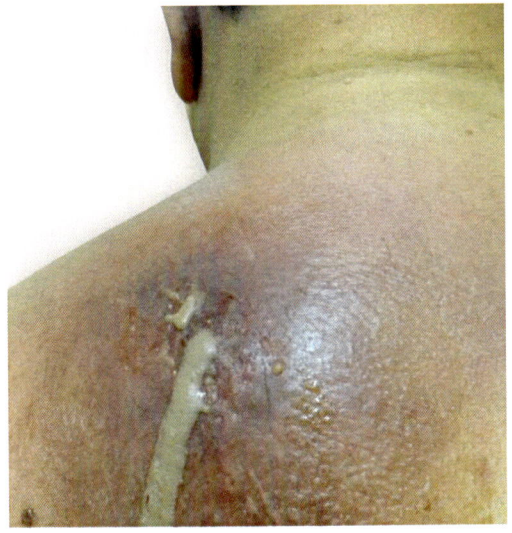

**FIG. 5:** A large carbuncle on the back. *(Chapter 19)*

## PLATE 8

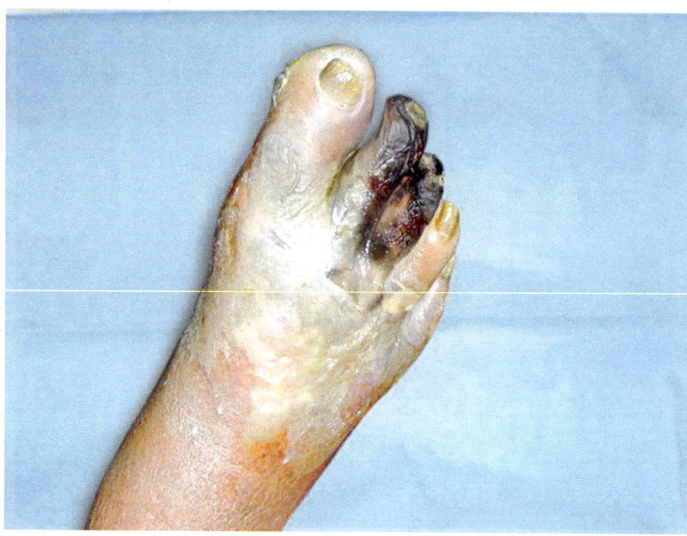

**FIG. 6:** Right foot abscess with gangrene of second and third toes. *(Chapter 19)*

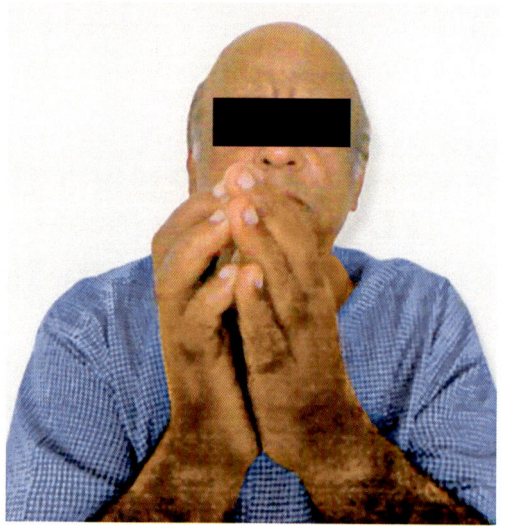

**FIG. 7:** *Namaste* sign: Cheiroarthropathy and limited joint mobility in a long-standing diabetic, leading to inability to fully extend the fingers at interphalangeal joints. This is best demonstrated as in picture above, by asking the patients to place the palms of both hands together. *(Chapter 19)*

*Note:* Inability to attain classical *Namaste* posture.

# PLATE 9

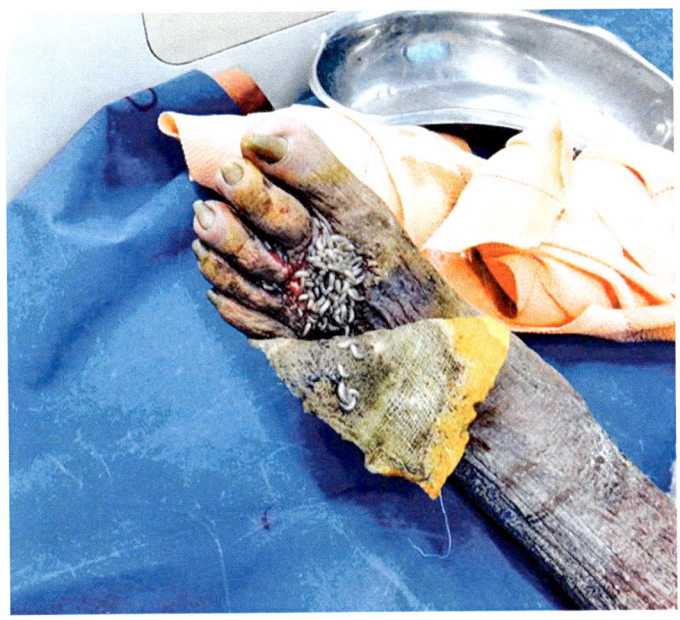

**FIG. 1:** Diabetic foot infested with maggots. *(Chapter 20)*

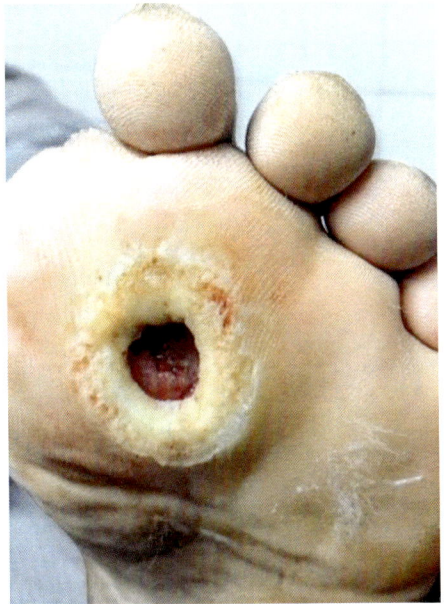

**FIG. 2:** A classical neuropathic foot ulcer on left sole. *(Chapter 20)*

# PLATE 10

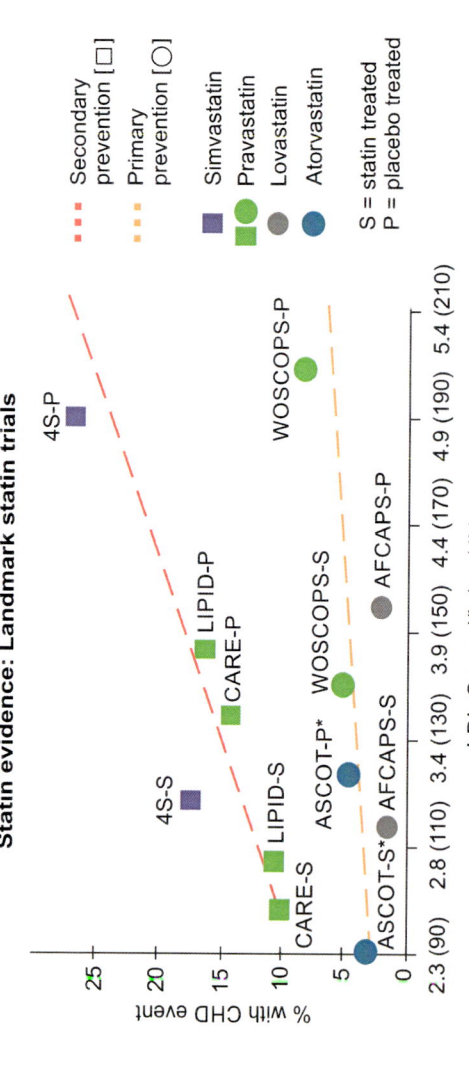

*Extrapolated for 5 years.

**FIG. 2:** Landmark statin trials for primary and secondary prevention of CHD. *(Chapter 22)*

(CHD: coronary heart disease; LDL-C: low-density lipoprotein cholesterol)

*Source:* Adapted from Kastelein JJ. The future of best practice. Atherosclerosis. 1999;143 (Suppl 1):S17-21.

# PLATE 11

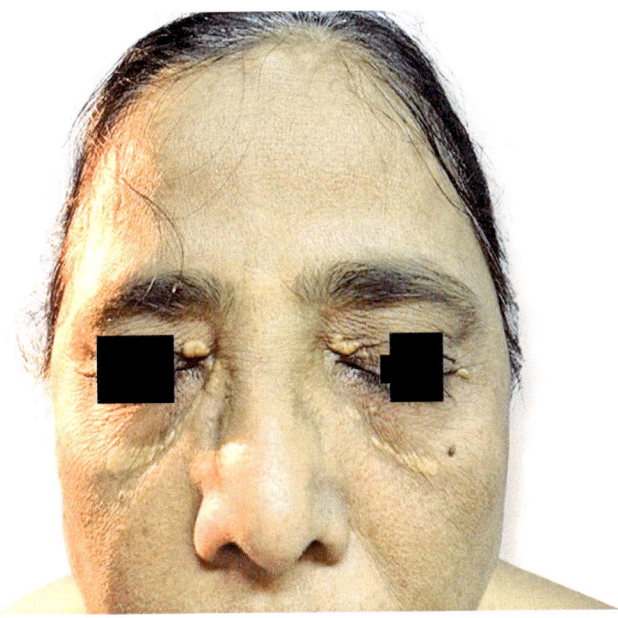

**FIG. 3:** Typical "butterfly rash" around eyes in middle-aged type 2 diabetic patient with dyslipidemia. *(Chapter 22)*

# PLATE 12

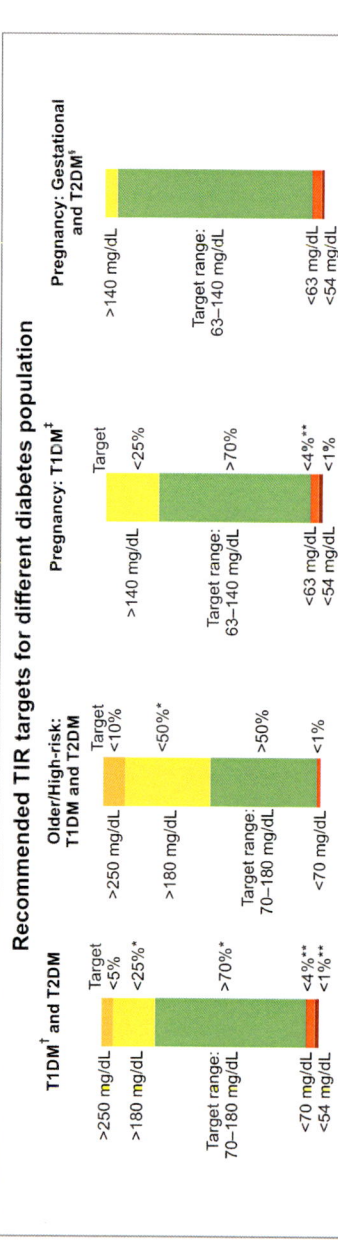

**FIG. 1:** Recommended time in range. *(Chapter 26)*

(TIR: Time in range; T1DM: type 1 diabetes mellitus; T2DM: type 2 diabetes mellitus)

†For age <25 years, if the A1C goal is 7.5%, then set TIR target to approximately 60% (See clinical applications of time in ranges section in the text for additional information regarding target goal setting in pediatric management).
‡Percentages of time in ranges are based on limited evidence. More research is needed.
§Percentages of time in ranges have not been included because there is very limited evidence in this area. More research is needed. Please see pregnancy section in text for more considerations on targets for these groups.
*Includes percentage of values >250 mg/dL (13.9 mmol/L).
**Includes percentage of values <54 mg/dL (3.0 mmol/L).

*Source:* Battelino T, Danne T, Bergenstal R, et al. Clinical Targets for Continuous Glucose Monitoring Data Interpretation: Recommendations From the International Consensus on Time in Range. Diabetes Care 2019;42:1593-1603.

# CHAPTER 1

# Introduction

Diabetes mellitus (DM) is not a single disease but a syndrome consisting of different subtypes of diabetes with hyperglycemia due to insulin deficiency, either absolute or relative, as a common factor. Its prevalence is increasing rapidly and has already reached an epidemic proportion in India. With >74 million adult diabetics, India has second largest population of diabetics, while China with 141 million adult diabetics is the diabetes capital of the world (World Diabetes Atlas, IDF, 2021). In our country, particularly in rural and semiurban settings, >90% of diabetic patients are treated by primary care physicians. Hence, every family physician and general duty medical officer should be proficient in basic management of diabetes and knowledge of when to seek expert help. If one's basics are strong, it is very easy to take correct decisions regarding ordering precise investigations, advising about diet, and exercise and selecting appropriate oral antidiabetic drugs (OADs); noninsulin injectable antidiabetic agents [glucagon-like peptide-1 ($GLP_1$) agonists]; and insulin in correct dosages. Various complications of diabetes, including macrovascular and microvascular complications, impair quality of life, reduce life expectancy by 5–10 years and drastically increase the cost of treatment (Key statistics on Diabetes, published by Diabetes UK, 2010). Thus, simultaneous implementation of preventive and therapeutic strategies for various risk factors and complications of diabetes is vital. Even more vital is early diagnosis of diabetes.

Type 2 diabetes mellitus (T2DM) can remain undiagnosed and thus uncontrolled for up to 5 years after the onset. This is the main reason for many of these patients having complications of diabetes on the day of diagnosis. Large scale studies have conclusively proved that early diagnosis and tight blood glucose control established soon after the diagnosis is immensely beneficial as regards prevention of dreaded complications of diabetes. Hence, it is sometimes too late if a clinician thinks that his duty starts only after a patient comes to him for the treatment of diabetes. We as responsible members of the community should be proactive in community education on the importance of early diagnosis of diabetes and arrange camps for diagnosis of diabetes aiming at youngsters for their first blood glucose tests and other adults for periodic repeat blood glucose tests.

The aim of this book is to provide concise information required by a family physician or general duty medical officer to let him confidently handle his diabetic patients on his own and manage them successfully over a period of time. It will also be useful to the general physicians and residents in medicine. In our country's sprawling rural and semiurban areas, general surgeons, and gynecologists are often the first consultants to move in, and in absence of physicians and diabetologists, or even otherwise, they often treat diabetes cases. They also need periodic updates.

This book would serve their basic requirements. The focus of "Practical Diabetes" is on T2DM [previously known as noninsulin-dependent diabetes mellitus (NIDDM) or maturity onset diabetes], and its management in an outpatient clinic setup. It may be noted that >96% of diabetic patients in our country have T2DM. The author has extensively drawn from his vast experience as a clinician, medical teacher, and writer for writing this book in simple, user-friendly, and easy to understand language.

Introduction | 3

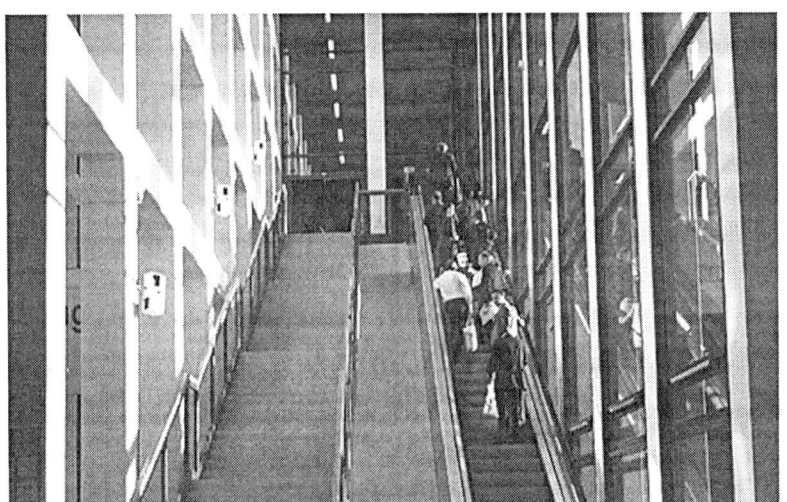

Diabetologists preach about exercise, but they do not practice. Picture is taken at a major international conference of diabetologists.

*Note*: All diabetologists are riding elevator, none climbing the stairs.

 **Highlights**
In 2021, IDF estimates show that:

 International Diabetes Federation

 **1 in 10**
Adults (20–79 years) has diabetes
537 million people

 **1 in 16**
Adults (20–79 years) has impaired fasting glucose
319 million people

 **3 in 4**
People with diabetes live in low and middle-income countries

 **1 in 2**
Adults is undiagnosed
240 million people

 **1 in 6**
Live births (21 million) affected by hyperglycemia in pregnancy, 80% have mothers with GDM

 **11.5%**
Of global health expenditure spent on diabetes (USD 966 billion)

 **1 in 10**
Adults (20–79 years) has impaired glucose tolerance
541 million people

 **1.2 million**
Children and adolescents below 20 years have type 1 diabetes mellitus

 **6.7 million**
Deaths attributed to diabetes

*Source*: IDF Diabetes Atlas 2021, 10th edition. www.idf.org. @IntDiabetesFed.

# CHAPTER 2

# Classification and Clinical Manifestations

## INTRODUCTION

Diabetes mellitus (DM) has been classified in the following categories (**Box 1**).

## TYPE 1 DIABETES MELLITUS: PREVIOUSLY KNOWN AS INSULIN-DEPENDENT DIABETES MELLITUS OR JUVENILE DIABETES

Less than 2% of the diabetic patients in our country belong to this class. Onset of type 1 diabetes mellitus (T1DM) is usually very acute and in childhood or adolescents.

These patients depend on insulin for their survival and withdrawal of insulin leads to ketoacidosis. T1DM occurs due to autoimmune or idiopathic destruction of insulin-producing β-cells in islets of Langerhans in the pancreas, resulting in inability to produce endogenous insulin, which is vital for control of blood glucose and other metabolic functions. These patients usually require at least two shots of short-acting and long-acting

---

**BOX 1** | **Classification of diabetes.**

- Type 1 diabetes mellitus
- Type 2 diabetes mellitus
- Other specific types of diabetes
- Gestational diabetes

or intermediate-acting insulin every day. Majority of the T1DM patients require more intensive insulin therapy such as multiple subcutaneous insulin injections or continuous subcutaneous insulin injections through an external insulin pump. One must note that not all young diabetic patients on insulin are necessarily type 1 diabetics. Many young diabetic patients in our country require large doses of insulin for adequate blood glucose control, e.g., those who have diabetes secondary to pancreatic destruction, following fibrocalculous pancreatitis or those type 2 diabetic patients who had severe malnutrition in intrauterine or infantile period. These patients are very often wrongly labeled as "insulin dependent" just because they are young and they are on insulin. Some of these patients stop insulin when they go to their native place for a long stay and report back in poor metabolic state, but the fact that they are still surviving is a confirmation that they are not type 1 or "insulin dependent" for life but insulin-requiring type 2 diabetic patients. Next time you see such a patient, confidently rule out T1DM in him, even if he has a discharge card mentioning "insulin-dependent diabetes" in the slot for diagnosis from a general medicine unit of a teaching hospital. The tendency among doctors to label all young diabetics on insulin as T1DM patients is akin to tendency among sports journalists and cricket lovers to call a mediocre medium paced bowler, a "fast bowler". Genuine fast bowler belongs to a rare species. However, please remember that these patients will usually require insulin for control of blood glucose, though they are not dependent on it for their survival.

Initial presentation of type 1 diabetic patients is usually dramatic. They present with severe symptoms such as polyuria, polydipsia, polyphagia, weight loss, and in some cases, superadded with symptoms of diabetic ketoacidosis such as vomiting, deep rapid breathing characteristic of acidosis, and deteriorating level of consciousness. If there is an underlying cause which has triggered metabolic deterioration, its symptoms are also superadded, e.g., cough and fever in case of pneumonia or tuberculosis. T1DM usually presents in children or in young adults. Occasionally, it strikes middle-aged patients. In some middle-aged patients, initial presentation of T1DM is similar to type 2 diabetes mellitus (T2DM), which is several times more common in that age group. They may show some response to oral agents initially, thus they are wrongly labeled as T2DM patients. However, they become insulin dependent over a shorter period as compared to average type 2 diabetic patients and they are positive for glutamic acid decarboxylase (GAD) and other antibodies, which confirms T1DM. These patients are labeled as latent autoimmune diabetes in adults (LADA). Thus, whenever you come across a middle-aged diabetic patient who was never controlled or who has lost glycemic control within a short time (several weeks to a few months), in spite of use of oral antidiabetic agents in optimal dosages and combinations, and in spite of not having other associated conditions, such as severe infections, corticosteroid intake, etc., suspect LADA.

You can confirm or rule out the diagnosis by doing GAD antibody test.

As far as initial management of type 1 diabetic patients is concerned, this requires experience. Hence, family physicians should consult diabetologists/endocrinologists as regards policy decisions and management.

Type 1 diabetic patients require insulin for lifetime and those who are severely symptomatic or with ketoacidosis should be admitted.

Severe hyperglycemia, recurrent vomiting, and unpredictable food intake are indications for intravenous insulin infusion while others can be put on multiple subcutaneous insulin injections. Besides insulin, fluid and electrolyte replacement should be carried out. A search for the underlying precipitating cause should be made and if found, should be appropriately treated, e.g., appropriate parenteral antibiotic for pneumonia. Before discharge, patient should be trained for insulin injection technique and educated on various aspects of diabetes with a focus on importance of persistent tight blood glucose control, weight maintenance, control of blood pressure, and cholesterol. He should be also trained on prevention and treatment of hypoglycemia, meal planning, and appropriate physical exercise. At least one additional member of the family should be trained along with the patient. Common sense should be used while selecting the family member for training. Those not requiring hospitalization should be trained on all the above mentioned aspects on outpatient basis in phased manner. In our country, many doctors, particularly family physicians, are unlikely to have services of trainers and dietitians on a daily basis.

In such situations, it is prudent to reserve once a week, a 2-hour slot for "diabetes clinic". It is convenient to call diabetic patients for training and follow-up during this slot. It is very important to know that unless and until the diabetic patient is well educated and trained, he will not be motivated to aim for and achieve persistent tight metabolic control. Dr Joslin, a pioneer American diabetologist who had devoted a large part of his working time to education of diabetic patients, had stated in 1930s: *"The diabetic who knows most, will live the longest"*.

## TYPE 2 DIABETES MELLITUS: PREVIOUSLY KNOWN AS NONINSULIN-DEPENDENT DIABETES MELLITUS OR MATURITY ONSET DIABETES MELLITUS

This subtype of diabetes is the most common type of diabetes all over the world more so in our country. Around 95–96% of diabetic patients in India belong to this subclass. In the 90s, it was labeled as noninsulin-dependent diabetes because unlike T1DM patients, these patients are not dependent on insulin for survival, even though many require insulin for adequate control of blood glucose a few years after maintaining good control on oral pills. Till 80s, T2DM was called maturity onset diabetes because it was usually diagnosed in the middle age. Unless associated with acute stressful conditions such as severe infection, acute myocardial infarction, etc., these patients are asymptomatic for a long period and onset of symptoms is very gradual. Very often, diagnosis is made accidentally during periodic health checkups, preinsurance checkups, and pre-employment or preoperative checkups. If one bypasses all these checkups, he may present with severe symptoms of diabetes such as weakness, weight loss, polyuria, polydipsia, polyphagia, itching, etc. It takes up to 5 years after the beginning of diabetes to reach this state. Rarely, T2DM patients present with symptoms typical of diabetic ketoacidosis, i.e., deep rapid breathing, deteriorating level of consciousness, vomiting, etc., in addition to above mentioned symptoms. Such patients usually have severe insulin resistance due to severe underlying stressful condition such as infection (diabetic foot, pneumonia, and tuberculosis), myocardial infarction, etc.

In T2DM, there is an interplay between environmental and genetic factors leading to a chain of events, ultimately leading to diabetes. Most of the patients have varying degrees of dual defects, β-cell dysfunction and insulin resistance. Both these pathogenic factors have contributions from genetic and acquired factors. For example, many type 2 diabetic patients have inherited β-cell defect to which acquired dysfunction of β-cells due to infantile or intrauterine malnutrition and transient dysfunction due to toxic effect of severe hyperglycemia (glucotoxicity) are superadded. Insulin resistance also has genetic as well as acquired components. Obesity is associated with insulin resistance and has acquired as well as genetic components. Acquired insulin resistance can be multifactorial. Stress, drugs, and sedentary lifestyles are some of the factors leading to acquired insulin resistance.

Type 2 diabetes mellitus is more common in obese people because of insulin resistance which is associated with obesity. If obese people have absolutely healthy β-cells, they never become diabetic because their β-cells have the capacity to produce extra insulin to override insulin resistance. Thus, all the obese people do not become diabetic. In the USA, 25% of the nondiabetic adults are insulin resistant. They do not become diabetic because their β-cells do not have any genetic defect and thus are able to respond to increased demand of insulin by producing more insulin to counteract insulin resistance. However, in those who have β-cell defect, inherited or acquired, their capacity to override insulin resistance by producing additional insulin is limited, thus they cannot cope up with body's demand for extra insulin and become diabetic **(Table 1)**.

It is now accepted that T2DM is a multihormonal and multi-locational disease. In addition to insulin resistance and β-cell dysfunction, there are many other pathophysiological alterations in type 2 diabetic patients.

Some of the pathophysiological defects are mentioned here:

*Alpha cell defect*: There is an inappropriate postprandial hyperglucagonemia in type 2 diabetic patients due to inability of α-cells to suppress glucagon release in response to rising blood glucose in postprandial period. This leads to excessive hepatic glucose production in the postprandial period.

*Reduced glucagon-like peptide-1 ($GLP_1$) levels*: The physiological role of $GLP_1$ is to combine with its receptors on β-cells and facilitate

| TABLE 1: Risk factors for type 2 diabetes mellitus (T2DM). ||
|---|---|
| T2DM is caused by a combination of lifestyle and genetic factors ||
| These risk factors are classed as modifiable or nonmodifiable ||
| *Modifiable risk factors* | *Nonmodifiable risk factors* |
| Overweight and obesity | Family history |
| Sedentary lifestyle | Gender |
| Dietary factors | History of gestational diabetes |
| Metabolic syndrome | Ethnicity |
| Previously identified IGT/IFG | Age |
| Adverse Intrauterine environment | Polycystic ovary syndrome |
| Inflammation | |
| (IFG: impaired fasting glucose; IGT: impaired glucose tolerance) ||
| *Source*: Alberti KG, Zimmet P, Shaw J. International Diabetes Federation: a consensus on Type 2 diabetes prevention. Diabet Med. 2007;24(5):451-63. ||

release of insulin from the β-cells. Type 2 diabetic patients have impaired postprandial rise in $GLP_1$ in response to food (incretin defect). This defect contributes toward hyperglycemia, particularly postprandial hyperglycemia.

Those with T2DM, obesity, and other insulin-resistant states have reduced dopaminergic tone in suprachiasmatic hypothalamic region in early morning, thus disturbing the physiological circadian rhythm. This is associated with excessive release of neurotransmitters, such as noradrenaline, which in turn leads to inadequate suppression of hepatic glucose production and inadequate suppression of adipose tissue lipolysis.

More glucose is reabsorbed from renal tubules in diabetic patients as compared to nondiabetic patients due to upregulation of sodium-glucose cotransporter-2 ($SGLT_2$) enzyme **(Fig. 1)**.

## TYPE 2 DIABETES MELLITUS IN CHILDREN AND ADOLESCENTS

Recently, increasing prevalence of T2DM has been reported in children and adolescents from all over the world including India. These patients are overweight, have significant insulin resistance

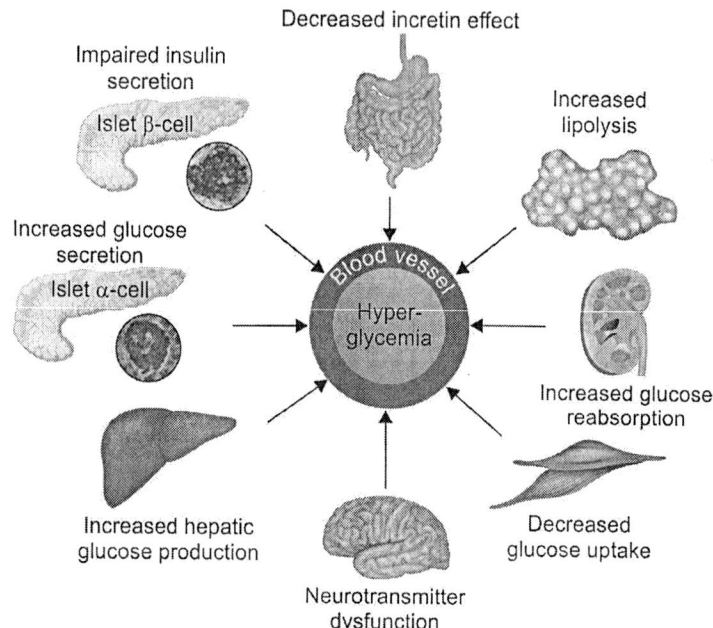

**FIG. 1:** Sites of pathophysiological defects contributing to hyperglycemia.

*Source*: Defronzo RA. Banting Lecture. From the triumvirate to the ominous octet: a new paradigm for the treatment of type 2 diabetes mellitus. Diabetes. 2009;58(4):773-95.

and unlike type 1 diabetic patients, are ketosis resistant. They respond well to diet, exercise, and metformin.

Thus, even though T2DM presents most commonly in adults, it can present in childhood; similarly, not all T1DM patients present in childhood; occasionally, they can present in middle age.

Please refer to next chapter on T2DM in children and adolescents for details.

## MATURITY-ONSET DIABETES OF THE YOUNG

While, a classical T2DM has polygenic inheritance; maturity-onset diabetes of the young (MODY) has monogenic inheritance. The distinct clinical features of MODY include following: onset before the age of 25 years, mild hyperglycemia, good response to sulfonylureas, absence of vascular complications, absence of obesity as well as features of metabolic syndrome, other than dysglycemia; and autosomal dominant inheritance. One of the essential clinical features of MODY is affection of at least three generations consecutively. Absence of GAD and anti-islets cells antibodies, reasonable plasma C-peptide levels, and good response to sulfonylureas are the features leading to exclusion of T1DM from the differential diagnosis. Molecular genetic studies should be done in suspected cases to clinch the diagnosis. MODY has six subtypes (MODY 1-6). The reliable pan India prevalence data about MODY in India is not available. In white European population, MODY forms 0.5-1.0% of type 2 diabetic populations.

## OTHER SPECIFIC TYPES OF DIABETES

There are many rare conditions which are associated with or which lead to diabetes. The list is given here:
- Monogenic diabetic syndromes such as neonatal diabetes and maturity onset diabetes in the young.
- Genetic defects of β-cell function (e.g., glucokinase gene mutation)
- Genetic defects in insulin action (e.g., leprechaunism)
- Diseases of exocrine pancreas [e.g., pancreatitis, fibrocalculous pancreatic diabetes (FCPD)]
- Endocrine disorders (e.g., Cushing's syndrome, acromegaly, and thyrotoxicosis)
- Drug-induced or chemical-induced diabetes (e.g., thiazide, corticosteroids, statins)
- Infections (e.g., congenital rubella)
- Immune-mediated diabetes (e.g., due to anti-insulin antibodies)
- Other genetic syndromes associated with diabetes (e.g., Down's syndrome).

### Gestational Diabetes

Diabetes first diagnosed during pregnancy is called gestational diabetes. It occurs in about 4% of pregnancies in western countries. In a study done in Chennai and nearby rural areas in 2003, a prevalence of 16.7% and 10.7% was reported, respectively. Gestational diabetes mellitus results from insulin resistance of pregnancy, interacting with β-cell defects. Usually, blood glucose is normalized after the delivery. Since significant insulin resistance of pregnancy develops only in third trimester, gestational diabetes sets in only in this period. Presence of glucose intolerance in early pregnancy indicates preexisting T1DM or T2DM. Women having gestational diabetes are at higher risk to develop T2DM during the later part of their life.

## A NOTE ON OLDER CLASSIFICATION OF DIABETES

The above mentioned classification of diabetes was initially put up by American Diabetes Association in 1997 and subsequently adopted by World Health Organization (WHO) in 1998. The earlier classification of diabetes which was in use till 1997 had a subtype called malnutrition-related DM (pancreatic diabetes).

The patients who were earlier classified in this type of diabetes are seen in many of the developing countries including India, particularly in southern and eastern states. Usually, young adults are affected in their second or third decades. They are usually malnourished and they require relatively large doses of insulin for metabolic control. With a few exceptions, all of them require insulin for control but at the same time, discontinuation of insulin does not lead to diabetic ketoacidosis because they do not have total insulin deficiency and a small amount of endogenous insulin, though insufficient for metabolic control is still sufficient to prevent significant fat breakdown and generate ketoacidosis unless severe stressful conditions coexist.

Hence, these patients are insulin-requiring but not insulin dependent. Pancreatic diabetes was further divided in two subtypes.

### Fibrocalculous Pancreatic Diabetes

In this condition, diabetes develops following recurrent and chronic pancreatitis associated with destruction and stone formation in the pancreatic duct. Symptoms of diabetes are associated with recurrent severe upper abdominal pain and in some cases, symptoms of malabsorption due to associated deficiency of digestive enzymes produced in exocrine part of the pancreas.

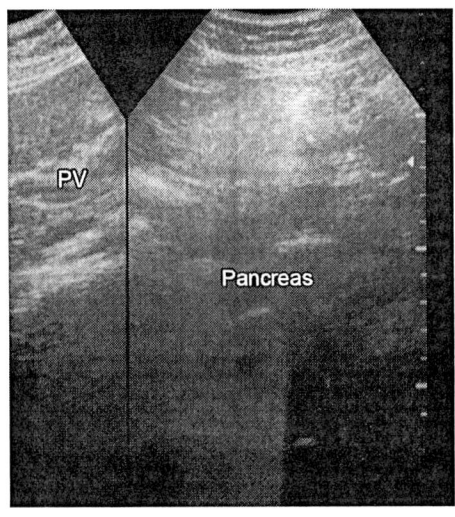

**FIG. 2:** An ultrasound (USG) scan of pancreas of a patient suffering from fibrocalculous pancreatic diabetes, depicting areas of calcification.

Plain X-ray of the abdomen and ultrasound (USG) of abdomen reveal pancreatic stones and calcification. In addition in many patients, ultrasonography shows pancreatic ductal dilatation.

Fibrocalculous pancreatic diabetes is now reclassified under "other specific types of diabetes" because according to current thinking it is secondary to pancreatic destruction (**Fig. 2**).

## Protein-deficient Diabetes Mellitus

Many of these patients have suffered from severe protein deficiency in their intrauterine period, infancy, or early childhood, leading to damage of β-cells in the pancreas. Many of the protein-deficient diabetes mellitus (PDDM) patients have current or old signs of under nutrition.

According to the current classification of diabetes, PDDM does not warrant a separate class and is included in T2DM.

Hormonal and clinical profiles in these two subtypes of pancreatic diabetes are slightly different. However, further details are beyond the scope of this book. These patients usually require twice a day or more complex insulin regimens.

## PECULIARITIES OF DIABETICS IN INDIA

- India has second largest number of diabetic patients.
- Percentage of type 2 diabetic patients among the diabetic population is higher than the developed countries, except Asian developed countries such as Japan.
- Incidence of T1DM increases as one travels from the South Pole to the North Pole, and is highest in Nordic countries such as Finland. Even in Europe, as one travels from North to Southern European countries, such as Portugal, Spain, incidence of T1DM is reduced. Incidence in our country is low.
- T2DM presents at least 10–15 years earlier than western countries.
- Obesity, as defined by body mass index (BMI) criteria, is not as commonly associated with Indian type 2 diabetic patients as compared to West; however, central obesity with BMI in normal range is very common, so is insulin resistance.
- Hereditary component in pathogenesis of T2DM is strong, particularly in South India.
- Secondary diabetes following destruction of pancreas due to FCPD is seen in a small percentage of patients. This variety of secondary diabetes is restricted to developing countries such as India.
- Prevalence of T2DM in children and adolescents is increasing very rapidly in India.

## A NEW WAY OF CLASSIFYING DIABETES IN CLUSTERS

A recent Swedish study looked at six variables [age at diagnosis, presence of GAD antibodies, β-cell function, insulin resistance as assessed by HOMA β-cell model, BMI, and glycated hemoglobin (HbA1c)] in a diabetic population of 8,980 patients. These parameters were prospectively correlated with development of complications and use of antidiabetic medications. Based on the data analysis, patients were classified into five different replicable clusters with significantly different patient characteristics and risk for complications.

These clusters are as follows:
- *Cluster 1*: Severe autoimmune diabetes (SAID)
- *Cluster 2*: Severe insulin-deficient diabetes (SIDD)
- *Cluster 3*: Severe insulin-resistant diabetes (SIRD)
- *Cluster 4*: Mild obesity-related diabetes (MORD)
- *Cluster 5*: Mild age-related diabetes (MARD)

Researchers argue that classifying the patients in five different clusters has therapeutic implications as those in cluster 2 and cluster 3 had high prevalence of retinopathy and nephropathy and thus precise antidiabetic medications can be chosen and specific strategies for prevention of complications can be implemented. Inclusion of patients from only one country was a limitation of the study as the data cannot be extrapolated universally.

A similar study was led by Dr V Mohan from Chennai on 19,084 type 2 diabetic patients. In this study, variables such as, age at diagnosis, HbA1c, BMI, waist circumference, fasting and poststimulation C peptide levels, triglyceride, and high-density lipoprotein (HDL) cholesterol levels in blood were correlated with complications and use of antidiabetic medications. Based on the data analysis, patients were classified into four different replicable clusters with significantly different patient characteristics and risk for complications. The clusters are as follows:

1. Severe insulin-deficient diabetes (SIDD)
   *Characteristic features*: Early onset, low BMI, sever insulin deficiency as well as insulin resistance, poor control, and high prevalence of retinopathy.
2. Insulin-resistant obese diabetes (IROD)
   *Characteristic features*: Obesity, high insulin resistance, high C-peptide levels, and high prevalence of nephropathy.
3. Combined insulin resistant and deficient diabetes (CIRDD)
   *Characteristic features*: Young age at onset, insulin deficiency, and insulin resistance intermediate between SIDD and IROD, high triglycerides and low HDL cholesterol levels, increased risk for retinopathy as well as nephropathy.
4. Mild age-related diabetes
   *Characteristic features*: Older patients, high HDL cholesterol, low risk of complications.

Like the Swedish study, subclassification of individuals in four different clusters can have potential benefits from the point of prognostication and choosing specific antidiabetic agents for specific clusters. Additionally, since the data was generated on a large number of Indian patients, the findings of this study are directly applicable for our patients.

The cluster-based classification of diabetic patients is a new exiting subject and after more intensive and extensive studies in globally representative diabetic patients, will have a say when official classification of diabetes is updated in future. The data generated from such studies will lead to further development of precision medicine in the field of diabetology.

# CHAPTER 3

# Type 2 Diabetes Mellitus in Children and Adolescents

## INTRODUCTION

Till two decades back, type 2 diabetes mellitus (T2DM) was considered as an exclusive disease of adults, mostly middle-aged people. In fact, till 90s, it was officially known as maturity-onset diabetes. It was known since long that average age at the diagnosis of T2DM in India was 10 years younger (in fourth and fifth decade and occasionally in third decade instead of fifth and sixth decade as in western population). However, over last two decades, more and more cases of T2DM are seen in children and adolescent. Such cases were first described from the western countries and soon they started appearing in India. In the USA, <3% of diabetics in children had T2DM, barely two decades back. At present 45% of children having diabetes have T2DM in the USA. In Japan, 80% of children with diabetes have T2DM. Precise figures are not available from our country even though our incidence and prevalence figures are closely following the advanced countries. The increased prevalence of T2DM in children and adolescents is mainly due to rapidly increasing prevalence of obesity in this age group.

Over entire last century, the prevalence of obesity was gradually increasing and over last two decades, the rate of increase has tremendously accelerated. In addition to increase in prevalence in middle-aged persons, the prevalence in children and adolescents has also increased considerably. In a recent survey done in Chennai, about 15% of children and adolescents were overweight. In India, socioeconomic changes are occurring at very rapid speed.

Urbanization, industrialization, and westernization have become unstoppable. While industrialization, is good and urbanization inevitable with industrialization, blindly following western habits are detrimental and hence should be avoided. Our food habits are changing rapidly. The frequency of eating in restaurants has increased. We are eating more refined, energy-dense fast food. The portion sizes of various dishes and readymade fast food items have increased as a result of aggressive marketing of "jumbo sized" food packages and multiunit packs at so called discounted prices inducing the consumers to buy and consume more than required. Even while eating at home, the food our children eat has undergone dramatic changes as compared to food prepared and eaten at home barely a generation ago. *Maida*-based preparations, such as *biscuits* and bread, have replaced rough cereal-based freshly cooked preparations, such as *roti* and *bhakri*. Nowadays, most of womenfolk are engaged in full time job or profession, pure homemaker woman is a rarity. Resultant lack of time and lack of additional help, which was available in a joint family a generation ago, has led to replacement of home-cooked traditional foodstuffs by ready-to-eat items such as *biscuits* and noodles. The readymade items contain refined raw material deficient in fiber and thus are energy dense (a unit volume contains more calories than homemade fresh preparations based on whole cereal flour and fresh vegetables and fruits). Coaching classes, smart phones, TV/internet, and computers take up whatever little free time children could use for physical activity on the playground. All these factors are responsible for rapidly increasing prevalence of obesity and diabetes.

## CLINICAL FEATURES

The common age of onset is during adolescence and teens.

The clinical features are similar to those of T2DM in adults. Most of the patients are obese, even morbid obesity is not rare in these patients. Signs of insulin resistance, such as acanthosis nigricans, are usually present **(Fig. 1)**. Strong family history of T2DM is often present. Like their adult counterparts, symptoms are usually gradual in onset. Weight loss, lethargy, tiredness, polyuria, polydipsia, and itching are some of the common symptoms. Sometimes T2DM in children presents with acute symptoms,

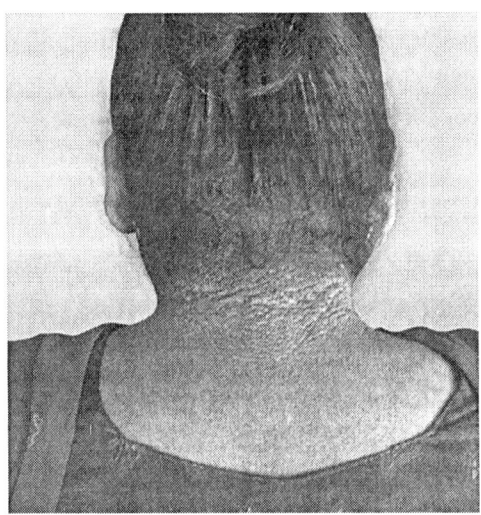

**FIG. 1:** The picture above depicts classical acanthosis nigricans. *(For color version, see Plate 1)*

*Note*: The hypertrophic dark brownish gray skin at the back of neck. Acanthosis nigricans is a sign of insulin resistance. Other manifestations of insulin resistance include hypertension, hypertriglyceridemia, and obesity. The patient depicted above had all these manifestations.

which resemble classical symptoms of type 1 diabetes mellitus. During the initial presentation, patients may be dehydrated and extremely weak and occasionally urine can be weakly positive for ketones. Under such circumstances, clinical differentiation between the two types of diabetes is difficult. These patients are initially treated with insulin and fluid and electrolyte replacement. After swift control of glucotoxicity with insulin, their insulin requirement is rapidly reduced. This serves as a clue for possibility of T2DM and absence of markers such as glutamic acid decarboxylase (GAD) and other antibodies in blood clinches the diagnosis. These patients can be subsequently maintained on lifestyle management and oral antidiabetic drugs (OADs).

## MANAGEMENT OF T2DM IN CHILDREN

The basic principles of management are same as those of T2DM in adults. Appropriate diet and exercise form the basic foundations of management. If and when these measures are not sufficient to reach glycemic goals, OADs are added. Since insulin resistance is predominant underlying pathophysiology in most of these patients, metformin, the time-tested insulin sensitizer is usually the agent of first choice. Since it is a new entity, large-scale randomized double-blind trials with metformin or any other OAD have not yet been performed in type 2 diabetic children. The general principles of subsequent management are same as in the adult counterpart. Insulin is used, if symptoms at diagnosis are severe and definite diagnosis is not established. There are some trials on liraglutide in children above the age of 10 years. Early diagnosis and prompt management to reach the glycemic and weight and waistline targets is vital, more so than even the adult counterpart because of the long life ahead of the patients who are struck with T2DM in childhood. If the targets are not reached and maintained, the vascular complications strike these patients in their youth. This affects their productivity at the prime of their lives leading to adverse effects on the socioeconomic aspects of the family. Thus besides diet, exercise and medications, patient education has vital central role. Patient must understand as early as possible that there is no alternative to tight metabolic control.

# CHAPTER 4

# Epidemiology of Diabetes

## INTRODUCTION

A study of prevalence pattern of a disease in a community is known as epidemiology.

*Prevalence* of a particular disease in any given community at any given time is expressed in percent and it represents percent of total population suffering from that disease. *Incidence* gives information on the number of new cases developing a particular disease in a community during a specified period, usually in a calendar year.

During the past 50 years, many countries in the world including India have experienced dramatic improvement in life expectancy due to improved nutrition, better hygiene, and control over many communicable diseases and malnutrition-related diseases. However, prevalence of noncommunicable diseases, such as diabetes, has dramatically increased leading to increasing burden and cost to the society. The term *epidemiological transition* is applied to describe these changes in disease pattern. This transition has catapulted diabetes from its former status as a rare disease at the beginning of last century, to its current position as a major global disease responsible for considerable mortality and morbidity.

The prevalence of diabetes has increased by leaps and bounds in India and has already reached epidemic proportions. India has >74 million adult diabetic patients, while globally there were 537 million adults with diabetes in December 2021. **Figure 1** gives region wise distribution of number of adults with diabetes. South East Asia region includes India, which has 74 million out of 90 million diabetic patients in the region.

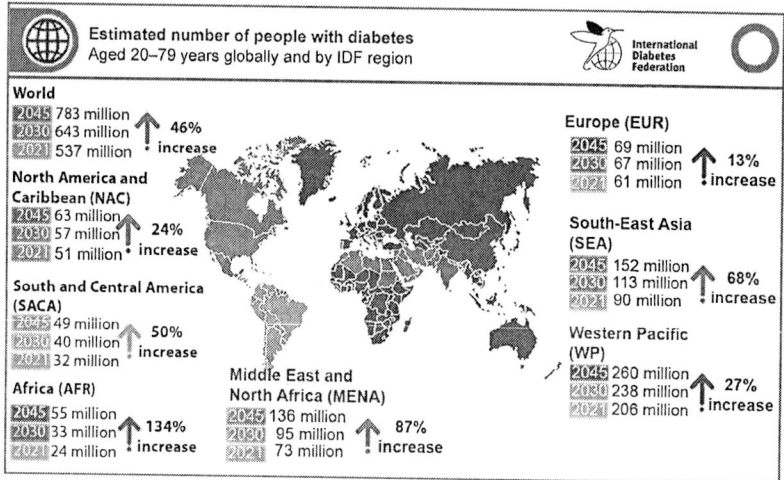

**FIG. 1:** Number of adults with diabetes in 2021, region wise distribution International Diabetes Federation (IDF) 2011. *(For color version, see Plate 1)*

Source: IDF Diabetes Atlas 2021, 10th edition. www.idf.org. @IntDiabetesFed.

Also note the global projections of number of adults with diabetes in **Figure 2**.

Thus, it is vital to collect epidemiological data on diabetes from all over the country so that it can be used to evolve prudent preventive and therapeutic strategies best suited for our socioeconomic situation.

Till early 70s, properly collected epidemiological data on diabetes from India was conspicuous by its absence. There were a few studies from different parts of India, most of them were spot surveys done during social gatherings and also hospital-based or practice-based studies. Such a data does not represent the prevalence rates in the community as only healthy people attend social gatherings, while hospital-based and practice-based data totally misses out on asymptomatic, undiagnosed patients. Even in an advanced country, such as the USA, it is estimated that for every known diabetic, there is one unknown (undiagnosed) diabetic. International Diabetes Federation (IDF) has estimated that in December 2021, there were 240 million undiagnosed diabetic patients in the world. In India, it is estimated that 56% of diabetic patients are undiagnosed. The era of community-based, scientific epidemiological studies on diabetes in our country began in early 70s, when Indian Council of Medical

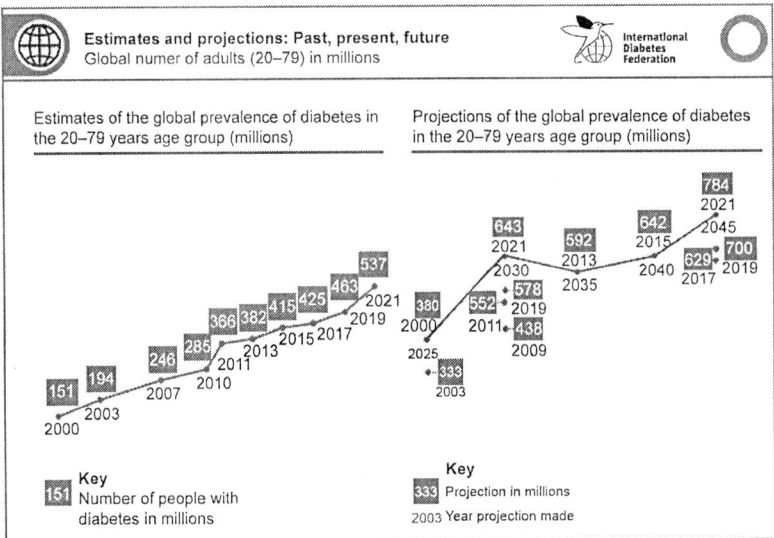

**FIG. 2:** Number of adults with diabetes in 2021 and projections for 2045-IDF (International Diabetes Federation) data. *(For color version, see Plate 2)*

*Source*: IDF Diabetes Atlas 2021, 10th edition. www.idf.org. @IntDiabetesFed.

Research (ICMR) conducted multicentric urban as well as rural studies from six different parts of our country. Subsequently, many more scientific studies have been conducted.

## EPIDEMIOLOGY OF TYPE 1 DIABETES MELLITUS

Definitive data from population-based studies on prevalence of type 1 diabetes mellitus (T1DM) is not available from India. As per the estimations of IDF, the yearly incidence in India is three cases per 100,000 population. T1DM is relatively rare in our country and <2% of the diabetic patients in India are having T1DM. Asian continent has lowest incidence rate of T1DM, approximately 0.5 cases per annum per 100,000 population. Some patients, who have onset of diabetes in the middle age and whose symptoms develop gradually and who develop either primary failure or early secondary failure to sulfonylureas, are actually suffering from late onset and slowly progressive subtype of T1DM. Immunological markers for T1DM are positive in these patients. There are a few studies on these patients from South India, but epidemiological studies are lacking.

Prevalence of T1DM increases as one travels from southern to northern hemisphere. About 15–20% of diabetic patients in Northern European countries are having T1DM. Among the countries in the European continent, there are significant north-south differences as regards incidence. Incidence rate of T1DM in Finland is 57.4 per 100,000 as against 3.9 per 100,000 in Macedonia in Southern Europe. In addition to geographical variation, there is a seasonal variation in incidence rates. More cases are diagnosed in winter. This is attributed to seasonal variation for viral infections which trigger autoimmune destruction of β-cells in pancreas, leading to acute onset diabetes. An interesting finding is that in the USA, incidence is much higher in white population as compared to blacks in the same area. Since the environmental factors are same for both the ethnic groups, the difference in incidence is probably based on genetic factors. Offspring of T1DM father are three times more likely to develop it by the age of 20 years as compared to those of T1DM mother (6% vs. 2%). It is postulated that exposure to diabetic environment in utero offers protection, perhaps by inducing immunological tolerance to the antigen involved in autoimmune destruction of pancreatic β cells. However, genetic factors are less important in pathogenesis of T1DM as compared to type 2 diabetes mellitus (T2DM). This has been amply proved by the studies done in twins.

*Relationship between T1DM occurrence and certain human leukocyte antigens*: In the early 70s, certain human leukocyte antigens (HLAs) were shown to be positively associated with T1DM but not with T2DM. Although, initially, certain HLA-B antigens were identified for association with T1DM, HLA-DR antigens have since been shown to have stronger association with the disease. In all the populations studied, T1DM has been confined largely to the individuals who carry HLA-DR3 or HLA-DR4 antigens.

## EPIDEMIOLOGY OF TYPE 2 DIABETES MELLITUS

As against incidence studies in T1DM, prevalence studies are more commonly done in T2DM. It has become epidemic in many developing and rapidly industrializing countries including India. In our country, around 95–96% of the diabetic patients have T2DM. Prevalence of T2DM, which was about 2% in early 70s, has sharply risen to >8% in late 90s and >14% in recent surveys in urban areas of our country. As per the pan India urban as well as rural prevalence study done by ICMR in 2011, India had 62.4 million diabetic patients and 72.2 million prediabetic patients. As per the estimates made by IDF in December 2021, 74 million out of global population of 537 million adult diabetic patients live in India. Prevalence rates of T2DM correlate with the degree of modernization, and many societies which are rapidly undergoing a transformation from traditional to modern lifestyles are experiencing some of the highest rates of diabetes. Noted diabetologist and epidemiologist Dr Paul Zimmet has termed the process leading to the epidemic of diabetes in developing countries as "Cocacolonization". Thus, globalization may be good for economy but it is a threat to civilization. "Westernization, industrialization, and cocacolonization have ruined civilization". Over the years, epidemiological studies done in different parts of the globe have shown that the Indian migrants settled abroad have a higher prevalence as compared to the local host population living in identical environment, as well as the population native in India. This has been reported from countries with long-established Indian populations such as Singapore, Fiji islands, South Africa, Tanzania, Uganda, Trinidad, and UK. Data generated over last four decades from our country have proved that the prevalence of T2DM is rapidly rising among urban native Indian population and is approaching the prevalence rates seen in the migrant Indian population.

While there is a drastic increase in prevalence rate in urban India, the prevalence in rural India has increased at slower rate. Consumption of traditional diet and relative absence of mechanization have protected the rural population to some extent.

However, as per recent survey done in Tamil Nadu, prevalence of diabetes is rapidly rising even in rural areas. In a study by Mohan and his group, prevalence of T2DM was 13.5% in rural Kanchipuram area in Tamil Nadu in 2019. Another very worrisome finding is reduction in prevalence rate of impaired glucose tolerance (prediabetes). It means faster conversion of these people to diabetes and thus more rapid rise is the prevalence of diabetes.

**Figure 3** shows prevalence of diabetes and prediabetes as per the study done by ICMR in 2011.

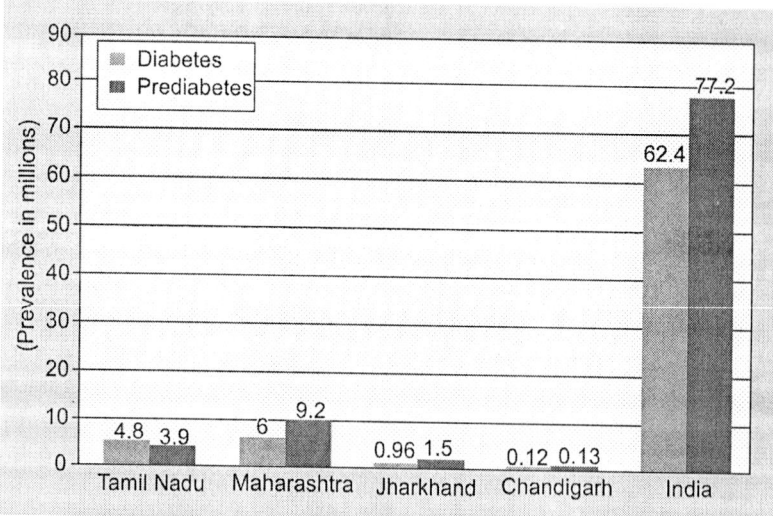

**FIG. 3:** Prevalence of diabetes and prediabetes in India: Indian Council of Medical Research (ICMR)-India study, number of people with diabetes and prediabetes in India, 2011.

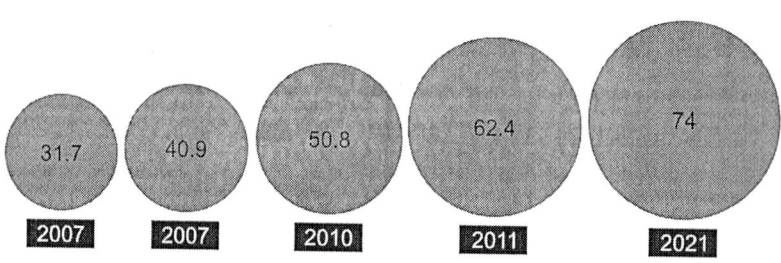

**FIG. 4:** Increasing prevalence of diabetes in India, persons with diabetes (millions).

By extrapolating IDF 2021 data for prediabetes for South East Asia, India was having 82 million prediabetics in 2021.

**Figure 4** shows rising prevalence of diabetes in India.

There is a large variation in prevalence of T2DM between the different ethnicities. The highest rates are found in some native American tribes such as the Pima Indians (over 50%), while low prevalence rates are found in least developed rural communities in many Afro-Asian countries (3%).

| TABLE 1: Prevalence of gestational diabetes in India. | | |
|---|---|---|
| Region | Prevalence in % | Year of report |
| Tamil Nadu | 17.9 | 2004 |
| Mysore | 6.2 | 2008 |
| Kashmir | 3.9 | 2014 |
| Punjab | 35 | 2015 |
| Lucknow | 41 | 2015 |
| Maharashtra | 9.5 | 2015 |

## EPIDEMIOLOGY OF GESTATIONAL DIABETES MELLITUS

Gestational diabetes mellitus (GDM) occurs in about 4% of the pregnancies in the Western World. It is more common in India. **Table 1** shows prevalence of gestational diabetes among pregnant women in India. Please note that surveys were done at different times and methodology varied from survey to survey. In the majority of cases of gestational diabetes, blood glucose returns to normal in postpartum period, but the lifetime risk for future diabetes is substantially increased in women who develop GDM. About 40% develop diabetes in next 10 years.

## CONCLUSION

The epidemics of interrelated lifestyle disorders have struck the globe like tsunami with its epicenter in rapidly developing and industrializing Asian countries such as India and China. The global epidemic of T2DM is particularly affecting developing countries and migrant population from these countries to more industrialized and westernized societies. Eighty percent of world's diabetic patients live in low- or middle-income countries. This epidemic has closely followed the epidemic of obesity. The epidemic of T2DM itself is being closely followed by that of cardiovascular disorders particularly coronary artery disease. Until recently, based on the available epidemiological data, which was outdated to some extent, it was believed that India had the dubious distinction of having more diabetic patients than any other country including China.

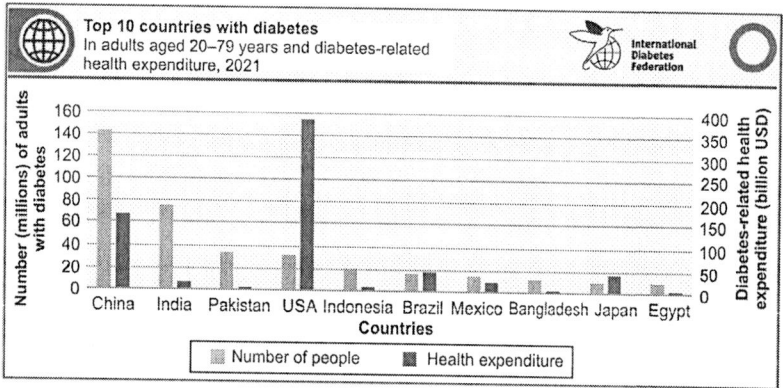

**FIG. 5:** Top 10 countries with adult diabetes and diabetes-related health expenditure as per International Diabetes Federation (IDF) 2021 data. *(For color version, see Plate 2)*

*Source*: IDF Diabetes Atlas 2021, 10th edition. www.idf.org. @IntDiabetesFed.

However, India is not the country with highest number of diabetic patients as on December 2021!, also note very meager expenditure on diabetes healthcare in India as compared to developed world **(Fig. 5)**.

# CHAPTER 5

# Diabesity

## INTRODUCTION

The onset of epidemic of obesity was closely followed by that of type 2 diabetes mellitus (T2DM) and at present, both these epidemics are in full force globally. The global epidemic of obesity is nicknamed as "globesity". Obesity and diabetes are closely interrelated. Obesity leads to insulin resistance, which in a person with genetic or acquired β-cell defect leads to T2DM at a stage when β-cells with limited functional capacity can no longer meet progressively increasing demand for insulin. Thus, diabetes follows obesity in those predisposed due to genetic or acquired β-cell defect. This dual epidemic of obesity with diabetes has been labeled as "diabesity". Dr C Everett Koop, a former US Surgeon General, coined the term diabesity.

Those obese persons who do not have β-cell defect can meet additional insulin requirement and thus do not become diabetic. Thus, obesity is not a prerequisite for development of T2DM. Insulin resistance can develop even in those who are not obese. Nonetheless, if one analyzes all those who are nonobese by body mass index (BMI) criteria, many of them, particularly those who are diabetic, would fall into central obesity category by waist circumference criteria. In short, obesity and diabetes run hand in hand and their coexistence is called diabesity, but not all obeses are diabetic patients and not all diabetic patients are obese. Diabesity has struck the world, particularly India as a double tsunami.

The association of risk of diabetes with increasing weight has been clearly demonstrated in several recently published reports.

In one such report, the incidence rate of diabetes increased from 13 to 104 per 100,000 person-years comparing women whose BMI was <22 to those whose BMI ranged from 25 to 26.9. Although this was a significant difference, the largest absolute increase in risk was found in obese range. From lowest BMI group in obese range of 27–28.9 to the highest group of >35, the incidence rate increased from 200 to 1,190 per 100,000 person-years. In the west, majority of type 2 diabetic patients are overweight. In India even though majority are having BMI in the normal range, they are centrally obese. Their waist circumference is above normal. According to one survey, only 20% of Indian type 2 diabetic patients are overweight by BMI criteria but around 50% are centrally obese as per waist circumference value. Indians have a tendency, which is partly genetically determined, to have excessive fat deposition in abdominal viscera. Since we do not have a strong muscle mass and since we have relatively less fat in subcutaneous tissues, our BMI is within normal range even in many of those who have significant central obesity. This type of fat distribution is present even in persons from lower socioeconomic class. Thus, many Indians are actually "*thin, but fat*" people. **Table 1** gives comparative figure for BMI and body fat percentage for Asian Indians and persons of white race.

**Figure 1** depicts a type 2 diabetic patient with classical central obesity.

From these figures, it is clear that Indians have excessive fat even when their BMI is within normal range. The association between central obesity as measured by waist circumference with diabetes and cardiovascular disease (CVD) is stronger than that of

**TABLE 1:** Comparison of body fat (%) and BMI in Asian Indians and in white race.

| Race | BMI (kg/m²) | Fat (%) |
|---|---|---|
| Asian men | 22 | 22.7 |
| White men | 25.2 | 21.2 |
| Asian women | 22.7 | 37.4 |
| White women | 23.3 | 30.3 |

*Source*: Snehalata et al. JAPI 1999;47:1164-7; Gallagher et al. Am J Clin Nutr. 1966; 60:23-8.

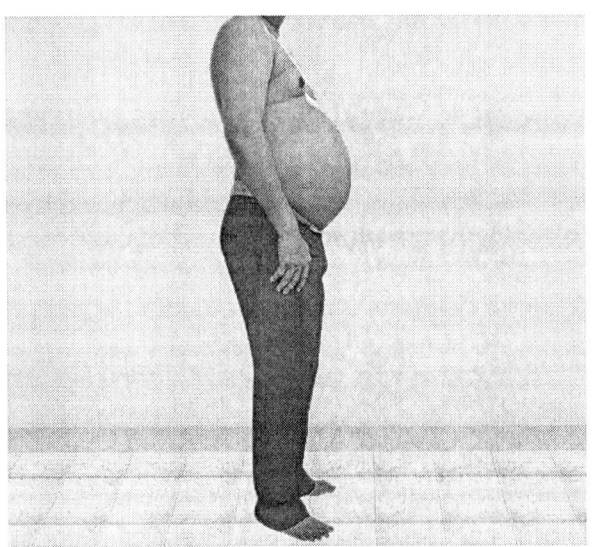

**FIG. 1:** A type 2 diabetic patient with classical central obesity.

general obesity with these two lifestyle disorders. Previously, fat tissue was looked upon as a mere storage organ. In-depth research on obesity has led us to understand fat tissue in more details. It is now clearly understood that fat tissue is an important endocrine organ. It forms and releases several vital substances including hormones, proinflammatory substances, and other proteins in circulation. Deficiencies and excess formation of some of these are associated with pathological states. For example, leptin deficiency is associated with an extreme form of monogenic obesity while deficiency of adiponectin is associated with insulin resistance. Visceral abdominal fat is more insulin-resistant than subcutaneous fat. Moreover, it secretes detrimental hormones and inflammatory substances in higher quantities than subcutaneous fat. These substances are directly carried to liver through enterohepatic circulation. Thus, abdominal visceral fat is more harmful than subcutaneous fat.

Over entire last century, the prevalence of obesity was gradually increasing and over last two decades, the rate of increase has tremendously accelerated. For the first time, we now have more overweight people in the world than underweight. In addition to increase in prevalence in middle-aged persons, the prevalence in children and adolescents has also increased considerably. In a recent survey done in Chennai, about 15% of children and adolescents were overweight. As per World Health Organization (WHO) and International Diabetes Federation (IDF) estimations, there are >650 million obese and 537 million diabetic people in the world. In addition, there are 1,200 million overweight but not obese (BMI between 25 and 30) people and about 550 million people with prediabetes. In India, socioeconomic changes are occurring at very rapid speed. Urbanization, industrialization, and westernization have become unstoppable. Our food habits are changing rapidly. Eating in restaurants has increased. We are eating more refined, energy-dense fast food. The portion sizes of various dishes and readymade fast food items have increased. Accelerated prevalence of obesity and diabetes is the result of these socioeconomic changes. In spite of weight control industry attaining multibillion dollar turnover, obesity epidemic has not shown even any remote signs of receding.

Obesity refers to increase in amount of body fat. Usually in a day-to-day practice, obesity is measured and classified as per individual's BMI value. BMI is defined as body weight in kg divided by square of height in meters. For example, a lady having a height of 150 cm or 1.5 m and weight of 50 kg, has a BMI of 50 divided by 2.25 (a square of 1.5) = 22.22. Based on BMI values, the overweight is divided into simple overweight and obesity and further subclassified as per the **Table 2**.

With the exception of highly muscular people such as weightlifters, BMI conveys the real fat mass and thus is a pragmatic

**TABLE 2:** Gradation as per body mass index (BMI).

| Gradation as per BMI | BMI |
|---|---|
| Underweight | <18 |
| Normal | 18–22.9 |
| Overweight | 23–24.9 |
| Mild obesity | 25–29.9 |
| Morbid obesity | >30 |

*Note:* The figures mentioned in the table are for Indian population. They differ from figures for western population, which are widely quoted in the literature.

**TABLE 3: Comparative prevalence figures of overweight and obesity in India, UK, and USA.**

| USA | UK | India |
|---|---|---|
| 66% adult are overweight | 60% adult are overweight (BMI >25) | 33% men and 55% women are overweight (Delhi survey) |
| 30% adults are obese (BMI >30) | 19% are obese, 1% are morbidly obese | 76% women in New Delhi have central obesity |
| (BMI: body mass index) | | |

indicator of general obesity, since it is very easy to calculate BMI. However, it is the abdominal obesity which is more important as regards lifestyle disorders such as diabetes.

**Table 3** gives comparative prevalence figures of overweight and obesity in India, UK, and USA.

## CENTRAL OBESITY

Obesity is an ancient problem. Hippocrates, the famous Greek physician had made detailed description of obesity and its management 2,500 years ago. In ancient Ayurvedic literature, obesity, and its coexistence with a subtype of diabetes has been very elaborately described. However, the subject of fat distribution started receiving attention barely five decades back. Professor Vague was first to demonstrate the significantly higher association between upper body obesity and diabetes and CVD as compared to lower body obesity. Based on measurement of body circumferences and skin fold thickness at different sites, he classified obesity in two different types: (1) upper body obesity (apple-shaped or android obesity) and (2) lower body obesity (pear-shaped or gynecoid obesity) **(Figs. 2A and B)**. His observation of stronger association of upper body obesity with diabetes and CVD was subsequently supported in early 80s by American and Swedish workers who used waist-hip ratio parameter to classify obesity. In the late 80s, association between upper body obesity or central obesity and insulin resistance and latter association with various other risk factors were described by Reaven. He called the association as "syndrome X". Subsequently, the same became synonymous with metabolic syndrome.

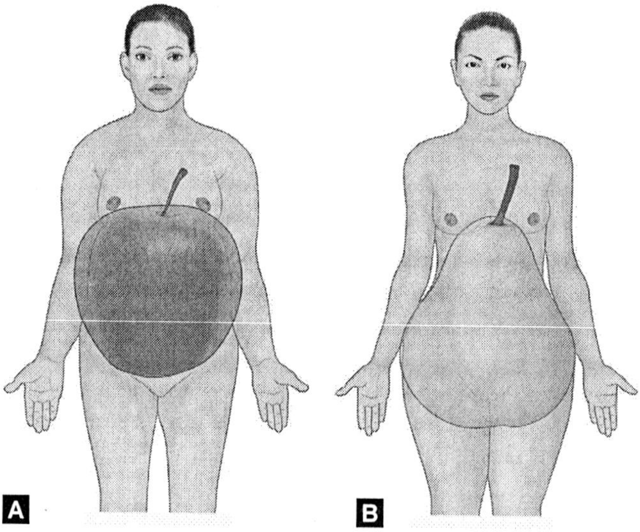

**FIGS. 2A AND B:** Upper body obesity and lower body obesity: (A) Apple-shaped upper body obesity and (B) Pear-shaped lower body obesity.

Since there are practical difficulties in precisely measuring hip circumference, more so in India, and since waist circumference has been a proven indicator of upper body obesity, it has replaced waist-hip ratio measurement for assessment of central obesity (upper body obesity). The cutoff points for Indians are 90 cm for men and 80 cm for women. **Figures 2A and B** indicate central obesity. In a commonly used method for measurement of waist circumference, a nonextensible tape (plastic or metallic) is used to measure the circumference at midpoint between iliac crest and the last rib. The instrumental methods to measure body composition, such as dual-energy X-ray absorptiometry (DEXA), bioelectric impedance, isotope dilution, CT, MRI, etc., are expensive and cannot be used at the bedside or in outpatient clinic and are thus used only in research settings.

## HOW DO WE BECOME FAT?

Baring few cases of purely genetic obesity such as leptin deficiency, most of the cases that we see in our day-to-day practice are due positive energy balance resulting from excessive energy intake and/or insufficient physical activity albeit with a genetic background.

Genes load the gun and environmental causes pull the trigger. In other words, genes make soil fertile while environmental causes plant the seeds. Rapidly progressing mechanization has led to free use of the industrial products in all walks of life including rural life. We use automobiles for transport, elevators to climb, washing machines and dish washers to clean, and various gadgets to cook. Even our farmers are using tractors to produce grains. TV, internet, and computers take up whatever little free time which we could use for physical activity. All of us are spending far less energy than our predecessors a few decades back. Moreover, instead of reducing our energy intake, we have increased it. Frequency of eating out and that too junk food-based meals has increased considerably even in average families. Even while eating at home, the food we eat has undergone dramatic changes. *Maida*-based preparations such as *biscuits* and bread have replaced rough cereal-based freshly cooked preparations such as *roti*. The readymade foodstuffs contain refined raw material deficient in fiber. In addition these preparations contain far higher quantities of fats, which provide 9 calories per gram as against 4 calories provided by carbohydrates and proteins. Thus, these dishes are energy-dense (a unit volume contains more calories than homemade fresh preparations based on whole cereal flour and fresh vegetables and fruits). One additional factor, particularly in India, is intrauterine malnutrition. Low-birthweight infants are more prone to develop obesity and associated metabolic disorders including diabetes in later part of their life when exposed to oversupply of nutrients. Their metabolism, which gets adopted to conserve energy more efficiently, cannot change when they go into positive energy balance in later part of their life due to overeating and less physical activity. Some endocrine disorders such as Cushing's syndrome are occasionally responsible for obesity, and this should be kept in mind during the workup of the patient. Several drugs including hormones and psychoactive drugs can cause obesity. Thus, obesity as we see in our diabetic patients can be occasionally multifactorial in origin.

## DISORDERS ASSOCIATED WITH OBESITY

Obesity is associated with increased prevalence of various disorders besides diabetes and CVD. Gallbladder disorders, certain malignancies such as carcinoma of colon, breast and endometrial cancer, obstructive sleep apnea, osteoarthritis, and some psychological disturbances are more common in obesity as compared with individuals with normal weight.

## MANAGEMENT OF DIABESITY (TABLE 4)

Management of diabesity essentially consists of simultaneous management of obesity and diabetes. Management of diabetes has been discussed in chapters on meal planning, exercise, oral antidiabetic drugs, insulin, and various antidiabetic drug combinations. Thus, management of obesity will be discussed in this chapter and the emphasis will be on behavioral therapy and pharmacological management of obesity as meal planning and exercise have been dealt with elsewhere in the book. When obese people lose weight, they derive considerable benefits. Twenty percent reduction in all-cause mortality has been reported in one study done by Williamson et al. In another study, 20–30% reduction in mortality due to diabetes has been associated with weight reduction. Thus, weight reduction is extremely cost-effective.

*Setting weight-loss goals*: Setting realistic achievable goals is important. In severely obese patient, the first goal should be to prevent further weight gain. Subsequently, one should plan for 5–15% weight loss in first 1–2 years and subsequently, emphasis should be on weight maintenance. This much weight loss will reduce most of the risk factors associated with obesity.

**TABLE 4:** Guidelines for selecting therapeutic modality depending upon the gradation of obesity and presence of comorbidities.

| Treatment | BMI category (kg/m$^2$) | | | | |
|---|---|---|---|---|---|
| | 23–24.9 | 25–27.9 | 28–32.4 | 32.5–37.49 | >37.5 |
| Diet, exercise | + | + | + | + | + |
| Behavioral therapy | + | + | + | + | + |
| Pharmacotherapy | – | + if comorbidities | + | + | + |
| Surgery | – | – | – | + if comorbidities | + |

## Behavioral Treatment

Behavioral treatment includes various methods and strategies that are used in coordination to bring about the changes in lifestyle. Behavioral strategies are the cornerstone of treatment of obesity. Several behavioral strategies are applied simultaneously. Keeping food diaries and activity records: patients are taught to enter each and every food item before they eat and to assess and record calorie content. They are also taught to note down the situation or trigger, which led to eating. The records are kept continuously for 4-6 months. Similarly, details of all the activities are also recorded. The analysis of data generated from this record keeping is very useful to get tips regarding change of behavior as regards food intake and physical activity. Slowing down the act of eating helps to reduce weight. It gives a feeling of fullness earlier than usual, thus reducing the food intake. Concentrating on the taste of food and savoring food while eating helps to slow down the speed of eating. Social support should be enhanced by including a family member's or a friend's help. Using wearable Apps on the smart phones to feed activities such as food intake and to set the goals and track activities such as physical exercise and sleep is a smart way of applying behavioral treatment in a day-to-day practice. Behavioral therapy does not work in isolation; it has to be integrated with lifestyle changes and medications.

## Pharmacotherapy

Reduction of weight and maintenance of reduced weight is extremely difficult and often nonpharmacological modes of management such as behavior therapy and lifestyle changes are not sufficient to bring weight down to set goals. Bariatric surgery is the treatment of choice for morbid obesity and severe obesity with comorbidities. However, when majority of overweight and obese people do not reach their weight reduction goals with lifestyle changes alone; pharmacotherapy is required in such situations. There is a paucity of safe and effective antiobesity agents. Older drugs such as sibutramine and rimonabant have been banned, even a recently introduced agent, lorcaserin has been banned in India, soon after USA, the country of its origin banned it within years after its introduction in USA market. Today, orlistat is the only antiobesity drug available in India. High strength (3 mg) liraglutide, which is available in western countries, is not yet marketed in India.

Pharmacotherapy does not cure obesity. Drugs work as long as they are taken and help to reduce weight by about 5–10%. The action starts slowly and the peak effects are usually seen around 18–24 months after the beginning of therapy. Some patients get frustrated after weight loss plateaus off and there is no further weight loss. At this juncture, they tend to discontinue therapy resulting in weight regain and further frustrations and depression. Thus, it is prudent to have frank in-depth discussion before prescribing weight reducing agent to brief them about what to expect from the drug.

### *Orlistat*

It is a potent and selective inhibitor of pancreatic lipase. It works by inhibiting fat digestion in small intestine in dose-dependent manner. Up to 30% of digestion of fat is inhibited. The undigested fat is excreted in fecal matter. Since it has a specific action on fat digestion, it is of no use in patients who consume small amounts of fat. It is administered in the doses of 120 mg three times a day before each meal. Gastrointestinal (GI) side effects are common initially and they gradually reduce or subside after few weeks. It is prudent to put the patients on multivitamin supplement while on orlistat as it leads to malabsorption of fat soluble vitamins in some patients. Leakage of fat globules through rectum and staining of underwear is another side effect. Orlistat has been clinically tested in obese diabetic patients as well as in those with metabolic syndrome and obesity and has been found to be effective and reasonably tolerated. Orlistat has also been successfully tested in obese patients with impaired glucose tolerance to prevent diabetes. Among all the antiobesity agents, orlistat is the only one which is available across the globe and which is not under the scanner of regulatory authorities for adverse effects. 60 mg strength of orlistat is available over-the-counter in USA.

### New Antiobesity Agents

#### Liraglutide

Liraglutide is an injectable agent and is routinely used in the dosage of 0.6–1.8 mg daily in a single daily subcutaneous injection in the management of type 2 diabetic patients. Significant weight reduction and freedom from bothersome side effects like hypoglycemia has made liraglutide extremely popular antidiabetic agent in western countries where cost of treatment is usually borne by insurance companies as in USA or Government as in Europe. Being costly, liraglutide has had a limited success in our country, where in majority of cases, the patient has to bear the cost of treatment. However, it is an excellent choice for obese diabetic patients who can afford it. Besides efficient antidiabetic action and weight reduction, it protects cardiovascular system from atherosclerotic CVD, offers some renoprotection; and safety from hypoglycemia, which is common with insulin and sulfonylurea based oral antidiabetic pills. After successful completion of clinical trials in >3,000 patients, in which 3 mg of liraglutide given once a day in subcutaneous injection in nondiabetic obese people resulted in mean 8 kg weight loss, it has been introduced as an antiobesity agent in USA and Europe under brand name Saxenda (it is sold under brand name Victoza as an antidiabetic agent). I have been regularly prescribing it in affording obese diabetic patients particularly those with associated atherosclerotic CVD's or high risk for them, and getting satisfactory results on both the fronts, blood glucose control as well as weight reduction. With the help of some periodic free samples from the manufacturers, the monthly cost can be reduced to Rs. 5,000–6,000. Liraglutide formulation, specifically designed for weight reduction is not yet available in India.

Newer glucagon-like peptide-1 ($GLP_1$) agonist, semaglutide is at being tried as an antiobesity agent once a week.

### Phentermine + Topiramate oral combination: (Qsymia)

Phentermine, an appetite suppressant and topiramate, an anticonvulsant in a fixed dose combination of 3.75 mg and 23 mg respectively, was introduced in USA in 2013 for the management of obesity. The combination needs to be given once a day in morning. Pregnant women should not use it. Kidney stones, depression, and insomnia are occasionally observed in patients on this combination.

A specifically formulated fixed dose combination of phentermine and topiramate in a single tablet is not yet available in India.

***A combination of bupropion and naltrexone (Contrave):*** This new drug combination has been recently introduced as an antiobesity agent in USA, the only country where it has received marketing approval. While bupropion is an antidepressant, naltrexone blocks the effects of narcotic agents and alcohol. This combination is not to be used by those having uncontrolled high blood pressure, epilepsy, kidney failure, and pregnant and breastfeeding women.

***Other agents:*** Besides the mainline agents described above, there are many agents used in a day-to-day practice for management of obesity. Some of these agents like phentermine are approved by the United States Food and Drug Administration (US FDA) only for short-term use while others like fluoxetine and sertraline are used as "off the label drugs" (officially indicated for depression but doctors prescribe them for management of obesity also, even though they are not officially recommended for use in obesity). Metformin, which is a mainline antidiabetic agent having weight stabilizing properties, is occasionally used as an antiobesity agent even in nondiabetic obese people. For those who are obese and diabetic, recently introduced new antidiabetic medications such as those from sodium-glucose cotransporter-2 inhibitor ($SGLT_2I$) group (dapagliflozin, canagliflozin, and empagliflozin) and $GLP_1$ analog group (liraglutide, exenatide, dulaglutide, and oral semaglutide) offer weight reduction in addition to blood glucose reduction. Because of many other advantages, which are described at appropriate place in this book, these agents are gradually replacing sulfonylurea-based pills in the management of diabetes.

## Bariatric Surgery (Metabolic Surgery)

Since a combination of nonpharmacological methods and weight-reducing agents does not reduce weight by >10% in majority of patients, those who are morbidly obese and those who are bordering on morbid obesity associated with comorbid conditions such as hypertension, diabetes, dyslipidemia, etc., one of the surgical procedures should be considered.

### Indications for Bariatric Surgery

- Body mass index >32.5 with comorbid conditions such as diabetes and failure of nonsurgical methods
- Body mass index >37.5% and failure of nonsurgical methods

In last few years, there has been a tremendous increase in the number of bariatric surgical procedures performed all over the world, including India. Many organizations have changed the guidelines of indications for bariatric surgery and the new indications include: (1) BMI >30 with comorbid conditions such as diabetes and failure of nonsurgical methods; (2) BMI >35 and failure of nonsurgical methods.

In patients who have undergone Roux-en-Y gastric bypass surgery, blood glucose is reduced soon after the surgery, much before weight loss. There are many mechanisms through which this is achieved.

Altered hormonal and neural signals from GI tract to brain and other organs lead to dramatic effects on hunger and satiety. Both $GLP_1$ and glucose-dependent insulinotropic peptide (GIP) levels increase after surgery. Thus, bariatric surgery is sometimes referred to as metabolic surgery. Some of the other mechanisms contributing toward weight loss after bariatric surgery include:
- Reduced absorption of food due to bypassing areas of intestine where normally food is digested and then absorbed.
- Less consumption of food due to fullness and loss appetite resulting from reduced stomach volume following restrictive procedures on stomach such as sleeve gastrectomy
- Change in composition of intestinal bacterial flora
- Increased concentration of bile in lower small intestine

Some of the commonly used surgical procedures are described here in brief:
- *Roux-en-Y gastric bypass with pancreaticobiliary diversion (distal stomach, duodenum, and jejunal bypass)*: Best procedure with far superior results than other procedures (100% improvement in glycemia and 82% resolution of diabetes, 40% weight loss, half of it is regained after 10 years). No weight loss in normal weight or underweight persons who underwent this surgery. Normal weight gain during the pregnancy. 40% reduction in mortality at 7.1 years mainly due to reduction of CVD, diabetes and malignancy.
- *Adjustable gastric banding*: Reduces food intake and slows the transition of food. Direction of food is normal. It leads to 20% weight loss, 50% of it will be regained at 10 years.

- *Vertical sleeve gastrectomy*: Greater curvature of stomach is excised. Food passes in normal direction and speed of onward transmission is increased. This procedure has been increasingly used as the procedure of choice in many centers of late.

Thus many diabetic obese patients undergoing bariatric surgery have beneficial effects on their blood glucose. Most diabetic patients have significant reduction in their antidiabetic medications and many do not need them at all. Those who do not have diabetes, bariatric surgery, by substantially reducing weight, will prevent diabetes. A study was done on >1,600 obese people with BMI >35, who did not have diabetes at the start of the study. They were divided in two groups; one group was put on intensive diet plus exercise, while the other was subjected to one of the abovementioned bariatric surgical procedures. When reviewed 15 years later, 395 and 110 people in diet plus exercise group and bariatric surgery group had diabetes respectively. Thus those in later group developed diabetes in significantly lesser number. Of course they had several other advantages such as prevention of other obesity-related disorders such as high blood pressure, osteoarthritis, accidents, etc.

Now let us look at the largest study on bariatric surgery. It was done in Sweden and they studied 4,000 patients up to 10 years after the surgery. It was called SOS study. 10 years after surgery, 74% of patients who underwent gastric bypass surgery had still maintained weight loss of >20%, while only 4% of those who did not undergo surgery but implemented lifestyle changes could sustain 20% weight loss. In the same study, it was observed that at 2 years and 10 years after surgical procedures, 20% and 10% of those on lifestyle measures were in remission of diabetes, but the corresponding figures for those who underwent bariatric surgery were 70% and 35%.

Thus, in properly selected people, bariatric surgery is an excellent tool, not merely for treatment of obesity and diabetes, but also for prevention of diabetes.

Bariatric surgery should not be considered in those who are mentally unstable and in those with short life span due to major incurable underlying disease. Bariatric surgical procedure should not be taken lightly as like any other surgical procedure bariatric surgery is associated with side effects, though they are negligible in properly selected patients under a surgeon specifically trained and experienced in bariatric surgery.

In short, obesity is a common lifestyle disorder, the prevalence of which is increasing rapidly. It predisposes the affected person to several comorbid conditions including diabetes. All these comorbidities work in tandem and reduce the life span of the affected person. Thus obesity needs to be tackled on the war footing. Various modalities of treatment are available and one needs to combine them judiciously. The results of appropriate treatment are encouraging.

Thus, if your BMI is 24, you should follow diet, exercise, and behavior therapy, if you have BMI of 26.5, you should consider one of the pills to reduce your weight in addition to diet, exercise, and behavior therapy, in case you also have diabetes or other comorbidities. If your BMI is 29, even if you do not have associated comorbidities, you should use pills in addition to lifestyle changes, and if your BMI is 33, you should consider bariatric surgery if associated comorbidities are present. And if you are morbidly obese, i.e., BMI >37.5, you can opt for bariatric surgery even if associated comorbidities are absent.

Comorbidities = Associated disorders like diabetes, high blood pressure, high cholesterol, etc.

Recently, a mega trial on obesity called "Look Ahead" study was completed. It has taught many important lessons and given strong take-home messages. The synopsis of Look Ahead study is given here.

## Look Ahead Study

Recently, a more than decade long study, Look Ahead study was concluded in USA. 5,145 morbidly obese people participated in this study. They were divided in two groups: (1) group subjected to intensive lifestyle changes and aiming 10% reduction in body weight, and (2) group following conventional lifestyle. People in both the groups had similar characteristics at the beginning of the study. The median follow-up was for 9.6 years while the longest follow-up was for 11 years. The primary endpoints studied were death from cardiovascular causes, nonfatal myocardial infarction, and stroke. Those in group A lost 8.6% and 6% weight at the end of 1st and 6th year respectively. There was significant improvement in glycated hemoglobin (HbA1c), systolic blood pressure (BP) and high-density lipoprotein (HDL) cholesterol in this group as compared to group B, while diastolic BP and triglycerides were similar in both the groups at the end of trial. Low-density lipoprotein (LDL) cholesterol rose in group A, probably because fewer patients were on statins as compared to those in group B. The surprising and disappointing observation was that there was no difference in cardiovascular mortality between the two groups. What are the possible explanations? 8.6% weight loss could not be sustained for long term and 6% weight loss was not sufficient. The training for intensive lifestyle changes was inadequate. Rise in LDL cholesterol could have partly nullified good effects of weight loss. Weight loss late in life did not benefit because by that time legacy effect of overweight was firmly established. These are some of the possible explanations. Sustained weight loss achieved at younger age would probably help to reduce mortality and morbidity associated with obesity.

> *"The chief cause of premature development of arteriosclerosis in diabetes is an excess of fat, an excess of fat in the body (obesity) and excess of fat in the diet, and an excess of fat in the blood. With an excess of fat diabetes begins and from excess of fat diabetics die, formerly of coma, recently of arteriosclerosis".*
>
> —Dr Elliot Joslin, 1927

# CHAPTER 6

# Metabolic Syndrome

## INTRODUCTION

Metabolic syndrome (MS) is a name given to a cluster of metabolic and anthropometric features that include central obesity, glucose intolerance or diabetes mellitus (DM), hypertension, and dyslipidemia. Other laboratory findings include hyperuricemia, microalbuminuria, hemostatic derangements, and increased concentrations of inflammatory markers. Reaven first described MS in 1988. It was initially known as syndrome X or Reaven's syndrome or syndrome of insulin resistance. Different renowned bodies, such as World Health Organization (WHO), International Diabetes Federation (IDF), National Cholesterol Education Program (NCEP), have formulated their own criteria for diagnosis of MS and these vary from each other. While central obesity is an obligatory requirement in IDF definition, glucose intolerance is mandatory for the diagnosis of MS in WHO definition. The criteria recommended by some other bodies require investigations to measure insulin resistance. These investigations are costly and time-consuming and thus are impractical and not discussed here. The diagnostic criteria recommended by NCEP are most suited for the day-to-day practice **(Table 1)**.

*Note*: The criteria for central obesity described in **Table 1** are for Caucasians. For Indians, waist circumference >90 cm in men and 80 cm in women is taken as an indicator of central obesity.

**TABLE 1: Diagnostic criteria for Metabolic syndrome.**

| Criteria | NECP | WHO | IDF |
|---|---|---|---|
| Central obesity waist circumference in centimeter or waist-hip ratio | Waist circumference<br>• >102 (men)<br>• >88 (women) | Waist-hip ratio<br>• >0.9 (men)<br>• >0.85 (women) and/or BMI >30 | Waist circumference<br>• >94 (men)<br>• >80 (women) |
| Fasting plasma glucose | >110 mg% | • >120 mg% or 2 hours post glucose<br>• >140 mg% or known diabetic | >100 mg% or known diabetic |
| Blood pressure (mm Hg) | >130/85 | >140/90 | >130/85 |
| Fasting triglyceride concentration HDL concentration | • >150 mg%<br>• <45 mg% (men)<br>• <39 mg% (women) | • >150 mg%<br>• <50 mg% (women)<br>• <40 mg% (men) | • >150 mg%<br>• <35 mg% (men)<br>• <50 mg% (women) |
| Minimum criteria for diagnosis of MS | Any three of above criteria | One of the glycemic abnormalities mentioned above + two more | Central obesity + two more |

(BMI: body mass index; HDL: high-density lipoprotein; IDF: International Diabetes Federation; MS: metabolic syndrome; NECP: National Cholesterol Education Program; WHO: World Health Organization)

## PREVALENCE OF METABOLIC SYNDROME

In the USA, in population aged above 20 and 40 years, the prevalence of MS is 20–25% and 44%, respectively, while it is 86% in diabetic persons. Depending upon the definition used, the prevalence of MS in general population in Europe varies between 7 and 39%. In Chennai, 23% of general population had MS; while in a survey done in Mumbai, prevalence of MS was 77% among the diabetic patients. In a study done on policemen in Kolkata, 56% of policemen had MS.

## THE IMPORTANCE OF METABOLIC SYNDROME

The persons fulfilling the criteria of MS are at higher risk to develop coronary artery disease (CAD) and other macrovascular diseases, as well as DM in future as compared to a person who does not fulfill the criteria of MS, when other factors such as age, sex, race, etc., are similar. This is not at all surprising as MS is a condition in which several risk factors for CAD and DM coexist. Both CAD and DM are chronic, progressive, noncurable diseases, which have high morbidity and mortality. The treatment of both is very expensive. Both strike the population at their creative peak and thus carry tremendous economic burden to the patient, his family, and to the country. Unfortunately, our country is simultaneously struck by the mega epidemics of CAD as well as DM. Considering all these factors, it is mandatory for a family physician to periodically carry out routine health checkup, which should include measurement of blood pressure, height, weight, waist circumference, and laboratory investigations such as blood glucose estimation and lipid profile in their patients and family members so that cases of MS are identified at an early stage and lifestyle measures and pharmacological treatment, whenever appropriate, are started in order to revert those with MS back to non-MS status in order to reduce their risk of developing CAD and DM **(Fig. 1)**.

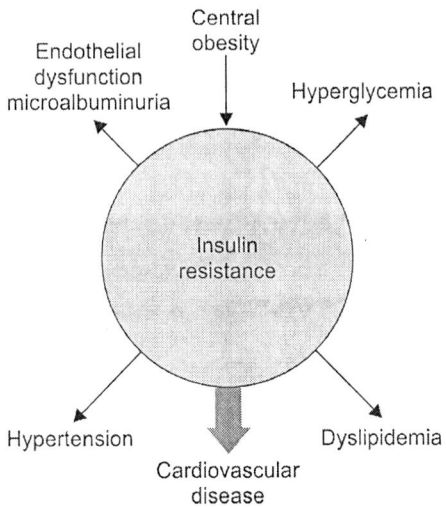

**FIG. 1:** Insulin resistance syndrome.

## MANAGEMENT OF METABOLIC SYNDROME

Each individual risk factor should be aggressively managed. The criteria of management of each risk factor in MS are the same as those for individual risk factors when they exist in isolation or in groups of more than one, but still short of diagnosis of MS. Lifestyle measures, such as appropriate meal planning and increased physical activity in the form of regular dynamic exercise, are the basic foundations of management of MS. If these measures are not sufficient to reduce the waist circumference, blood pressure, triglycerides, high-density lipoprotein (HDL) cholesterol and blood glucose values to the desired levels, appropriate pharmacological therapy should be initiated. The details about lifestyle measures as well as pharmacotherapy are given in chapters on diabesity, prevention of diabetes, blood pressure, and dyslipidemia and thus will not be repeated here.

## THE CONTROVERSY ON METABOLIC SYNDROME

Some experts object the very existence of MS. They feel it is not at all a real syndrome but just a cluster of some risk factors. Lack of a single underlying etiology for all the risk factors, existence of multiple definitions, and several alternative names describing similar conditions, periodic additions of new risk factors to expand the definition of MS are some of the points in their favor. This school of thoughts believes that no purpose is served by labeling some coexisting risk factors of CAD and DM as MS. According to them, every risk factor, whether it is existing in isolation or in a group of more than one, but still outside the ambit of MS, needs to be identified and aggressively treated. Thus, no additional purpose is served by labeling these risk factors as MS. They also feel that a wrong signal is being sent to the family physician that the management should start only after the diagnosis of MS is established and individual risk factors should be left untreated. The author of this book agrees with this school of thoughts to a great extent. The proponents of MS feel that by creating a separate entity of MS, practitioner's attention will be focused on the risk factor management and thus prevention of CAD and DM will be more successful.

# CHAPTER 7

# Diagnosis and Laboratory Investigations

## INTRODUCTION

It goes without saying that a prerequisite for proper management of diabetes is precise diagnosis. However, in practice, in mild or borderline cases, many times a wrong diagnosis is made due to various factors such as misconceptions, use of nonspecific tests, too much reliance on urine sugar reports, etc. Misconceptions in the minds of laboratory staff add to the problems instead of solving them! For example, it is not uncommon to get a report from the laboratory in a 75-year-old patient, not yet confirmed diabetic, with postprandial blood glucose of 145 mg% with a red underline below 145 mg% or the values are mentioned in red. Unfortunately, sometimes these patients are straightaway put on oral hypoglycemic agents leading to severe hypoglycemia.

Just as over diagnosis of diabetes leads to over enthusiastic treatment, more often, the late diagnosis is the cause of worry. The time gap between the onset of type 2 diabetes mellitus (T2DM) and development of symptoms can be as long as 5 years. During this period, vascular complications set in. Thus, it is not uncommon to come across a patient having diabetic retinopathy on the day of diagnosis of diabetes mellitus (DM). In short, early and correct diagnosis of DM, as well as avoidance of over diagnosis, both are vitally important.

## CRITERIA FOR DIAGNOSIS OF DIABETES

*For nonpregnant persons*:
- In a person with classical symptoms of diabetes, one reading of unequivocal hyperglycemia, i.e., random venous plasma glucose ≥200 mg% is sufficient to make diagnosis of diabetes. For example, if a person has polyuria, polydipsia, weight loss, and random blood glucose of 315 mg%, he is diabetic and no other test is required to confirm the diagnosis. In such a situation, full glucose tolerance test (GTT) is a definite waste of time and money and hence need not be done.
- Fasting venous plasma glucose of 126 mg% or more on more than one occasion is sufficient for diagnosis of diabetes even in the absence of symptoms. If another blood glucose value on the same day is also in diabetes range repeat fasting blood glucose test is not required. Fasting means no calorie intake for 8 hours.
- A 2-hour venous plasma glucose of 200 mg% or more after oral glucose load of 75 g on more than one occasion. If another blood glucose value on the same day is also in diabetes range repeat postglucose load test is not required.
- Glycosylated hemoglobin (HbA1c) ≥6.5%. It should be measured by method certified by NGSP (National Glycohemoglobin Standardization Program) and standardized to DCCT (Diabetes Control and Complications Trial) assay.

In nondiabetic persons, fasting and 2 hours post oral 75 g glucose values of venous plasma glucose are lower than 100 and 140 mg% respectively and HbA1c is <5.7%.

If fasting venous plasma glucose level is between 100 and 125 mg% and if 2 hours post 75 g glucose venous plasma glucose level is below 140 mg%, the condition is called *impaired fasting glucose (IFG)*; and if 2 hours post 75 g oral glucose challenge values are between 140 and 199 mg%, the condition is known as *impaired glucose tolerance (IGT)*.

These two conditions represent an intermediary state between normal on one side and diabetes on other side *(prediabetes)*. Some people have isolated IFG/IGT, while others have combined IFG and IGT. Prediabetes is also diagnosed if HbA1c is between 5.7 and 6.5%.

As regards microvascular complications of diabetes, people in IFG and IGT are not at significant risk and in this respect both the conditions are equivalent. However, as regards macrovascular diseases associated with diabetes, people in IGT are at a higher risk as compared to those in IFG ("The clock for cardiovascular disease starts ticking when blood glucose values enter IGT range"). With control of weight, prudent diet, and physical exercise, approximately 50% of people with IGT revert back to normal. Some remain in IGT range while others slip into clear diabetic range over a course of time. On an average, every year 18% of people with IGT in India become diabetic. The conversion rate for IGT to diabetes is much lower (5–10%) for people in western countries. It should be remembered that in IGT group, there is no urgency to put them on oral antidiabetic drug (OAD); they need proper diet control, exercise, and 6 monthly follow-up with blood glucose estimation. Those who are unlikely to follow diet and exercise regimen can be put on metformin or acarbose. It is not uncommon to see an IGT patient, recently and wrongly diagnosed as a diabetic and put on a stiff dose of sulfonylurea, to present with OAD-induced repeated hypoglycemia as the presenting symptom.

While interpreting results of laboratory tests, remember to verify the following:
- Is it true glucose estimation or sugar estimation (Folin and Wu)? The latter method gives 10–15% higher values.
- Is it a plasma value or whole blood value? Whole blood glucose values are lower by about 20%.
- Is it capillary glucose value or venous glucose value? While there is no difference in the fasting state between the two methods, postprandial values are higher in capillary blood as compared to venous blood.

All values mentioned under diagnostic criteria in this book are venous and plasma true glucose values **(Table 1)**.

## DIAGNOSIS OF GESTATIONAL DIABETES MELLITUS

Historically, criteria for the diagnosis of gestational diabetes mellitus (GDM) have always been intensely debated and more than one school of thoughts has always existed. We will bypass the details of these debates and rationales put forward by the various schools of thoughts and follow the 2010 recommendations of the International Association of Diabetes and Pregnancy Study

**TABLE 1: Diagnostic glucose concentrations for diabetes, IFG and IGT in mg%.**

|  | Whole blood | | Plasma | |
| --- | --- | --- | --- | --- |
|  | Venous | Capillary | Venous | Capillary |
| *Diabetes mellitus* | | | | |
| Fasting | ≥110 | ≥110 | ≥126 | ≥126 |
| Two hours postglucose load | ≥180 | ≥200 | ≥200 | ≥220 |
| *IGT* | | | | |
| Two hours postglucose load | ≥120 and <180 | ≥140 and <200 | ≥140 and <200 | ≥160 and <220 |
| *IFG* | | | | |
| Fasting | ≥90–<113 | ≥90–<126 | ≥100–<126 | ≥100–<126 |

(IFG: impaired fasting glucose; IGT: impaired glucose tolerance)

**TABLE 2: Diagnosis of GDM in pregnancy-threshold values.**

| Glucose value | Mg% |
| --- | --- |
| FPG | 92 |
| 1 hour OGT-PG (75 g) | 180 |
| 2 hours OGT-PG (75 g) | 153 |

(FPG: fasting plasma glucose; GDM: gestational diabetes mellitus; OGT-PG: oral glucose tolerance-plasma glucose)

Groups, which were adopted by the American Diabetes Association (ADA) in 2011 **(Table 2)**.

GDM = one or more values ≥ threshold (all are venous plasma glucose values)

In addition to the abovementioned method of diagnosis of GDM, World Health Organization (WHO) definition is also commonly followed in some countries. As per WHO, GDM is diagnosed when 2 hours post 75 g glucose challenge plasma glucose equals or exceeds 140 mg%.

## Limitations of Urine Glucose Estimation

As regards urine glucose estimation, it should never be solely relied upon for diagnosis of diabetes. It can only be used for getting a very rough idea of control on a day-to-day basis, provided the patient or his physician interpreting the results is thoroughly conversant with limitations and pitfalls.

While doing urine tests, observe the following:
- Use the dry strip method (e.g., Diastix) which is specific for glucose instead of Benedict's test, which gives many false-positive results. In order to reduce the cost by 50%, cut the test strip vertically in two equal halves.
- Ask the patient to completely empty the bladder 15 minutes before the time of urine estimation so that when the second sample is collected for estimation, freshly formed urine is obtained. Such urine glucose estimation will give a more realistic idea about the spot blood glucose value.

  In many diabetic patients, glucose is invariably spilled over in urine during the postprandial period but they can still have a normal fasting blood glucose and absence of urine glucose in fasting state. However, in such patients, urine voided first thing in the morning is actually a mixture of urine formed over several hours overnight and hence it can show glycosuria even though urine actually formed in the morning does not contain glucose. Hence, it is important to always collect freshly voided urine for glucose estimation.
- Every time you order blood glucose, insist for a glucose test on freshly voided urine so that you get some idea of the patient's renal threshold (i.e., blood glucose level beyond which glucose starts spilling in urine). Normally, the threshold for glucose is 180 mg%. However, many diabetic patients have a low renal threshold in the initial stages, i.e., glucose appears in their urine at blood glucose levels <180 mg%. Hence, one should be careful while increasing the dosage of OADs in such patients solely on estimation of the urine glucose value. On the other hand, many long-standing diabetic patients have a high renal threshold for glucose. In other words, glucose in urine is absent even when blood glucose is >180 mg%.

In short, urine glucose tests should be used by patients who do not have access to glucometer for day-to-day self-monitoring in-between his visits to the doctor for getting a rough idea about control and he should report back to the doctor prior to his next appointment date if there is a persistent change in the pattern of urine glucose.

In addition to the various points mentioned above, it may be worthwhile to remember the following:
- Absence of glucose in the urine does not rule out diabetes as in many mild diabetics, fasting urine could be negative for glucose but postprandial urine is more likely to be positive for glucose.
- Presence of sugar or glucose in the urine does not necessarily mean that the person is a diabetic.
- Even if you have a reasonably good idea of a given patient's urine threshold for glucose, urine glucose estimation still cannot differentiate between normoglycemia and hypoglycemia. Hence, it cannot replace a blood glucose test (absence of glucose in the urine does not mean the patient is "well controlled"; he could be "overcontrolled").
- Do not rule out hypoglycemia in a patient in whom a spot urine test is positive for glucose, if the patient had not voided urine for several hours.
- A new class of drugs known as sodium-glucose cotransporter-2 inhibitors ($SGLT_2Is$) has emerged. These agents reduce blood glucose by blocking renal reabsorption of glucose. Thus patients on these medications will always have glucose in their urine even if they have normal or low blood glucose.

Considering several limitations of urine glucose estimation and easy availability of glucometers and laboratory tests, urine glucose estimation has extremely limited utility in the current scenario and should be used only if glucometers are not available or not affordable.

## Urine Examination for Ketones

It is very important to examine urine for ketones in certain specific situations such as:
- When patient has excessive thirst, hunger, and urination.
- Whenever there is vomiting with or without deterioration in general condition.
- Whenever a diabetic patient is drowsy or unconscious and urine is loaded with glucose and blood glucose is above 250 mg% (in such a case close relative should perform urine ketone examination).

In abovementioned situations, presence of ketones in urine indicates diabetic ketosis and the patient should be instructed to seek immediate medical attention.

Method for examination of ketones in urine is simple and essentially same as that for glucose estimation. A dry strip for urine ketone examination, e.g., Keto-Diastix, which is designed to simultaneously examine glucose and ketones in urine is available in the market.

## INVESTIGATIONS IN DIABETICS AND SUSPECTED DIABETICS

For the diagnosis of diabetes, one should order fasting and post 75 goral glucose challenge, venous plasma glucose. GTT is usually not required. One should order fasting and postglucose challenge blood glucose tests in the following situations:
- Those having symptoms of diabetes.
- Those having tuberculosis, peripheral neuropathy, hypertension, coronary artery disease, obesity, cerebrovascular disease, peripheral vascular disease, eczema, premature cataract, etc.
- As a preoperative checkup
- Those above 30 years, as part of a routine medical checkup (above 20 years in case of those with a very strong family history of T2DM).
- These tests should be done every 6 months in those who have prediabetes, and every 3 months in those who are known diabetics provided they are well controlled. In known diabetics, instead of postglucose blood glucose, postmeal blood glucose should be ordered. In the initial period and in those who have unstable control, blood glucose tests should be repeated more frequently whereas in emergencies, such as diabetic ketoacidosis, hypoglycemic coma, etc., blood glucose should be done several times a day.

In a newly detected diabetic patient, the following additional baseline investigations should be ordered:
- Lipid profile (at first follow-up)
- Serum creatinine
- Full urine examination and test for microalbuminuria, if routine urine examination shows absence of albuminuria. If urine is positive for microalbuminuria, repeat the test on two more occasions in next 6 months. If two out of three tests are positive, microalbuminuria is confirmed.

- Electrocardiogram
- Detailed ophthalmic checkup (5 years after the diagnosis in type 1 patients)

Subsequently, serum creatinine, ophthalmic checkup, and urine for microalbuminuria should be repeated every year. If the patient develops proliferate retinopathy, he should be further evaluated with fluorescein angiography and treated with laser photocoagulation to prevent blindness.

If a patient develops diabetic nephropathy, his OAD should be reassessed, and use of nephrotoxic drugs, e.g., aminoglycoside antibiotics (Gentamicin, Amikacin, etc.), and nonsteroidal anti-inflammatory drugs (NSAIDs) should be avoided. Whenever a diabetic patient loses control and in those who are difficult to control from the beginning, a thorough search should be made for occult tuberculosis and other infections and X-ray chest and other appropriate investigations should be ordered. Whenever a long-standing diabetic gradually requires lesser dosage of OAD or insulin or he goes into hypoglycemia with the same dosage, suspect diabetic nephropathy.

## GLYCOSYLATED HEMOGLOBIN ESTIMATION

This blood test is useful to estimate the average control of blood glucose in the previous 90 days.

The blood can be drawn any time of the day. If done by a reliable laboratory, it provides important information which blood glucose estimation cannot provide. Ideally, it should be done at every 3–6 monthly interval, in addition to blood glucose estimation. The two values together give vital information.

*For example*:
- *Normal HbA1c, high fasting blood sugar (FBS)-interpretation*: Overall control over the last 90 days was okay and it is possible that either control was lost recently or the patient did not take the previous evening's medication. One should verify before increasing the dosage of medication under such circumstances.
- *High HbA1c, normal fasting, and postlunch blood glucose*: Other postprandial values need to be checked. Some people take small working lunch but a large dinner, their postdinner blood glucose values are much higher than postlunch blood glucose values.

- *High HbA1c but normal blood glucose interpretation*: Overall control over the last 90 days was poor and control was achieved in the last few days. If such results are obtained in pre-employment checkup, one should suspect the possibility of a diabetic person hastily achieving control through treatment from a private doctor so as to pass the pre-employment medical examination.

Estimation of HbA1c has become an integral part of routine laboratory tests in a day-to-day management of diabetes in economically advanced countries and also in many centers in our country. HbA1c has very good correlation with microvascular complications of diabetes. However, it has certain limitations which preclude its widespread use in our country, such as cost of estimation and lack of standardization.

## Principles of HbA1c Test

In circulating blood, glucose is constantly getting attached to hemoglobin through nonenzymatic process (glycation of hemoglobin). This attachment is irreversible and percentage of HbA1c out of total hemoglobin in circulation depends upon blood glucose level. Thus in a diabetic patient, depending on the degree of hyperglycemia over previous 90 days, higher percentage of hemoglobin is glycated as compared to normal persons in whom around 4–5.7% of hemoglobin is glycated. In other words, HbA1c levels are in the range of 4–5.7% in nondiabetic and normal persons. Thus, a diabetic with persistent poor control will have very high level of HbA1c while a diabetic with persistent tight blood glucose control will have his HbA1c values near those for normal persons. Diabetic patients should aim to keep their HbA1c constantly between 6.5 and 7%.

## Glycosylated Hemoglobin as a Diagnostic Test for Diabetes Mellitus

Diabetes mellitus is a metabolic and vascular disease with hyperglycemia and specific microvascular complications in those who are poorly controlled over a long-term period as its characteristic features. However, there is no well-defined threshold level of blood glucose beyond which microvascular complications develop and below which there is a complete immunity from complications. Thus fasting venous plasma glucose value of 126 mg% and 2 hours post 75 g oral glucose load value of 200 mg% are somewhat arbitrary diagnostic values for DM. At present, for the want of better diagnostic test, blood glucose values are used as the only criteria for the diagnosis of diabetes, however, these have certain limitations.

Among the microvascular complications of diabetes, diabetic retinopathy is the most extensively studied complication as regards its corelationship with fasting and postglucose load blood glucose values. Till 1997, fasting venous plasma glucose and 2 hours post 75 g oral glucose load cutoff points for diagnosis of diabetes were 140 and 200 mg%, respectively. These points were based on symptoms of diabetes and not on risk for development of microvascular complications. Even though there is no clear-cut threshold blood glucose value for retinopathy, some people with fasting blood glucose values between 126 and 140 mg% have evidence of early nonproliferative diabetic retinopathy; however, retinopathy is very rare in those having fasting venous plasma glucose value below 126 mg%. Thus, in 1997 criteria for diagnosis of diabetes based on fasting blood glucose were lowered from 140 to 126 mg (venous plasma glucose). Moreover, fasting value of 126 mg% has better correlation with postglucose load value of 200 mg% as regards microvascular complications. Even though, lowering of diagnostic fasting blood glucose value was seen as a definite improvement, using blood glucose values for diagnosis of diabetes still have some limitations, such as (1) poor reproducibility due to analytical variance, (2) need to remain in fasting state for 8 hours, (3) false lower values if the blood sample is not analyzed within 1 hour due to glycolysis. Laboratory methods for estimation of HbA1c and instruments used for estimation have been standardized in the advanced countries by the NGSP of USA. Ninety-nine percent of the laboratories estimating HbA1c are NGSP certified in the USA. HbA1c values are reproducible. Storage of collected blood for few hours does not lead to faulty estimation. In addition, HbA1c has a better corelationship with microvascular complications as compared to blood glucose values. While the former is an indicator of average glycemic control over preceding 12 weeks, the later gives information about glycemic control at the precise point of time of drawing glucose from the body. Thus HbA1c is relatively unaffected by acute stressful conditions. Moreover, blood for its estimation can be drawn at any time of the day.

Considering above-listed advantages of using HbA1c test, some diabetologists in advanced countries are of the opinion that it should be used as an additional option for the diagnosis of diabetes in nonpregnant persons. In 2008, the ADA along with International Diabetes Federation (IDF) and European Society for Study of Diabetes had jointly set up a committee of experts to study the current and future means of diagnosing diabetes in nonpregnant adults. The International Committee's report was discussed in a symposium held during ADA's Annual Congress in June 2009 and published in July 2009 issue of diabetes care.

## RECOMMENDATIONS AND CONCLUSIONS OF INTERNATIONAL COMMITTEE

- At present, there is no single "gold standard" test for the diagnosis of diabetes.
- The measure to capture chronic exposure to glucose is more likely to be informative regarding presence of diabetes than single measure of glucose.
- HbA1c is a reliable measure of chronic hyperglycemia and has a better corelationship with chronic microvascular complications.
- HbA1c estimation done by the method certified by NGSP has several advantages over blood glucose estimation.
- Properly performed HbA1c is a better test for diagnosis of diabetes than blood glucose estimation.
- Diagnosis of diabetes is made if HbA1c is ≥6.5%.
- Diagnosis of diabetes should be confirmed by repeat HbA1c estimation unless there are gross symptoms of diabetes and random blood glucose is above 200 mg%.
- In those suffering from hemoglobinopathies and anemia interfering with HbA1c estimation and interpretation, and if HbA1c estimation is not available, current conventional tests should be used for the diagnosis of diabetes.
- In pregnancy, blood glucose estimation should be continued to be used for the diagnosis of diabetes as changes occurring in red cell turnover rate during the pregnancy could affect HbA1c estimation.

**TABLE 3:** Average blood glucose levels over last 90 days for a range of glycosylated hemoglobin (HbA1c) values.

| HbA1c in % | Mean blood glucose in mg% |
|---|---|
| 4 | 60 |
| 5 | 90 |
| 6 | 120 |
| 7 | 150 |
| 8 | 180 |
| 9 | 210 |
| 10 | 240 |
| 11 | 270 |
| 12 | 300 |
| 13 | 330 |

- Individuals with HbA1c values between 6.0 and 6.5% are likely to have higher risk for progression to diabetes and thus should be kept on follow-up and screened for other risk factors. Subsequently, in January 2010, ADA ratified the recommendations of the International Committee as regards the use of HbA1c for the diagnosis of DM in its position statement issued in supplement to diabetes care (January 2010).

**Table 3** gives average blood glucose levels over last 90 days for a range of HbA1c values.

## Fructosamine Test

Like HbA1c, it is a blood test in which glycated plasma proteins are measured and expressed as percentage of total plasma proteins. It gives information on average metabolic control over the previous 2 weeks. It is not yet regularly done in our country. It is more useful than HbA1c to access metabolic control during pregnancy.

Today, HbA1c, in spite of some limitations mentioned above, is considered as the best parameter to assess long-term glycemic control. At the same time continuous interstitial fluid monitoring [continuous glucose monitoring (CGM)] technology has made a significant progress and metrics derived from it such as "time in range", "time below range", and "time above range" are being increasingly used in day-to-day practice for assessment of glycemic control. The information provided by them is complementary to that provided by HbA1c estimation; these parameters should not be used as alternative to HbA1c.

## Estimated Average Glucose, a Patient-friendly Concept of Expressing Metabolic Control

Glycosylated hemoglobin is expressed in percent value. Even though, it is an indicator of average blood glucose control, since the unit of expression is not in mg%, and since the values are at variance with blood glucose values, the expression is not patient friendly, but is confusing to the patient (HbA1c of 7% indicates average blood glucose of 154 mg%). Furthermore, some patients have confusing questions such as "it is same as hemoglobin?", "why it cost me 10 times as compared to hemoglobin?"

In order to express average blood glucose in patient-friendly and meaningful manner, a large multicentric, multinational work was carried out in 700 persons (300 each had type 1 diabetes mellitus and T2DM and 100 were normal controls). Originally, 11 centers spread across North America, Europe, Africa, and Asia were included. One center dropped out due to technical reasons. Those having conditions, such as anemia, hemoglobinopathies and renal impairment, were excluded from the study. A large amount of data on glycemic control was generated in these people by studying them for 4 months.

In this period, all were subjected to continuous interstitial fluid glucose monitoring for 48 hours every month for 4 months. In addition, they were subjected to HbA1c estimation five times at a central laboratory in Europe. Participants also underwent self-capillary glucose monitoring seven times a day and three times a week for 4 months. From this data (2,400 interstitial fluid measurements, 300 capillary measurements, and five HbA1c measurements per patient), average glucose value was calculated and its correlation with HbA1c was worked out and a mathematical formula to convert HbA1c into average glucose value was developed. Interstitial fluid values were scaled up by 5% to derive capillary glucose values. A total of 507 participants completed the entire study.

# CHAPTER 8

# Use of Glucometer in Family Practice

## INTRODUCTION

In a day-to-day practice of a family physician or a general duty medical officer, he commonly has to deal with routine management including dosage adjustments and also handle emergencies in a diabetic patient. Thus, a reliable and properly functioning glucometer with all the accessories is a must for him both in the clinic and in the emergency bag. Glucometer is as essential to a clinician as a stethoscope, blood pressure apparatus, and a torch.

*Applications of glucometer in family physician's clinic:*
- When a patient walks in with symptoms suggestive of diabetes. Even though, one should not solely rely on glucometer readings when hyperglycemia is detected for the first time, availability of on the spot blood glucose value will definitely help in planning of further line of action including the investigations.
- When a known diabetic patient visits the clinic for routine checkup on the eve of his departure from the city and thus does not have a time for formal laboratory tests in near future.
- When a known diabetic patient attends the clinic with symptoms, which may or may not be related to diabetes and does not have a recent laboratory blood glucose report.
- On emergency visit, on the spot blood glucose estimation is a must at every emergency.

Symptoms, such as hunger, palpitations, sudden sweating, giddiness, etc., could be due to hypoglycemia. Random blood glucose on the spot helps to detect or rule out hypoglycemia.

In case of hypoglycemia, one should immediately correct the low blood glucose level by serving a carbohydrate snack like biscuits or refined sugar-containing liquids and subsequently reduce dosage of his antidiabetic medications, if required. In case the patient is semiconscious or unconscious, 50 mL of 25% glucose should be injected intravenously. Hypoglycemia in patients on α-glucosidase inhibitors (acarbose and voglibose) should be treated by administering oral or intravenous glucose as it does not respond to carbohydrate snacks or sucrose or table sugar (α-glucosidase inhibitors slow down the breakdown of carbohydrates, including sucrose to glucose). On the spot blood glucose estimation with glucometer also helps to rule out hypoglycemia and think of alternative condition. Sudden sweating could be a symptom of acute myocardial infarction.

Since hypoglycemia is more common, there is a tendency in patients to assume that they are having hypoglycemia and to consume two teaspoons of sugar every 10 minutes. In case of heart attack, it leads to late diagnosis and loss of vital time before the patient is admitted in intensive care unit. Thus, timely on the spot blood glucose estimation can save precious time and life, as well as lots of money by avoiding delay in hospitalization in case of serious condition, such as acute myocardial infarction or other cardiac emergencies, or by avoiding unnecessary hospitalization in case of simple hypoglycemic episode. Prompt use of glucometer and swift appropriate action in only one episode will more than compensate for the entire investment cost of glucometer.

## EQUIPMENT REQUIRED FOR HOME BLOOD GLUCOSE MONITORING

- Reliable glucometer
- Chemically treated strips compatible with the meter
- Lancets or fine needles to prick the finger for a drop of blood
- Cotton swabs
- Methyl alcohol or medicated spirit

*Glucometer:* It is a small electronic instrument which analyzes the concentration of glucose in a drop of blood transferred on chemically treated plastic strip from patient's finger. The strip is inserted in a slot on the meter. Glucometer runs on batteries. Several brands are available in our country.

The cost of the meter varies from ₹850 to 3,000. For those with high consumption of strips, many companies offer free glucometers. The high-end meters have additional features such as varying memory capacity to store previous readings along with date and time, automatic calculation, and display of mean blood glucose value of last 7 and 14 days, warning beep and message if the values are out of range on either side, facility to download the readings to computer, bluetooth connectivity, coding free operations, etc.

Once a drop of blood from finger after a prick with the lancet or needle is deposited on the designated area on the plastic strip, which is inserted in the slot on the meter, the blood glucose value is digitally displayed on the meter screen in 5 seconds. One plastic strip is required for each test. The cost of strip works out to be in the range of ₹14 to 25, depending upon the meter and the number of strips purchased at a time. These strips are available in vials; usually each vial contains 25 strips. They have unopened expiry period of about 18 months and a separate independent expiry period, usually of 6 months, after the seal is opened. The disposable lancets and needles cost approximately ₹1 to 4. The pain following finger prick, particularly when spring-loaded lancet device is used, is minimal and easily bearable. All meters come with a spring-loaded lancet device at no extra cost.

## RELIABILITY OF GLUCOMETER

More than 40 years have elapsed since the introduction of glucometers. During this period, technology has been continuously updated and deficiencies found in earlier meters have been gradually overcome. The modern meters are reliable provided one understands and follows the instructions mentioned in the manual, stores the strips properly, and avoids using outdated strips (expiry dates of unopened and opened vials are mentioned on the vial). It must be noted that with glucometer, capillary whole blood is tested for glucose; while during laboratory test, venous plasma component of blood is tested for glucose. While in fasting state, glucose levels in capillary whole blood and venous plasma are more or less equal; in the fed state, level in former is about 20 mg% higher than the latter. Even after accounting for the abovementioned difference, up to 15% difference between capillary whole blood values and laboratory test is acceptable. Thus, one need not doubt reliability of glucometer if the values of laboratory test and reading done at the same time are not identical.

However, glucometer requires periodic calibration. This can be done every 2-3 months by simultaneous testing of blood glucose in laboratory and with glucometer. One should also remember that hypoperfusion and anemia affect capillary blood glucose. Former gives false low values while latter results into false high values. Family physicians should also strongly recommend glucometer to all the diabetic patients for self-monitoring of blood glucose (SMBG).

## TRAINING THE PATIENTS USING GLUCOMETERS

### Frequency of Self-monitoring of Blood Glucose

The frequency of SMBG depends on several factors such as subtype of diabetes, degree of stability of blood glucose, presence of special situations (pregnancy, perioperative period, emergency situations, etc.). In stable and well-controlled type 2 diabetics, SMBG is required once or twice a week; while in type 1 diabetics, those diabetics on multiple insulin injections daily, those with brittle blood glucose control, and in pregnant diabetic women, at least three tests per day are required. These are rough guidelines which will require modifications in an individual case.

### Timing of Blood Glucose Examination

#### Routine Tests

The timing of blood glucose will depend on individual case. The usual test timings are premeals (before breakfast, lunch, and dinner), and postmeals (2 hours after breakfast, lunch, and dinner). Usually, initially, emphasis is on premeal monitoring and adjustment of dosages of antidiabetic medications based on premeal blood glucose values. Once these are stabilized, attention is shifted to postmeal monitoring. One also has a choice of estimating premeal and postmeal values on the same day. One can plan to test the blood glucose at different times in a rotating manner, e.g., on Monday, prebreakfast, postlunch, and predinner blood glucose estimation; on Tuesday, prebreakfast, prelunch, and postdinner blood glucose estimation. In addition to premeal and postmeal estimation, occasionally, particularly in those on insulin (once a week in those on multiple insulin injections and once a month in those on one long-acting or intermediate-acting injection), one should test at 3 AM. These values give more precise idea about the level of overnight control and help in taking correct decision regarding adjustment of predinner and bedtime insulin dosage. In some patients, particularly with relatively large dose of predinner intermediate-acting insulin, (NPH insulin such as Insulatard) early morning (around 3 AM) blood glucose dips in hypoglycemic range and reactive hyperglycemia occurs in morning (around 8 AM), as a result of early morning hypoglycemia. Detecting early morning hypoglycemia and making appropriate changes in insulin dosage can break this vicious cycle.

### *SOS Tests*

In addition to the test timings mentioned above, patients should be advised to do random blood glucose estimation in following circumstances: during symptoms such as hunger, palpitations, sudden sweating, giddiness, etc. These symptoms could be due to hypoglycemia, which needs to be confirmed or ruled out on the spot. However, anxiety-related nonspecific symptoms are also common in the community including diabetic patients. Anxious diabetic patients, who do not have glucometer or do not use it during sudden symptom, are likely to be caught in a trap if they interpret their anxiety-related symptoms as those due to hypoglycemia and reduce the dose of their antidiabetic medications without consulting their doctor and avoid doing a laboratory blood glucose test. They also eat snacks every time they get these symptoms. Symptoms disappear on their own; however, since they have taken a snack, they assume that they really had hypoglycemia. These two uncalled-for actions lead to hyperglycemia and expose them to the complications of diabetes.

# Five Important Points for Mastering Your Blood Glucose Estimation Technique

*Choose Good Glucometer*

Modern glucometers give results in 5 seconds; they require extremely small amount of blood; the area on the strip containing blood remains outside the meter and thus meter does not get clogged with the blood. Moreover, many of these meters do not require coding when you change over to blood glucose estimation strips manufactured in different batch. Thus, these meters are far superior to older meters, which required longer time to flash blood glucose values on their screens, and which required coding and a larger amount of blood drop. If you are still using one of the older meters, changeover to modern glucometer. Bayer's "Contour", Johnson and Johnson's "OneTouch" and Roche's "Accu-Chek" are some of the leading brands. Each of these leading brands has more than one model. Ensure that you select one in which coding is not required as there is a likelihood of forgetting to do recoding whenever you start using new vial manufactured in different batch. Always purchase glucometer locally from formal sources so that servicing and continuous supply of strips are available. Do not depend on relatives, sending or bringing glucometers from the western countries as these are not serviceable and their strips are often not available locally. Remember, strips of one manufacturer are never compatible with meters of other manufacturers and most of the manufacturers have several models of meters and strips of one model are not compatible with all the models of same manufacturer.

*Care of Blood Glucose Estimation Strips*

Store the strips properly; avoid contact with moisture by immediately closing the vial stopper tightly after taking out a strip. Do not use strips after their expiry. These strips have two expiry periods, which are mentioned on the vials. There is an unopened expiry period, which means that all the strips should be discarded at the end of that period. There is another expiry period, the period after breaking the seal. This is usually shorter, about 6 months. This means that once the seal is broken you can use the strips for

6 months after which remaining strips should be discarded even if they are still within their unopened expiry period.

### *Clean and Dry Fingers Properly*

Wash patient's hands with soap and water and dry them before pricking. If remnants of sweet eaten by the patient a few minutes back are still on his fingertips, you will get high result. If fingertips are not dry after cleaning, water will get mixed with the blood drop and thus the result will be lower. You can use alcohol instead of soap and water. In that case, wait for a few seconds to allow alcohol to get evaporated otherwise you will end up doing test on diluted drop of blood. Eau de cologne, aftershave lotion, and medicated alcohol, which are available with the chemists, are the substitutes which can be used in place of alcohol (spirit), which is not easily available in our country.

### *Get Proper Blood Drop for the Test*

Generate adequate-sized blood drop by using just adequate force with lancet or number 24 needles. Do not squeeze with excessive pressure as during such process body fluids, which contain a slightly lesser concentration of glucose, get mixed with a drop of blood before it comes out on fingertips. Always wipe out first drop of blood, gently squeeze the finger again, and use second drop of blood for the test as it is less likely to be contaminated.

### *Periodically Cross-check the Meter Readings*

Do not have a total blind faith on the readings obtained with glucometer. It is not a substitute for periodic laboratory blood glucose testing. Always cross-check glucometer reading with laboratory readings. Do not expect exact reading, up to 15% difference is acceptable. Also, periodically cross-check with control solution provided by the manufacturer along with glucometer, after ensuring that control solution is not out of date.

## CONCLUSION

Every family physician and general duty medical officer must have his own properly calibrated and functioning glucometer all the time with him in the clinic as well as on the emergency visits.

**TABLE 1:** Format for storing self-monitored blood glucose (BG) data.

| Date | Fasting BG | Prelunch BG | Postlunch BG | Predinner BG | Post-dinner BG | 3 AM BG | Random BG |
|------|------------|-------------|--------------|--------------|----------------|---------|-----------|
| 15/6 |            |             |              |              |                |         |           |
| 16/6 |            |             |              |              |                |         |           |
| 17/6 |            |             |              |              |                |         |           |

*Note:* All blood glucose values are in mg%.

He should also encourage SMBG by the patients. Depending upon type of diabetes, degree of glycemic control, and type of antidiabetic treatment used, give them a structured plan about frequency of testing and properly recording the data. Emphasize that generated data needs analysis and timely action **(Table 1)**.

# CHAPTER 9

# Metabolic Memory (Legacy Effect)

## INTRODUCTION

In last three decades, several large well-planned long-term longitudinal studies comparing aggressive management for glycemic control as well as for blood pressure and lipid control with conventional management were completed [DCCT (Diabetes Control and Complications Trial), UKPDS (United Kingdom Prospective Diabetes Study), Steno-2]. In DCCT, aggressive insulin therapy was compared with conventional insulin therapy in type 1 diabetics; in main UKPDS, aggressive therapy for blood glucose control was compared to conventional therapy in type 2 diabetic patients; while in Steno-2 study, simultaneous aggressive management of hyperglycemia, hypertension, and hyperlipidemia was compared with conventional management of above mentioned risk factors in type 2 diabetic patients. As expected and as is well-known, aggressively managed patients in DCCT and UKPDS had better glycemic control and fewer microvascular complications at the end of study period (**Fig. 1 and Table 1**). Similarly, aggressively treated patients in Steno-2 study had better control of blood glucose, blood pressure, and lipids and all these factors resulted in lesser cardiovascular events. The differences in two groups in all the studies were statistically significant. At the end of these studies, patients were given a choice to continue same treatment or cross over [the second part of DCCT study was called EDIC (Epidemiology of Diabetes Interventions and Complications) study]. Both the groups were closely observed till the end of further predetermined

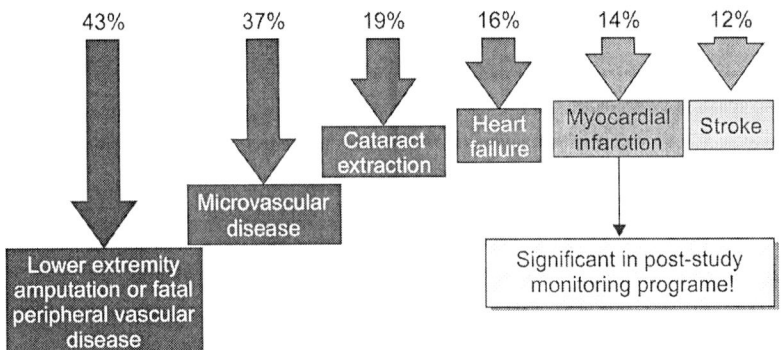

*Note:* Every 1% drop in HbA1c can reduce long-term diabetes complications.
**FIG. 1:** Benefits of intensive glycemic control in type 2 diabetes mellitus.
(HbA1c: glycated hemoglobin; UKPDS: United Kingdom Prospective Diabetes Study)

| TABLE 1: Good glycemic control (lower HbA1c) reduces complications. | | |
| --- | --- | --- |
| HbA1c | DCCT 9→7% | UKPDS 9→7% |
| Retinopathy | 76% | 17–21% |
| Nephropathy | 54% | 24–33% |
| Neuropathy | 60% | – |
| Macrovascular disease | 41% | 16%* |

*Not statistically significant.
(DCCT: Diabetes Control and Complications Trial; HbA1c: glycated hemoglobin; UKPDS: United Kingdom Prospective Diabetes Study)

*Sources:*
1. Diabetes Control and Complications Trial Research Group. The effect of intensive treatment of diabetes on the development and progression of long-term complications in insulin-dependent diabetes mellitus. N Engl J Med. 1993;329:977-86.
2. Ohkubo Y, Kishikawa H, Araki E, Miyata T, Isami S, Motoyoshi S, et al. Intensive insulin therapy prevents the progression of diabetic microvascular complications in Japanese patients with non-insulin-dependent diabetes mellitus: a randomized prospective 6-year study. Diabetes Res Clin Prac. 1995;28:103-17.
3. Intensive blood-glucose control with sulphonylureas or insulin compared with conventional treatment and risk of complications in patients with type 2 diabetes (UKPDS 33). UK Prospective Diabetes Study (UKPDS) Group. Lancet. 1998;352:837-53.

long-term period. Over the period of time, the differences in their values gradually reduced [difference in glycated hemoglobin (HbA1c) in DCCT and UKPDS studies and in HbA1c, blood pressure, and lipid levels in Steno-2 study]. This occurred because majority of patients in conventional arm in the original studies opted for aggressive treatment after they received the briefing about study results, while there was some slackening as regards lifestyle changes as well as drug compliance in those who were originally in aggressive arm. However, patients, who were in aggressive arm in the first half of the respective studies, continued to receive the benefits of tighter controls and achievements of target values in first half of the respective studies. Thus, at the end of second half of the study, the difference in the rate of developing microvascular complications was maintained in spite of similar HbA1c values in the DCCT and UKPDS studies, while cardiovascular mortality was further reduced as compared to at the end of first half of the Steno-2 study in those who received aggressive management in first half of the study. Similar findings were also observed in HOPE study. This was a large study which ran for four and half years in its first part. People with risk factors for cardiovascular disease or having type 2 diabetes mellitus (T2DM) were divided in two groups. One group was put on 10 mg of ramipril daily in addition to their routine medications for diabetes, hypertension, hypercholesterolemia, and antiplatelet medications. This group was compared with a group on placebo (for ramipril); oral antidiabetic drugs (OADs), antihypertensive, antiplatelet medications, and statins were given as required. The group on ramipril had statistically significant reduction in macrovascular and microvascular events. At the end of four and half years, those on placebo were given an option of taking ramipril while those on ramipril in the first half were given the option of discontinuation. Majority in placebo group started ramipril while some in ramipril group discontinued it. At the end of second half of the study (HOPE-2 study), those originally on ramipril continued to get vascular protection and the gap between relative rate of reduction of vascular complications between the two groups widened. This phenomenon of extension of metabolic and vascular benefits is coined as "legacy effect or metabolic memory effect".

With the early animal experimental findings supported by several clinical trials in type 1 diabetic patients as well as type 2 diabetic patients including the trials and their extended observation period arms quoted above, it is accepted that metabolic memory or legacy effect is not only a hypothetical concept but has a strong underlying biological mechanism **(Table 2)**.

### TABLE 2: Clinical trials supporting metabolic memory hypothesis.

Interventional and extended observational phases

| Trial | Interventional phase mean duration (years) | Extended observational mean duration (years) |
|---|---|---|
| DCCT/EDIC | 6.5 (DCCT) | 11 (EDIC) |
| UKPDS | 10 (insulin/sulfonylurea) | 10 |
| UKPDS | 10.7 (metformin) | 10 |
| Steno-2 | 7.8 | 5.5 |

(DCCT: Diabetes Control and Complications Trial; EDIC: Epidemiology of Diabetes Interventions and Complications; UKPDS: United Kingdom Prospective Diabetes Study)

It has been observed that legacy effect is more pronounced in type 1 diabetic patients as compared to type 2 diabetic patients and the reasons for these observations are obvious. Due to explosive nature of symptoms, type 1 diabetes mellitus (T1DM) is diagnosed soon after the onset and thus the treatment is started immediately, while T2DM can remain silent for a long time and thus even if treatment is started immediately after the diagnosis of diabetes, variable time gap exists between the onset of hyperglycemia and the onset of symptoms, during which some amount of bad metabolic memory can be generated.

## PATHOGENESIS OF METABOLIC MEMORY

Some of the key factors in genesis of vascular complications of diabetes are generation of excessive free oxygen radicals and advanced glycated end products (AGEs) in the mitochondria of endothelial cells. Hyperglycemia leads to intracellular hyperglycemia in endothelial cells. This leads to generation of excess of free radicals in mitochondria of endothelial cells. Availability of these free oxygen radicals to mitochondrial respiratory chain leads to activation of pathways such as protein kinase C (PKC), increased polyol and hexokinase pathway fluxes and excessive generation of AGE. Additionally, free radicals alter the expression of many genes involved in pathogenesis of diabetes mellitus. Activated PKC intensifies expression of various adhesive molecules, proinflammatory cytokines, and growth factors such as tumor necrosis factor, interleukin (IL)-1, IL-6, IL-8, cyclooxygenase 2, and nitric oxide synthase. Increased oxidative stress also leads to increased synthesis of extracellular matrix and plasminogen activator inhibitor-1 and reduced production of prostacycline. Activation and migration of leukocytes to subendothelial area lead to further oxidative stress and release of proinflammatory factors. Intracellular protein glycation and AGE formation modify transcription of many genes, which further increase mitochondrial free radical formation. AGE binds to receptor for AGE (RAGE) leading to expression of various genes associated with vascular complications of diabetes. Thus, a vicious cycle sets in during which oxidative stress, AGE formation, interaction of AGE with RAGE aggravate each other and also lead to activation of several other proinflammatory pathways, ultimately leading to permanent endothelial damage. EDIC study showed positive correlation between level of AGE and retinopathy and neuropathy.

## THERAPEUTIC IMPLICATIONS AND FUTURE PROSPECTS

There is a dire need of "switching off" metabolic memory before it could produce permanent endothelial damage leading to subsequent vascular complications, before it is too late. Since oxidative stress works as initial trigger, antioxidants could be used from theoretical point of view to "switch off" metabolic memory. However, available antioxidants have miserably failed to produce any beneficial effect. Thus, an alternative strategy to prevent generation of excessive free radicals and AGE should be worked out. Very early diagnosis followed by aggressive treatment to simultaneously and quickly achieve glycemic, lipid, and blood pressure goals is the foundation of therapeutic approach. Swift control of hyperglycemia by itself will control free radical overproduction and AGE formation to considerable extent. Some novel agents to reduce free radical generation and AGE formation or to increase AGE degradation are under investigations. Currently used antihyperglycemic agents such as metformin and pioglitazone have shown some ability to block the formation of AGE. Telmisartan has been shown to down regulate RAGE mRNA levels. Antioxidant property of gliclazide, a sulfonylurea used in intensified treatment arm of the ADVANCE (Action in Diabetes and Vascular Disease: Preterax and Diamicron

MR Controlled Evaluation) trial, has been demonstrated. Some work on benfotiamine, a vitamin B1 derivative, has been done as regards its ability to reduce AGE formation. While considerable time will be required to prove or disprove putative antioxidant, AGE blocking or AGE degradation enhancing and RAGE mRNA regulating actions of various above mentioned agents, one should concentrate at prompt and aggressive management of hyperglycemia, blood pressure, and lipid disturbances to significantly reduce vascular complications of diabetes.

## SUMMARY

Poor metabolic control in the initial period of diabetes leads to excessive production of free oxygen radicals in mitochondria of endothelial cells and overproduction of AGE. These changes lead to activation of many pathways leading to microvascular and macrovascular damage. The good news is that the metabolic memory can be "programmed" by establishment of tight glycemic control in the initial phase of diabetes. It is also vital to simultaneously establish tight blood pressure and low-density lipoprotein (LDL) cholesterol control to significantly reduce long-term vascular complications and thus morbidity and mortality associated with diabetes.

**Figure 2** explains the concept of metabolic memory. It shows the time since the diagnosis of diabetes on Y-axis and HbA1c on X-axis. The two broken black lines depict response to treatment as measured by HbA1c. The broken black line on right (upper broken line) shows actual response obtained in aggressive arm of Veterans Affairs Diabetes Trial (VADT). This trial was initiated in elderly, long-standing type 2 diabetic patients. The trial included those with mean duration of diabetes for 11 years. Notice following: (1) After very good initial response in first 2 years, HbA1c gradually rose till the patients were inducted in trial. This is a common observation in a day-to-day practice and is due to progressive deterioration in β-cell function and clinician's reluctance to aggressively up titrate the therapy. (2) After the patients were inducted in aggressive arm of the trial, HbA1c rapidly fell down and remained well under control throughout the entire period of the trial. However, in spite of such a tight control over a long-term period, these patients did

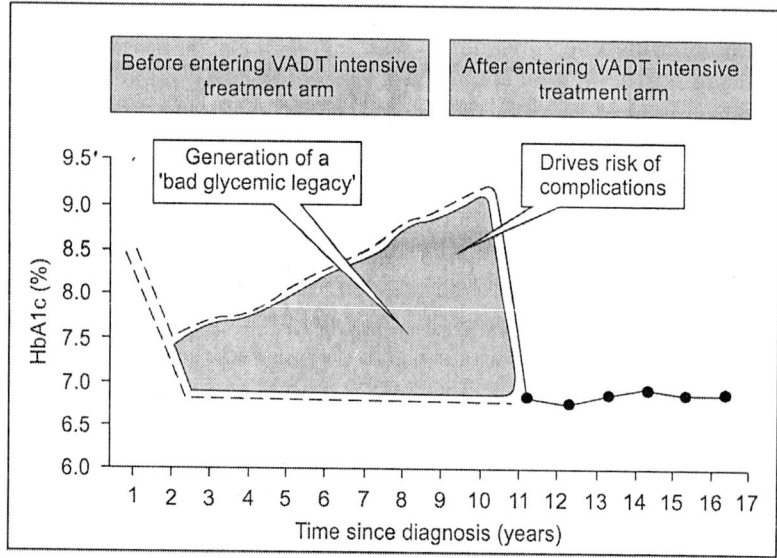

**FIG. 2:** Predictions from Veterans Affairs Diabetes Trial (VADT): Impact of bad glycemic legacy.

Source: Del Prato S. Megatrials in type 2 diabetes. From excitement to frustration? Diabetologia. 2009;52:1219-26.

not get any benefit as regards risk reduction in macrovascular complications, as compared to the patients in control group, who were conservatively treated and had higher HbA1c.

Now observe broken black line on the left (lower broken line). This line depicts imaginary HbA1c response to treatment, had these patients been treated aggressively throughout, right from the diagnosis of diabetes. Notice steep initial fall in HbA1c in first 2 years and subsequent persistent maintenance in normal range. The solid gray area in the **Figure 2** depicts the duration and severity of metabolic derangement as measured by HbA1c, which could have been avoided, had patients been aggressively treated throughout the 11-year period. The metabolic derangement, which prevailed over a long duration and which is depicted by the solid gray area, is responsible for lack of protective effects on macrovasculature observed in aggressively treated patients in VADT trial. This is "legacy effect".

The implications of these studies are very important. There is a strong case for early diagnosis of diabetes and aggressive management of blood glucose without wasting time immediately after diagnosis of diabetes. Prompt treatment soon after the diagnosis of diabetes is not sufficient to prevent complications because if a patient waits till he becomes symptomatic, he will loose vital years while his undiagnosed diabetes is gradually progressing and establishing bad metabolic memory. The medical community should be duty bound and proactively hold educational and diabetes detection camps to enable prompt diagnosis and treatment to prevent vascular complications of diabetes. Similarly, associated risk factors should be promptly identified and quickly brought under control. This will help in our endeavor for primary or secondary prevention of vascular complications of diabetes.

In 1935, the pioneer American diabetologist Dr Elliott Joslin made a statement "aim of therapy in diabetes is to bring down blood sugars to as near normal as possible". Most diabetologists disagreed with him at that time. We now understand farsightedness and vision of Dr Joslin!

Thus, clinicians should devote a lot of time explaining the importance of persistent tight blood glucose control to the patients and their relatives in order to motivate them to follow the advice and come for regular follow-up. If they understand "a stitch in time saves nine" and also the fact that there is absolutely no alternative to persistent tight blood glucose control, they will do a regular follow-up which will lead to better glycemic control and also better control of other risk factors such as hypertension, hyperlipidemia, and obesity. Even in a general practice setup, you can reserve a separate time slot away from peak hours to manage your diabetic patients, say for example, you can hold once a week Diabetic Clinics in your own dispensary. Such a practice is common in advanced countries like the UK.

> *"The aim of treatment of diabetes is to bring blood sugars as close to nondiabetic state as is feasible".*
>
> —Joslin 1935

# CHAPTER 10

# Management of Diabetes

## WHY CONTROL DIABETES?

It has now been proved beyond doubt that dreaded microvascular complications of diabetes can definitely be prevented or at least considerably postponed if persistent metabolic control is maintained. Microvascular complications are specific for diabetes and are responsible for considerable morbidity and mortality. For example, affliction of the capillaries in the retina (diabetic retinopathy) can ultimately lead to blindness (most common cause of blindness in the developed world and well-off patients in our country), thus making the affected patient dependent. Affection of capillaries in the kidneys (diabetic nephropathy) ultimately leads to end-stage renal failure, the most common cause of renal failure, needing either renal transplantation or permanent thrice-a-week dialysis. Both are extremely expensive and beyond the reach of an average Indian.

Diabetic neuropathy leads to pain which can be unbearable in some cases and paresthesia in the feet which interferes with the day-to-day activities and sleep, and can be totally incapacitating. Moreover, impaired sensations over the feet are one of the major underlying factors responsible for "diabetic foot" lesions, which can lead to gangrene and amputations.

If blood glucose is kept under control persistently, one can also prevent infections such as tuberculosis, pneumonia, skin and soft tissue infections, fungal infections, etc., which can affect morbidity.

Macrovascular diseases (cerebrovascular disease leading to stroke; coronary artery disease leading to myocardial infarction, cardiac failure; and peripheral vascular disease leading to gangrene) are commonly associated with diabetes due to accelerated atherosclerosis. This process can be slowed down with prudent management of diabetes.

Moreover, the mortality and morbidity are definitely less in those diabetic patients who are metabolically well controlled as compared to those who are uncontrolled, when they develop macrovascular emergencies.

The only way to prevent all these complications is to meticulously and persistently manage diabetes.

Till the mid-90s, we did not have concrete proof based on properly designed long-term clinical research as regards beneficial effects of persistent tight blood glucose control. Diabetologists used to debate a lot on pros and cons of tight blood glucose control. However, the scenario has totally changed since the publication of *DCCT (Diabetes Control and Complication Trial)* in 1993. This trial was done in the USA and Canada on type 1 diabetic patients. DCCT was a prospective, randomized trial that assessed the effect of intensive versus conventional insulin therapy on the incidence of microvascular complications of diabetes (retinopathy, nephropathy, and neuropathy) in 1,441 patients over a mean follow-up period of 6.5 years. Intensive therapy consisted of at least three insulin injections daily and at least four capillary blood glucose examinations daily with frequent communications with the investigators. Conventional therapy consisted of 1-2 insulin injections and one capillary blood glucose estimation daily with less frequent communication with the investigators. At the end of the trial it was found that the relative risk reduction as regards development of retinopathy, nephropathy and neuropathy, or progression of these microvascular lesions in those who had mild involvement at the beginning of trial, was >50% in those type 1 diabetic patients on intensive treatment as compared to those on conventional treatment. This difference was highly significant statistically. Subsequent to publication of DCCT trial, which was a very major milestone in the field of diabetes research, *UKPDS (United Kingdom Prospective Diabetes Study)* was published. This was the biggest clinical research ever undertaken in the field of diabetes till that time, and it proved that better blood glucose control through intensive management of diabetes led to statistically significant relative risk reductions as regards all the three diabetic microangiopathies as compared to conventional treatment. The relative risk reduction was 24% for all the microangiopathies taken together. More than 5,000 newly diagnosed type 2 diabetic patients participated and were followed up for a mean of 7 years. In another side study in the UKPDS, it was proved that in those diabetic patients who also had hypertension, intensive therapy with antihypertensive medications led to significant reductions in mortality and morbidity as compared to conventional antihypertensive therapy. One thousand one hundred forty-eight patients participated in this substudy. Mean blood pressure (BP) achieved in intensive and conventional treatment groups was 144/82 and 154/87 mm Hg, respectively. Atenolol and captopril were the antihypertensive drugs used in intensive arm. Both fared equally.

## DIFFERENCE BETWEEN ONSET AND PROGRESSION OF MICROVASCULAR AND MACROVASCULAR COMPLICATIONS

It is important to study and understand the major differences between onset, progression, and arrest of microvascular and macrovascular complications of diabetes. Microvascular complications start after the onset of diabetes; they can be prevented by tight glycemic control established soon after the onset of diabetes and maintained over a long-term period. Even in those who have microvascular affection due to inadequate glycemic control in the initial stages, establishing good glycemic control later in life can arrest further progression. Thus, good glycemic control always helps irrespective of stage of diabetes. The reason for less spectacular results in UKPDS as compared to DCCT as regards prevention of microvascular complications was significantly higher time gap between onset and diagnosis of type 2 diabetes mellitus (T2DM) as compared to type 1 diabetes mellitus (T1DM). Macrovascular complications start in prediabetes stage. Establishing tight glycemic control right from the period of diagnosis helps to prevent onset and progression of macrovascular disease, only if diagnosis is established soon after the onset of diabetes and if associated with good control of blood pressure and lipids. In those with long-standing diabetes, who had inadequate glycemic control in the initial years, and who already have macrovascular disease, establishing tight glycemic control in pursuit of preventing complications of diabetes is not productive as regards macrovascular complications. Though, progression of microvascular complications can be avoided; progression of macrovascular complications cannot be arrested by tight glycemic control established at this stage. In fact, episodes of hypoglycemia developed in pursuit of establishing tight glycemic control could precipitate serious acute cardiovascular events including fatal events. This difference between behavior of microvascular and macrovascular complications of diabetes is due to bad metabolic legacy of previously uncontrolled diabetes. This was amply brought out by three mega milestone trials done in elderly, long-standing type 2 diabetic patients in first decade of this century and published in 2008. Let us have a brief overview of these trials.

## ACCORD TRIAL

The American trial was done on >10,000 elderly type 2 diabetic patients, many with diabetes of >10 years duration and with established macrovascular disease. The aggressively treated patients reached tight glycemic goals and had lesser microvascular complications, but no reduction in risk of macrovascular complications. Incidence of sudden death, presumably due to sudden cardiac death triggered by hypoglycemia, was slightly higher in aggressively treated patients.

## ADVANCE TRIAL

This was a multinational trial and included patients from India. The setting of trial as regards number of patient, their characteristics and study design was more or less similar to the Action to Control Cardiovascular Risk in Diabetes (ACCORD) trial. Aggressively treated patients reached aggressive glycemic goals and had risk reduction as regards microvascular complications but not macrovascular complications. There was no increased incidence of sudden deaths. The glycemic goals were a bit less ambitious and were reached a bit more gradually as compared to ACCORD trial. These were probable reasons for absence of significant increase in hypoglycemic episodes and sudden deaths.

## VADT TRIAL

This was comparatively smaller trial done in American war veterans. The patient characters, design, and outcomes were more or less similar to ADVANCE (Action in Diabetes and Vascular Disease: Preterax and Diamicron MR Controlled Evaluation) trial.

## TAKE HOME MESSAGE

Type 2 diabetes mellitus should be diagnosed as early as possible and glycemic control should be established soon after the diagnosis and maintained throughout. This will prevent all vascular complications. In long-standing elderly diabetic patients with established macrovascular and microvascular disease, tight glycemic control at that stage will still prevent progression of microvascular but not macrovascular complications. Episodes of hypoglycemia, which can develop in pursuit of tight glycemic control in those with established and unstable macrovascular disease, could potentially bring out serious and occasionally, even fatal cardiovascular episodes. Thus, such patients should have individualized less aggressive glycemic goals. Glycemic control is important even in elderly patients with comorbidities, but one should have individualized targets depending upon presence and severity of comorbidities and the state of physical fitness and cognitive capabilities **(Table 1)**.

## MANAGEMENT OF DIABETES

Management of diabetes revolves around four pillars as shown in the **Figure 1**.

All the four modalities of management are equally important and to be successful, all the modalities should be implemented

| Study | Microvascular | | Macrovascular | | Mortality | |
|---|---|---|---|---|---|---|
| UKPDS (T2DM) | ↓ | ↓ | ↔ | ↓ | ↔ | ↓ |
| DCCT/EDIC (T1DM) | ↓ | ↓ | ↔ | ↓ | ↔ | ↔ |
| ACCORD (T2DM) | ↓ | | ↔ | | ↑ | |
| ADVANCE (T2DM) | ↓ | | ↔ | | ↔ | |
| VADT (T2DM) | ↓ | | ↔ | | ↔ | |

**TABLE 1: Impact of intensive therapy for diabetes: Summary of major clinical trials.**

▨ Initial trial   ☐ Long-term follow-up

(ACCORD: Action to Control Cardiovascular Risk in Diabetes; ADVANCE: Action in Diabetes and Vascular Disease: Preterax and Diamicron MR Controlled Evaluation; DCCT/EDIC: Diabetes Control and Complications Trial/Epidemiology of Diabetes Interventions and Complications; T1DM: type 1 diabetes mellitus; T2DM: type 2 diabetes mellitus; UKPDS: United Kingdom Prospective Diabetes Study; VADT: Veterans Affairs Diabetes Trial)

*Sources:*
1. Effect of intensive blood-glucose control with metformin on complications in overweight patients with type 2 diabetes (UKPDS 34). UK Prospective Diabetes Study (UKPDS) Group. Lancet. 1998;352(9131):854-65.
2. Holman RR, Paul SK, Bethel MA, Matthews DR, Neil HA. 10-year follow-up of intensive glucose control in type 2 diabetes. N Engl J Med. 2008;359(15):1577-89.
3. The effect of intensive treatment of diabetes on the development and progression of long-term complications in insulin-dependent diabetes mellitus. The Diabetes Control and Complications Trial Research Group. N Engl J Med. 1993;329(14):977-86.
4. Nathan DM, Cleary PA, Backlund JY, Genuth SM, Lachin JM, et al. Intensive diabetes treatment and cardiovascular disease in patients with type 1 diabetes. N Engl J Med. 2005;353(25):2643-53.
5. Action to Control Cardiovascular Risk in Diabetes Study Group, Gerstein HC, Miller ME, Bylington RP, Goff DC Jr, Bigger JT, et al. Effects of intensive glucose lowering in type 2 diabetes. N Engl J Med. 2008;358(24):2545-59.
6. ADVANCE Collaborative Group, Patel A, McMahon S, Chalmers J, Neal B, Billot L, et al. Intensive blood glucose control and vascular outcomes in patients with type 2 diabetes. N Engl J Med. 2008;358(24):2560-72.
7. Duckworth W, Abraira C, Moritz T, Reda D, Emanuele N, Reaven PD, et al. Glucose control and vascular complications in veterans with type 2 diabetes. N Engl J Med. 2009;360(2):129-39.

simultaneously. Addition of insulin in the prescription in hitherto oral antidiabetic drug controlled patient does not mean that now he can relax diet and exercise.

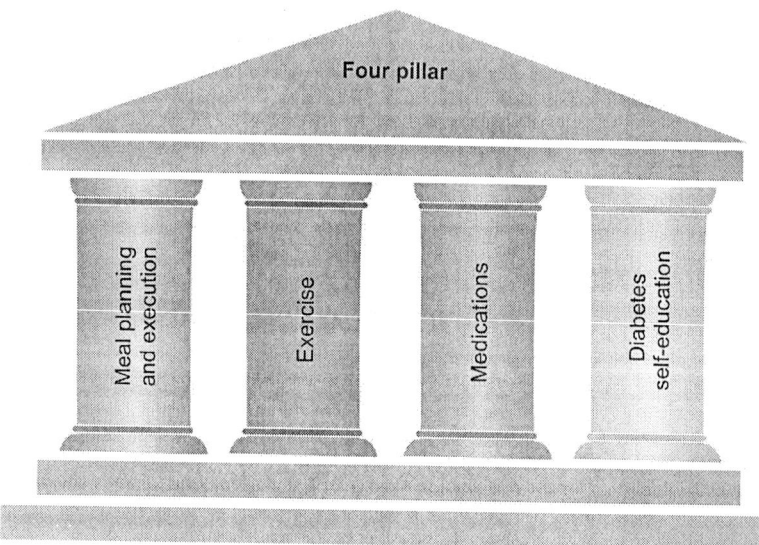

**FIG. 1:** Four pillars of diabetes management.

# CHAPTER 11

# Role of Exercise in the Management of Diabetes Mellitus

## INTRODUCTION

Exercise means different things to different people. It means sweat and tears on the hockey field, several sweaty bodies pounding flesh in the gym, the runner crossing long tracks or just plain and simple walking. However, there are no two opinions about one thing: all of us, whether perfectly healthy or suffering from some disease, we all need exercise to become fitter and healthier. Exercise improves our health, reduces stress and slows down aging process. Exercise makes us feel good. What is most important is that to enjoy all these benefits, it does not have to be arduous, simple walk for 30 minutes a day is good enough. Younger and fitter diabetic patients and those who have stiff weight reduction targets can be prescribed higher intensity exercise, of course after thorough physical and laboratory assessment. In addition to aerobic exercises such as walking, jogging, running, swimming, etc., one needs to prescribe muscle strengthening and stretching exercises.

Along with diet, medicines [insulin and other injectable or oral antidiabetic drugs (OADs)] and education, exercise forms the four cornerstones in the management of diabetes mellitus (DM). However, it is the most neglected aspect of management. If undertaken properly, diabetic patients are immensely benefited from exercise. Some of the beneficial effects have been discussed hereunder.

## BENEFITS OF EXERCISE

Appropriate exercise leads to improvement in metabolic control because during the exercise, glucose and fat are spent up to provide energy. During low intensity exercise both glucose and fat are burned in presence of adequate oxygen at level of mitochondria (aerobic exercise), during high intensity exercise, there is inadequate oxygen supply at mitochondrial level (anaerobic exercise) and under such circumstances only glucose can be burnt to produce energy. Long-term regular exercise leads to gradual expenditure of fat from the adipose tissue, leading to weight loss, and thus, reduction in insulin resistance, which is often significant contributor in the pathogenesis of diabetes. Reduction in degree of insulin resistance leads to better utilization of endogenous and/or exogenous insulin and thus, better blood glucose control, often with reduction of insulin/OAD dosage.

## OTHER BENEFITS

- Exercise helps in weight reduction.
- Appropriate exercise and diet control together are sufficient to control blood glucose levels in many mild type 2 diabetes mellitus patients, thus avoiding drug treatment.
- Exercise leads to lowering of blood pressure, which is commonly elevated in diabetes.
- Exercise helps in reducing blood levels of very-low-density lipoprotein (VLDL) and low-density lipoprotein (LDL) and increase the blood level of high-density lipoprotein (HDL) cholesterol.
- Exercise improves blood circulation in the legs (many long-standing diabetic patients suffer from poor blood circulation in the legs).
- Exercise leads to improved physical fitness and stamina.
- Resistance exercise (RE) leads to increased muscle mass, which in turn leads to weight loss through raising basal metabolic rate (BMR).
- Last but not the least, exercise imparts a sense of well-being and improves psychological status.

## WHAT ARE THE PRECAUTIONS TO BE OBSERVED BEFORE STARTING EXERCISE?

Inappropriate exercise can be hazardous. Hence, before prescribing exercise, you should carry out a detailed physical examination and certain laboratory investigations including electrocardiogram (ECG) to verify the following:
- The blood glucose level is reasonably controlled. Starting vigorous exercise in very poorly controlled diabetes, particularly in type 1 diabetes mellitus, could worsen blood glucose control and precipitate an emergency as insulin is required to facilitate entry of glucose into the cells where it is burned down as fuel. In severe insulin deficiency, glucose is unable to enter the cells and hence can accumulate in the blood to dangerous levels.
- The condition of cardiovascular system is stable. Ischemic heart disease is more common in diabetes and may remain silent or have atypical symptoms thus remaining undetected. Sudden vigorous exercise in such patients could precipitate serious problems such as acute myocardial infarction or left ventricular failure. Perform thorough physical examination including blood pressure (BP) measurement and get the BP in target range before showing green signal to exercise. Carry out ECG or go through recent ECG report if available. Depending upon individual situation, carry out 2D echocardiogram and further investigations whenever required.
- *Absence of advanced proliferative retinopathy*: This complication is present in some long-standing diabetic patients particularly those who are poorly controlled. If sudden vigorous exercise is performed by diabetic patients having proliferative retinopathy, vitreous hemorrhage, and retinal detachment can occur. Hence, fundoscopy is essential, particularly in long-standing diabetic patients having diminished vision, before they embark on an exercise program.
- *Prevention of hypoglycemia*:
  - Ask your patient to observe the following don't and do's to prevent hypoglycemia.
  - Do not exercise during peak insulin time, i.e., around 3 hours and 7 hours after plain- and intermediate-acting insulin, respectively.

- Do not inject insulin in the exercising arm as exercise hastens absorption of insulin and may precipitate hypoglycemia.
- Do remember that occasionally hypoglycemia unexpectedly occurs very late, e.g., late at nights, following morning exercise. Hence, assess your patient's blood glucose at different hours with the help of glucometer so that dietary supplements can be taken at proper time or the dosage of drugs (i.e., insulin or oral pills) can be adjusted. Such elaborate monitoring is only required initially to study the individual response pattern.

  The ideal time to perform exercise is in the morning after a light snack. This will prevent hypoglycemic reactions.
- Feet are healthy and there are no open wounds.
- Ensure that the patient is using properly fitting footwear while exercising.

## WHICH TYPE OF EXERCISE?

Various exercises are basically divided into two types:
1. Dynamic or aerobic
2. Static or anaerobic

In the former, the major muscle groups are stretched in a rhythmic pattern and the entire body is in motion while in the latter, muscles contract against the fixed objects and the body is static. Walking, jogging, cycling, swimming, etc., are examples of the former while pressing palms against the walls or weight lifting are examples of the latter. Dynamic exercise in which a large amount of energy is gradually spent over a period of time is ideal for diabetic patients. Depending upon the patient's age, sex, physical condition, and cardiovascular status, you should prescribe one of the dynamic exercises. For older diabetic patients, brisk walking is safe, easy to perform and an inexpensive exercise. All that they have to do is to invest in time and a pair of properly fitting and comfortable footwear.

Younger and fitter diabetic patients can choose from the following exercises—running, swimming, cycling, a game of tennis, etc.

All the abovementioned exercises are equally beneficial as compared to fancy or trendy things such as a work-up in a

## TABLE 1: Calories spent per minute.

| Type of exercise | | Calories spent/min |
|---|---|---|
| Brisk walking | | 3.6 |
| Cycling | | 4.5 |
| Jogging | | 4.5 |
| Running | | 5.0 |
| Swimming | | 6.0 |
| Tennis (singles) | | 7.0 |

gymnasium, health club, and yoga. The latter is not an exercise in its correct sense and helps in an indirect manner. Of course, there is no harm performing yoga in addition to exercise.

**Table 1** gives various dynamic exercises and approximate calories spent per minute while doing the given exercise.

## HOW LONG?

Ideally, 30–45 minutes of sustained dynamic exercise should be done in 24 hours. However, one should start gradually with 10 minutes daily in the first week and gradually go to 30–45 minutes daily in the next 2–4 weeks.

Remember, sustained exercise is important. The exercise should be strenuous enough to raise heart rate to 75% of maximal heart rate (MHR), for 10–15 minutes in the middle-third of exercise period. To calculate the target heart rate, use the following formula: subtract age of the patient in years from 220. For example, a man of 50 years should raise his heart rate to about 125 beats/min during peak exercise time, which should be one-third of the total duration of exercise (220–50 = 170, 75% of 170 is 127.5 or approximately 125 beats/min). Many housewives tell me they spend 2 hours shopping and do a lot of walking during this time but still it does not help them in achieving their goal. They obviously forget the several halts they make while shopping and the long casual talks with friends! If occasionally, your patient has to cancel the exercise program, ask him to make up during the course of the day by:

- Avoiding lifts
- Purposely parking the car away from the place of work.
- Getting down a bus stop or railway station earlier than the one nearest to the place of work/residence.

## HOW OFTEN?

If one wants to derive real benefit, exercise must be done at least five times a week.

## SOME WALKING TIPS

Give following tips to your patients:
- Use comfortable walking shoes, stick reflectors on front and back of shoes if you walk on roads and highways in the dark.
- Wear clean cotton socks.
- Wear loose cotton T-shirt and suitable shorts or track trouser depending upon weather.
- Keep your body straight while walking.
- Keep your chin parallel to ground; do not bend your head. Look straight in front.
- Push your elbow behind your body and then just let gravity and the momentum to push the arm forward, this action will help you increase your walking speed.

- To gain in speed further, roll your foot on your toes, pushing off the ball of your foot and toes as you go.
- Take short and fast steps to walk faster, avoid longer strides.
- If 30 minutes of brisk walking at a stretch is not possible, walk for 10 minutes at a time, three times a day. Do not simply shrug by saying "I do not have time".
- If you cannot walk briskly, compensate by walking for longer time.

## CROSS TRAINING

Doing same exercise repeatedly day in and day out can sometimes be boring. Thus, one should inculcate the habit of doing different exercise on some days. This is called cross training.

For example, a walker can do swimming, water walking, reverse walking, jogging, cycling, game of badminton, etc. Even yoga can be used as a variety of cross training.

Cross training provides following advantages:
- Change in type of exercise from time to time prevents overuse injury, muscle imbalances, and mental burnout.
- Change of exercise leads to strengthening the muscles not adequately exercised in your usual workout. For example, swimming and badminton provide good exercise to shoulder and upper limb muscles, furthermore swimming is a no impact all body exercise and is an excellent option for those having joint problems such as osteoarthritis of knee joint. Workouts such as water walking and reverse walking are also good alternatives, as they provide more workout to the group of muscles in lower limbs not adequately exercised while walking. There is a difference between walking and jogging. While in former, the landing impact is on the ball of foot, in latter the same is on heel. If you have an access to gym, you can use cross trainer instead of treadmill for cross training. It more actively involves your hip and thigh muscles as compared to walking or running on treadmill.

## RESISTANCE EXERCISE

Besides aerobic exercise, which is a mainstay of exercise for diabetic patients, 10 minutes of RE is recommended on alternate days. It provides following benefits:
- RE increases the muscle mass and tones up the body.
- RE increases basal metabolic rate (BMR), which leads to more energy expenditure, even at rest.
- Thus, RE leads to higher weight loss, which leads to reduction in resistance of tissues to insulin or in other words, increase in sensitivity of tissues to insulin. This leads to better blood glucose control. RE increases bone, mass and prevents osteoporosis in the long run.

There are different types of REs such as free weight lifting (dumb bells, weights), exercises with machines in gymnasium or using stretchable bands as shown in **Figure 1** or calisthenic exercises such as lunges, squat jumps, pull ups, etc.

Some examples of RE have been shown in **Figure 1**.

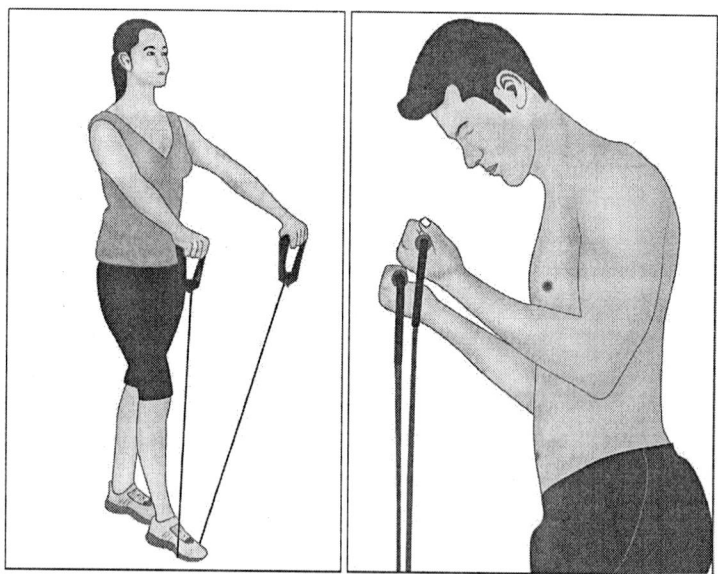

**FIG. 1:** Some examples of resistance exercise.

## STRETCHING OR FLEXIBILITY EXERCISE

Stretching exercise is a light to moderate physical activity. As one gets older, joint mobility gradually becomes limited. This interferes with daily activities such as getting up, walking fast, balancing, attaining correct posture, etc. It also makes one prone for backaches, injuries, and muscle soreness during and after exercise. In order to prevent these limitations and injuries one should regularly do 5 minutes of stretching exercise after aerobic exercise. At this time, when muscles are warmer, it is easier to increase muscle flexibility and range of motion. If you want to continue exercising even in your old age, maintenance of muscle flexibility and motion is vital. Thus, make sure that you always end your exercise session with 5 minutes of stretching right from young age. There are many stretching exercises, each meant for stretching individual muscle group. One should stretch all major muscles in rotation.

## CONCLUSION

Remember, proper exercise is very useful, safe, inexpensive, pleasant and an integral mode of management of diabetes, and should never be bypassed.

> *"Exercise is the most effective "antiaging pill" ever discovered".*
> —NIH, UK

# CHAPTER 12

# Meal Planning in Diabetes

## INTRODUCTION

Meal planning or judicious selection of food items as regards the type of foodstuff and the quantities to be consumed is an essential and primary step in the management of diabetes and by itself, along with prudent exercise, is sufficient to control blood glucose in many of those who have prediabetes and mild type 2 diabetes mellitus (T2DM). Those who require insulin or oral pills to control blood glucose should never neglect meal planning, just because they are on blood glucose lowering medicines.

I have purposely avoided the term "diet", because it carries different meanings to different people and is usually interpreted as restriction in quantity of foodstuff across the board. It has negative, restrictive or unfriendly connotation. In fact, people with diabetes and normal body weight need not reduce the calories consumed in 24 hours. What they need to do is to take small frequent meals, to avoid foodstuff containing refined sugar and reduce fatty food and red meat and to consume sufficient quantities of rough cereals and vegetables to provide for adequate fiber and feeling of satisfaction from eating adequate food.

If a diabetic patient understands the basic principles of sensible eating, he can consume food which is very near to his family's daily food and which does not require any special or separate preparation. All of us, including those having diabetes, require consuming well-balanced food for promotion of growth in our formative years as well as for maintenance of our body functions and repair of wear and tear of our tissues. While charting daily meal plan the objectives should be: (1) to provide the required calories to create energy and to attain and maintain ideal body weight; (2) to plan a well-balanced menu containing proteins, carbohydrates, fats, vitamins, minerals, and fiber in optimum quantities. Overweight people should purposely consume fewer calories than their daily requirement, so that extra deposits of visceral and subcutaneous fat are mobilized to bridge the gap between the required energy and that provided by the foodstuff. In this way, the patient is able to shed extra weight and this helps in improving insulin sensitivity of his tissues. In other words, insulin resistance is corrected. In this way, tissues get "extra mileage" out of externally administered insulin, as well as endogenous insulin. About 90% of type 2 diabetic patients and 24% of adult nondiabetics have insulin resistance.

## WHAT IS A BALANCED FOOD?

Well-balanced food contains all the constituents of food in ideal proportion. Now let us gather some basic information on various food constituents.

## Carbohydrates

Carbohydrates should provide the main source of energy. About 60–65% of energy should be supplied by carbohydrates, mainly complex carbohydrates, while simple sugar or items containing it should be avoided or very sparingly consumed.

Cereals and cereal-based foods supply complex carbohydrates, while sugar, honey, jams, etc., provide simple carbohydrates.

Cereal-based foodstuffs such as *chapati, roti, rice, bajra roti,* etc., form the bulk of the food in our country and are ideally suited for diabetic patients. Complex carbohydrates in these foodstuffs are slowly digested and converted into glucose in a gradual manner and hence their consumption is not associated with quick and sharp rise in blood glucose level. However, simple carbohydrates such as table sugar (sucrose), honeys, etc., are rapidly converted into glucose and quickly absorbed in circulation leading the sharp postprandial blood glucose peaks resulting in glycemic variability, which is liable to accelerate vascular damage.

## Proteins

Proteins are essential for growth as well as for repair of wear and tear. Milk and milk products, egg white, meat, fish, and dals are rich sources of proteins. About 15–20% of daily calories should come from proteins. Diabetic patients should consume 0.8–1.0 g of proteins per kilogram of body weight.

Patients with nephropathy should restrict protein consumption.

## Fats

Fats are important constituents of cell membrane and are storage centers for energy. Fats should provide 20% of daily energy requirement. Fats consist of fatty acids and glycerides. Depending upon the type of fatty acid it contains, fat is classified into following types:

*Saturated fat*: Animal fat, including fat in milk and milk products and *vanaspati* are rich in saturated fat. Animal fats are also rich in cholesterol. Among the oils, coconut oil is a rich source of saturated fats. Excessive consumption of saturated fats leads to rise in serum cholesterol level, which accelerates atherosclerosis. However, animal fats are also a source of vital omega-3 fatty acids and thus should be consumed in moderation. One-third of the energy from fat should be derived from saturated fats. Thus, a small amount of *ghee*, half to one teaspoonful per day is recommended.

*Monounsaturated fats*: Groundnut oil, mustard oil, and palm oil provide monounsaturated fats. One-third of the energy derived from fat should come from monounsaturated fat.

*Polyunsaturated fats*: Safflower oil, sunflower oil, corn oil, soybean oil, cottonseed oil, etc., are some of the rich sources of polyunsaturated fats. Remaining one-third of the energy provided by fats should be derived from polyunsaturated fats.

### Essential Fatty Acids

These are vital fatty acids, which cannot be made by the body, hence should be derived from food. Omega-6 ($\omega 6$) and omega-3 ($\omega 3$) fatty acids belong to this class. Each source of fatty food has different $\omega 6$ and $\omega 3$ fatty acids in different proportions. The ideal ω6/ω3 ratio should be 4:1. It should be noted that certain oils rich in polyunsaturated fats, such as sunflower oil and safflower oil are very aggressively marketed as safe oils because their consumption does not lead to rise in serum cholesterol. The advertisements even make an indirect claim that one can consume large quantities of these oils. However, these oils contain very unhealthy ω6/ω3 ratio thus should never be used as sole source of cooking medium. Moreover, all oils provide same calories, 9/g. Thus, excessive consumption of polyunsaturated oils is unhealthy.

In order to provide a better ω6/ω3 ratio, one should not solely depend upon polyunsaturated oils but use a judicious mixture of these oils with mustard oil, coconut oil, and *ghee*. However, *ghee* and coconut oil are rich in saturated fats thus should not be used as sole cooking medium. Fish oil is very rich source of ω3 fatty acids and it has been amply demonstrated that in countries where fish is a staple food, incidence of coronary heart disease is low. Thus, fish consumption is encouraged. Those who are vegetarians may consume 1–3 capsules of fish oil daily. However, it has not yet been proved that encapsulated fish oil is as good as consumption of natural fish. The normal weight diabetic should consume 3–4 teaspoonful of cooking oil daily (0.5 L/month). Besides, he should consume half teaspoonful of *ghee*. Overweight diabetic patients should consume less.

## Other Constituents of Food

### Fiber

Fiber is provided by indigestible plant cell components in our food. There are two types of fiber:

1. *Water-insoluble fiber:* Whole-wheat, whole grains, wheat bran, corn bran, brown rice, whole pulses, nuts, seeds, grapes, fruit, and root vegetable skin are rich sources of water-insoluble fiber. One should not peel off the skin of fruits before eating. Water insoluble fiber provides natural laxative action and adds bulk to the food.
2. *Water-soluble fiber:* It has a property of holding or adsorbing water and getting swollen. It delays stomach emptying and induces a feeling of fullness and helps in reducing food intake. Oatmeal, lentils, apples, oranges, pears, beans, flax seeds, etc., are rich in water-soluble fiber.

Traditional Indian vegetarian food rich in vegetables and cereals provide adequate fiber and hence supplementary medicated fiber preparations are usually not required for those eating adequate food. Moreover, such branded preparations are expensive. One can provide adequate fiber-rich and natural food to entire family at the same cost (provided of course the family has a reasonable size). Those who are poor eaters or eat predominantly nonvegetarian food are likely to have fiber deficiency in their diet and can take fiber supplements if they are unable to plan and eat high fiber food. Fiber-rich food provides following advantages:

- Digestion of carbohydrates to glucose and its absorption is delayed, thus a sharp postmeal rise in blood glucose is avoided.
- High fiber intake helps to reduce serum cholesterol and triglycerides.
- Due to bulk formation after water holding in the fiber, one gets a feeling of fullness in abdomen, thus limiting food intake.
- By preventing chronic constipation, risk for cancer of large intestine is reduced.

## *Water*

Water is an important constituent of food and is absolutely essential for survival. Sufficient amount of water is required for maintenance of blood volume and digestion of food. While dehydration should be avoided by ensuring adequate fluid intake, the tendency to drink excessive water, "because it flushes the toxins out of body and is good for health", should be avoided, particularly in those who have renal failure and heart failure. Water requirement of diabetic is similar to general population.

## *Vitamins and Minerals*

Persons with diabetes require vitamins and minerals in adequate quantities just as a normal person needs them. There is no difference in daily requirement. Well-balanced food provides all the vitamins and minerals in adequate quantities and regular lifelong vitamin supplements are not required for all the diabetic patients. However, those on low-calorie diet should take one tablet or capsule of B complex or multivitamin preparation.

Average diabetic, particularly a long standing diabetic usually requires several medications such as two or three oral antidiabetic pills, two antihypertensive pills, a statin to reduce his cholesterol or prevent heart disease even if cholesterol is normal, and aspirin. All these medicines are absolutely necessary, thus make the matters less complicated for the patient by avoiding vitamins and antioxidant pills. Remember lesser the number of pills, higher are the chances of compliance.

Thus, you may avoid prescribing a B1, B6, B12 preparation or a preparation containing methyl cobalamin in each and every diabetic.

## *Now Let us Plan Daily Menu in a Stepwise Manner*
### Step I: Calculate Desirable Body Weight
Take height in centimeters and subtract 100 or 109 in men and women respectively. For example, if height is 170 cm ideal body weight should be around 70 kg for men and 61 kg for women. The abovementioned simple mathematical formula gives a rough idea about ideal body weight. If one wants to be more specific, he should calculate patient's body mass index (BMI) by using following formula:

$$BMI = \text{Weight in kilogram} \div (\text{height in meters})^2$$

The normal range is 18–23 for men and 19–25 for women. One should keep his BMI in normal range. If it is high, he needs to shed weight.

*Waist circumference*: It is easy to measure and is very useful indicator of central obesity or upper body obesity. Central obesity is diagnosed if waist circumference is >90 cm in men and 80 cm in women.

A person with BMI in the normal range can still have central obesity.

Moreover since central obesity is more strongly associated with cardiovascular disease than general obesity, measurement of waist circumference and keeping it in normal range has attained great significance.

### Step II: Calculate the Calorie Requirement
**Table 1** shows how to decide about the calories required.

Growing children and pregnant and lactating women require extra calories.

**TABLE 1:** Calories per kilogram of desirable body weight based on physical activity.

| | Sedentary | Moderate | Heavy |
|---|---|---|---|
| Overweight | 20 | 30 | 35 |
| Normal weight | 30 | 35 | 40 |
| Underweight | 35 | 40 | 40–50 |
| Bedridden patient | | 25 | |

- *Physical activities carried out by following groups are classified as sedentary activity*: Teacher, doctor, nurse, tailor, peon, housewife, and retired people.
- *Physical activities carried out by following groups are classified as moderate activity*: Fisherman, agricultural labor, electrician, carpenter, welder, turner, industrial labor, automobile driver, etc.
- *Physical activities carried out by following groups are classified as heavy activity*: Stone cutter, mine worker, wood cutter, porter, etc.

### Step III: Convert Required Calories into a Meal Plan

To make a meal plan, one requires knowledge of composition of foodstuffs we eat and the calories provided by each gram of protein, carbohydrate, and fat, and also have some information on food exchange system.

Cereals (rice, wheat, etc.) are rich in carbohydrates, which form about 70% of their weight, but poor in proteins, while pulses (various *dals*) are comparatively richer in proteins.

Vegetables are a good source of carbohydrates, fiber, vitamins, and micronutrients but are a poor source of proteins. All these foodstuffs provide a small quantity of fat, which is known as "invisible fat". Meat and fish are rich in proteins while former, particularly red meat is also rich in fat. Meat and fish do not provide carbohydrates. Milk provides all the three proximate principles with quantity of fat varying depending upon the animal source and also whether it is processed to make it "low fat" milk. Cow's milk contains less fat as compared to buffalo's milk. Each gram of protein and carbohydrate provides 4 calories while each gram of fat provides 9 calories.

## THE FOOD EXCHANGE

A person with diabetes can and should make frequent changes in his menu, so that the monotony of eating same food is broken and he can actually enjoy his meals. While making changes, he should know that the total calories consumed in a day and the proportions of calories provided by proteins, carbohydrates, and fats should remain same. In other words, he must know the various alternatives he can consume in place of each food item on his menu. For example, if one does not want to consume a cup of cow's milk at breakfast, what are the various alternatives, which he can consume instead of milk? This information is provided by a list of food exchanges, which is given here.

### Cereal Exchange

Each exchange provides:
- Carbohydrates: 15 g
- Proteins: 2 g
- Calories: 70

One exchange is = any one of the following:
- Cooked rice: 75 g (3 tablespoons)
- Chapati: 20 g *atta* (flour)(1 small chapati)
- Roti: 20 g *atta* (*jowar/bajra*/corn/*ragi*)
- Idli: 1 medium
- Bread: 30 g (1 large slice/one and half average size)
- Corn flakes: 20 g (3 tablespoons)
- Dosa: 1 medium
- Porridge: 3/4 cup
- Marie/cream/craker biscuits: 3 pieces

### Pulses and *Dal* Exchange

Each exchange provides:
- Carbohydrates: 15 g
- Proteins: 6 g
- Fat: 1 g
- Calories: 90

One exchange is = any one of the following (in raw weigh):
- Rajma: 25 g
- Bengal gram: 25 g
- Black gram: 25 g
- Chawli: 25 g
- Mung: 25 g
- Kesari dal: 25 g
- Red gram: 25 g
- Masoor dal: 25 g

## Meat Exchange

Each exchange provides:
- Proteins: 7 g
- Fat: 5 g
- Calories: 70
- Carbohydrates: Nil

Our exchange = any one of the following:
- Mutton: 30 g
- Chicken: 50 g
- Fish: 60 g
- Pork: 30 g
- Ham: 20 g
- Beef: 50 g
- Egg: 50 g (1 unit)

## Milk Exchange

Each exchange provides:
- Carbohydrates: 7.5 g
- Proteins: 4.5 g
- Fats: 5 g
- Calories: 110

One exchange = any one of the following:
- Cow's milk: 150 mL
- Buffalo's milk: 90 mL
- Skimmed milk: 350 mL
- Skimmed milk powder: 30 g (3 tablespoons)
- Butter milk: 750 mL
- Cheese: 30 g
- Curds (cow's milk): 150 mL

## Fruits Exchange

Each exchange provides:
- Carbohydrates: 10 g
- Calories: 40

One exchange = any one of the following:
- Orange: 100 g (1 medium)
- Pear: 90 g (1 medium)
- Apple: 90 g (1 medium)
- Banana: 40 g (1 medium)
- Mango: 60 g (1/2 small)
- Water melon: 300 g (3 slices)
- Papaya: 120 g (2 slices)
- Grapes: 75 g (12 numbers)
- Figs: 100 g (3 medium)
- Pineapple: 90 g (5–6 thin round slices)
- Coconut water: 200 mL (1 glass)
- Guava: 100 g (1 medium)

## Vegetables A Group

All leafy and green vegetables except those mentioned in group B. They provide negligible calories.

## Vegetables B Group

100 g = 1 exchange = 1 *katori* provides:
- Carbohydrates: 7 g
- Proteins: 2 g
- Fats: Nil
- Calories: 35

*Examples:* Carrot, beetroot, green mango, beans, green peas, onion, lotus stem.

## Roots and Tubers

100 g = 1 exchange = 1 *katori* provides:
- Carbohydrates: 25
- Proteins: Nil
- Calories: 100

*Examples:* Potato, sweet potato (*Ratala*), yam (*Suran*), *Colocasia* (*Arbi*), tapioca (*Shimla Aloo*), *khamalu*.

*Note:* Roots and tubers should be avoided or taken in very small quantity only.

## Fat/Oil Exchange

Each exchange provides:
- Fat: 5 g
- Calories: 45

*Examples:* One teaspoonful (5 mL) of any cooking oils, e.g., safflower, sunflower, soya, mustard, groundnut, *til, vanaspati*; or 2 teaspoonfuls of cream.

> Some household measures:
> - Please ensure that your teaspoons, tablespoons, and cups have the following capacities:
>   - 1 teaspoonful (tsp)—5 mL
>   - 1 tablespoonful (tbsp)—15 mL
>   - 1 cup—150 mL

The 1,800 calories readymade menu which is suitable for persons with 60 kg ideal body weight and sedentary lifestyle is given in **Table 2**.

For a flexible meal plan to suit individual needs based on age, sex, weight, profession, and activities, refer to meal planning chart at the end of this chapter (**Table 4**) and plan a menu.

## GENERAL GUIDELINE

### Foods to be Consumed in Very Limited Quantity

- Fried snacks like *shev, chivda, farsan, papad, bhajiya, wafers*, chips, *batata vada*, etc.
- Saturated fats such as butter, *ghee*, cream, fatty meat (beef, lamb, organ meat, ham, and pork), coconut oil, and hydrogenated oil (*vanaspati*), yellow of egg, fatty gravies, nuts, and oil seeds such as cashew nut, *pista*, groundnut, etc.
- Beer, wines, whisky, and other alcoholic drinks are best avoided as far as possible. If total abstinence is not possible, intake should be limited to one peg per day and five pegs per week of

### TABLE 2: A sample of 1,800 calories diet.

| Time | Food items |
|---|---|
| Early morning | 1 cup tea/coffee (with 50 mL milk) |
| Breakfast | 2 small chapatis/2 large bread Slices/2 medium idlis<br>+ 1 cup cow's milk /1 egg<br>+ 1 tsp of butter/oil/*ghee* |
| Midmorning snack (at midpoint between breakfast and lunch) | 1 apple |
| Lunch | 3 chapatis or<br>2 chapatis + rice (3 tablespoonfuls)<br>+ 1½ *katori* dal + curds (100 mL)<br>+ 1–2 *katori* green leafy vegetables<br>+ 1 *katori* group "B" vegetables<br>+ 1 teaspoon oil for cooking |
| Afternoon tea time | 1 cup tea/coffee + 2 bread slices |
| Evening snack | 1 orange/apple |
| Dinner | Same as lunch |
| Bedtime | 1 cup milk + 2 biscuits |

*Note*: Nonvegetarians can replace curds at lunch/dinner time with chicken 50 g/fish 60 g.

hard drinks or one bottle per day and five bottles per week of mild bear or one small glass of wine per day. Sweat wines such as port wine should be avoided. Calories provided by alcohol should be accounted in the meal plan. 1 g of alcohol provides 7 calories. Avoid excess of salt as this can lead to hypertension, which as such is extremely common in diabetic patients. Both diabetes and hypertension are independent risk factors for coronary heart disease and cerebrovascular disease and when present together, the risk is compounded. Foods high in salt are *papad*, pickles, *chutney*, baking soda containing eatables, dried fish, processed food, preserved and canned food, cured meat, Chinese food, etc. There is no difference between rock salt and common salt. Salt intake should not exceed 5 g or 1 teaspoonful per day in diabetics who have concomitant hypertension, renal impairment, and heart failure

## Food Items to be Totally Avoided

Simple sugars such as glucose, sucrose (table sugar), dextrose, honey, jaggery, jam, jelly, syrups, marmalade, cakes, pastries, pies, puddings, ice cream, sweet biscuits, sweet meats, chocolates, condensed milk, fruit juices, aerated soft drinks such as Coca Cola, Limca, Thums Up, Pepsi, Gold Spot, tinned juices, sweat pickles, etc.

## Food Items Allowed in Unlimited Quantities

Condiments and spices, lime water (without sugar), tea and coffee (without sugar and using milk from the milk quota), thin butter milk, raw, and green vegetables, etc.

### *Fruits*

Fruits are a good source of vitamins, fiber, and antioxidants. One medium-sized fruit weighing roughly about 100 g or about 12–15 grapes can be safely consumed daily. One can change the fruit depending upon season, liking, etc. Among the fruit, *chikoo*, mango, and very ripe banana contain higher quantities of sugar and should be sparingly consumed.

### *Ready to Eat Cereals*

The market is flooded with several attractively packaged branded, ready to eat processed, and fiber deficient cereal preparations. These preparations contain various cereals in flakes form mixed with some vitamins and minerals. These marketed products are several times costlier than the homemade, freshly prepared cereal based dishes such as *poha, upma, idli, dosa*, etc. Those who consume a balanced diet do not require extra vitamins and minerals. However, the heavy advertisements sometimes misguide the consumers and many families with average household income spend heavily on these branded cereals. Moreover, these branded products invariably contain sugar and salt. Thus they are not recommended as preferred food choices.

### *Sugar Substitutes*

Aspartame and sucralose are two very commonly used sugar substitutes. They do not contain any significant calories. Thus their use can help in a small manner as regards weight control also. They are reasonably safe and recommended for use in diabetic patients by many National Diabetic Associations including American Diabetes Association. These are available in various forms such as pills, drops, and powder. They do not have any calories. Powder form of sucralose is heat stable, it can be mixed with raw material before it is subjected to high cooking temperature. We Indians, including our diabetic patients have a sweet tooth. Thus availability of sucralose will serve as a big boon for those who can now eat their favorite desserts such as *sheera, jalebi*, sweet cookies, cakes, pastries, *rasgulla*, etc. Of course these desserts should be consumed in very small quantities, even if they are prepared with sucralose instead of sugar as they usually contain cream and other substances which add to the weight problem, which can indirectly increase blood glucose. From time to time you will hear or read about side effects of artificial sweeteners. Be rest assured that if taken in small quantities up to 3–4 pills/drops/day, the artificial sweeteners available in the market are quite safe. Understand, respected and major international organizations in the field of healthcare and diabetes would not allow the use of these agents without thoroughly studying the data generated by safety studies. Of course pregnant ladies should refrain from using them. There is a tendency in some people to develop craving for extra food after preparations containing sugar substitutes, while some people develop a feeling that they are entitled for extra food since they have saved some calories by avoiding table sugar. Under these circumstances, one should avoid sugar substitutes.

## SOME TOOLS USED IN MEAL PLANNING

### Glycemic Index

Glycemic index (GI) is a meal planning tool which ranks carbohydrate-containing foods as per their potential to raise blood glucose compared to equivalent amount of glucose. Pure glucose has the highest GI of 100. In order to calculate GI of a given carbohydrate-containing food, rise in blood glucose at 2 hours following ingestion of 50 g of food under the test is compared with the rise in blood glucose following ingestion of 50 g of pure glucose. More than 600 food items have been assigned GI. In general, carbohydrate foods that breakdown quickly have high GI while the foods which are slowly broken down and digested over a time, have low GI. Thus, a flaked breakfast cereal or nan-made from *maida* has higher GI than whole wheat flour chapati. GI also depends on the amount of viscous fiber contained in a given food stuff, more the amount of fiber, lower is the GI. Thus, beans have low GI as compared to potato. Other factors include amount of fat present in a ready-to-eat dish. French fries have a lower GI as compared to mashed potato because of its fat content. However, even though based on GI, it is a better choice than mashed potato; higher fat content nullifies the advantage. GI depends on many variables including the degree of ripeness in case of fruits, method of cooking, amount of water and other liquids consumed during the meal, amount of fat eaten along with a carbohydrate-containing dish, etc. As per GI, foods have been classified as having high GI (mashed potato, ripe banana, honey, *maida*-based preparation), medium GI (french fries, rice, chapati), or low GI (*chana dal*, brown rice, chapatis with gram flour) **(Table 3)**. Thus, while meal planning, one should select food items with low GI to minimize postprandial blood glucose rise.

## Carbohydrate Counting and Carbohydrate-insulin Ratio

Carbohydrate counting (CC) is another tool for meal planning. It is used more commonly in USA than in other countries. Carbohydrate contents of food items to be consumed during the major meals and snacks are found out from the CC charts and tables, and accordingly the dosage of premeal insulin is decided, e.g., if one is planning to have 3 chapatis each weighing 20 g, he will consume 35 g of carbohydrates. In addition, if he is planning to go for 1 *katori mung dal* and 2 *katories* of green leafy vegetables, he will additionally consume 45 g of carbohydrates and thus total carbohydrate consumption during the meal would be 80 g. If you patient is on short-acting insulin before meals, he can calculate his insulin dose by using this information. On an average, one requires around 1 unit of insulin for 15 g of carbohydrates, thus his premeal insulin dose would be 5 units. If he planning to eat a bit more or less, or consume a different food item during next meal, he can refer to the CC tables, find out carbohydrates content of food he is

### TABLE 3: Glycemic index (GI) of some common food in % of GI of glucose which is 100.

| Food | GI | Food | GI |
|---|---|---|---|
| Glucose | 100 | Honey | 80–90 |
| Mashed potato | 80–90 | Potato chips | 50–59 |
| Beet root | 60–69 | Yam (*suran*) | 50–59 |
| Green vegetables | 10–19 | Tomato | 10–19 |
| Apple | 30–39 | Banana | 60–69 |
| Orange | 40–49 | Raw banana | 40–49 |
| Rice | 70–79 | Orange | 30–39 |
| Corn flakes | 80–89 | Orange juice | 40–49 |
| Bengal gram (*chana dal*) | 30–39 | Green gram (*mung dal*) | 40–49 |
| Black gram (*urad dal*) | 40–49 | *Rajma* | 20–29 |
| *Idli* | 80–89 | Curds | 30–39 |
| Brown bread/chapati | 70–79 | Whole milk | 30–39 |
| *Upma* | 70–79 | Ice cream | 40–49 |

*Note*: Fatty food has a lower GI as compared to food containing lower fat content (e.g., potato chips vs. mashed potato); thus, do not depend on GI as the sole factor for deciding about food choices. It helps you to select an item from the same food category (e.g., *chana dal*-based items over *urad dal*-based items, orange over banana, chapati over corn flakes, etc.).

planning to consume and adjust insulin dose accordingly. Thus, CC method offers some flexibility as regards consumption of the type and quantity of food.

Please note that carbohydrate-to-insulin ratio is not fixed but varies from person to person depending upon his sensitivity to insulin. Some will require 1 unit of insulin for each 10 g of carbohydrates while others will require 1 unit for each 12 g of carbohydrates. However, one can initiate insulin therapy with 1 unit per 15 g carbohydrates formula, monitor postmeal blood glucose and then fine tune or "titrate" insulin dosage as per the requirement.

## *How to Count Carbohydrates?*

It is mandatory for ready-to-eat food companies to declare details about the food content per serving size, on the package. The information includes amount of carbohydrates. For foods that do not have label, you have to make approximate estimates. Keeping general serving size in mind will help you to estimate the amount of carbohydrates in a food item you are planning to eat.

For example, following food items provide about 15 g of carbohydrate:
- 1 small fresh fruit
- 1 large-sized bread slice
- 1 small chapati
- One-third cup of rice
- 1 cup of vegetable soup
- Half a cup of oatmeal
- Half a cup of black beans or starchy vegetables
- Two-third cups of curds

Now use all the available data, refer to meal planning chart **(Table 4)**, and design your own menu.

## Bon Appétit

Enjoy your meal.

**TABLE 4: Meal planning chart.**

| Calories | 1,200 | 1,600 | 1,800 | 2,000 | 2,200 | 2,400 |
|---|---|---|---|---|---|---|
| **Bed tea/coffee** | 1 cup | 1 cup | 1 cup | 1 cup | 1 cup | 1 cup |
| **Breakfast** | | | | | | |
| Cereal exchange | 2 | 2 | 3 | 3 | 3 | 4 |
| Milk exchange | 1 | 1 | 1 | 1 | 1 | 1 |
| Fat exchange | 1/2 | 1 | 1 | 1 | 1 | 1 |
| **Mid-morning snack** | | | | | | |
| Cereal exchange | 1 | 1 | 1 | 1 | 1 | 1 |
| Milk exchange | – | – | – | – | 1 | 1 |
| **Lunch** | | | | | | |
| Cereal exchange | 2 | 2 | 3 | 4 | 4 | 5 |
| Pulse exchange | 1 | 1 | 1.5 | 1.5 | 1.5 | 1.5 |
| Curds | 50 mL | 100 mL | 100 mL | 100 mL | 100 mL | 100 mL |
| A group vegetables | Unlimited | Unlimited | Unlimited | Unlimited | Unlimited | Unlimited |
| B group vegetables exchange | 1 | 1 | 1 | 1 | 1 | 1 |
| Fat exchange | Nil | Nil | 1 | 1 | 1 | 1 |

*Continued*

*Continued*

| Calories | 1,200 | 1,600 | 1,800 | 2,000 | 2,200 | 2,400 |
|---|---|---|---|---|---|---|
| **Afternoon snack** | | | | | | |
| Tea/Coffee | 1 cup | 1 cup | 1 cup | 1 cup | 1 cup | 1 cup |
| Cereal exchange | 1 | 2 | 2 | 2 | 2 | 2 |
| Fat exchange | 1/2 | 1 | 1 | 1 | 1 | 1 |
| **Evening snack** | | | | | | |
| Fruit exchange | 1 | 1 | 1 | 1 | 1 | 1 |
| Milk exchange | – | – | – | – | 1 | 1 |
| **Dinner** | Same as lunch | Same as lunch | Same as lunch | Same as lunch | Same as lunch | Same as lunch |
| **Bedtime** | | | | | | |
| Milk exchange | 1 | 1 | 1 | 1 | 1 | 1 |

*Notes*:
- 1 egg can be exchanged for 1 milk exchange.
- Half cereal exchange can be exchanged with 1 fruit exchange at evening and at bedtime.

# CHAPTER 13

# Oral Antidiabetic Agents and Injectable GLP$_1$RAs

## INTRODUCTION

The ease of administration, relatively low cost [with the exception of oral Semaglutide], ability to control blood glucose levels in about 60% of type 2 diabetic patients at any given point of time in a clinic setting, and apprehensions to use insulin due to several misconceptions have made oral blood glucose-lowering agents immensely popular among the patients.

More than 96% of 74 million diabetics in our country have type 2 diabetes mellitus (T2DM). As in any other type of diabetes, the primary aim of treatment in T2DM is to achieve persistent tight blood glucose control. As long as the oral pills are effective to achieve this goal and if they are well tolerated and if there are no contraindications to their use in a given patient, oral antidiabetic drugs (OADs) can be used without any hesitation. However, one should also know their limitations. Hence, it is very important for an average general practitioner as well as a physician to have in-depth knowledge of OADs available in our country so that he can choose the appropriate agent in the correct dosage, depending upon the clinical situation.

## HISTORY OF DEVELOPMENT OF OADS

The history of oral antidiabetic agent therapy long antedates insulin, the first validated report being by Muller in 1877 on the effect of sodium salicylate on urinary glucose. In 1918, the blood sugar lowering influence of guanidine, the precursor of biguanides was described but the use of a series of somewhat toxic guanidine derivatives ceased a few years later as insulin became more rapidly available.

The modern OADs era began with the accidental discovery of the hypoglycemic activity of the sulfonamide, sulfonyl thiadiazole in 1942, and with the systematic study of their structure—activity relationships 2 years later by Loubatieres. The clinical introduction of sulfonylurea (SU) therapy followed in 1955 and after a re-examination of the chemistry and pharmacology of the guanidines, effective biguanide therapy became available 2 years later. OADs are in use for seven decades. Till mid-90s only two pharmacological classes of OADs were available namely SUs and biguanides. Subsequently acarbose, which acts at small intestinal brush borders and delays digestion of complex carbohydrates, was launched. In late 90s, repaglinide, first non-SU insulin secretagogue was made available and around the turn of century thiazolidinediones (TZDs), namely rosiglitazone and pioglitazone were on the market. In 2008, sitagliptin, the first dipeptidyl peptidase-4 inhibitor ($DPP_4I$) was launched, soon followed by vildagliptin and saxagliptin. In 2010, bromocriptine, which acts by resetting the reduced dopaminergic tone in hypothalamus, was introduced in clinical practice. Bromocriptine was the first OAD to undergo cardiovascular outcome study to prove its safety. Thus opened a totally new era in oral antidiabetic therapy. Subsequently in the first decade of twenty first century, injectable $GLP_1RAs$ were introduced starting with exenatide. In the mid second decade sodium-glucose cotransporter-2 inhibitors ($SGLT_2Is$) were introduced in clinical practice starting with dapagliflozin in Europe and canagliflozin in the USA. These modern agents are not merely "me-too" molecules but they represent totally different pharmacological classes of antidiabetic medications having a mechanism of action distinct from the older classes of OADs. These new agents have mechanisms of action, which are complementary to traditional agents with which they can be judiciously combined. In the meantime, while new molecules were being rapidly introduced in clinical practice, rosiglitazone was withdrawn from global market due to its alleged cardiac toxicity. We still have 23 agents from 8 broad classes of OADs. Thus, we have mind-boggling alternatives sometimes confusing a generalist. Let us look at how they act, how they differ with each other, complement each other; and what are the specific slots/niches of an individual agent.

## PHARMACOLOGY

The currently available agents fall into eight main groups, i.e.,
1. Insulin secretagogues subdivided into SUs and non-SUs
2. Biguanides
3. Thiazolidinediones, also known as glitazones
4. Alpha-glucosidase inhibitors (AGIs)
5. $DPP_4Is$ also known as gliptins
6. Oral and injectable $GLP_1RAs$
7. Dopamine agonists (bromocriptine)
8. Glimins, dual-acting agents working on β-cells as well as on insulin resistance. **Figure 1** shows various sites of action of antidiabetic agents.

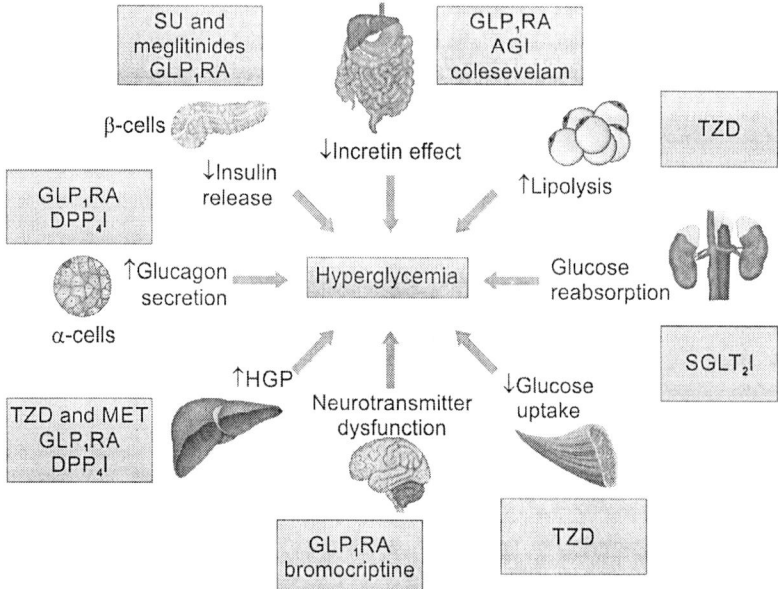

**FIG. 1:** Sites of action of noninsulin antidiabetic agents.

Based on sites of action, the abovementioned agents are grouped in following manner:

*Centrally acting agents*: These agents act on pancreas to stimulate release of insulin from β-cells (SUs and non-SU insulin secretagogues).

*Peripherally acting agents*: These agents increase the tissue sensitivity toward insulin. These agents are also known as insulin sensitizers. They are subdivided into biguanides acting mainly at liver and TZDs acting mainly at striated muscles and adipose tissues.

*Agents acting at intestinal mucosa*: These agents slow down digestion of carbohydrates and thus the absorption of glucose (AGIs).

*Agents acting through incretin axis*: $DPP_4Is$ increase the blood levels of $GLP_1$, a natural incretin secreted by small intestinal cells in response to food intake. $GLP_1$ reduces blood glucose through multiple actions. These agents act by reducing the effect of $DPP_4$, an enzyme secreted in small intestinal mucosa in close proximity to site of secretion of $GLP_1$ **(Fig. 1)**, by inhibiting it ($DPP_4Is$) or by being resistant to its action ($GLP_1RAs$).

*Agent acting on suprachiasmatic nuclei in hypothalamus*: Bromocriptine, the only member of this class, acts by resetting the lowered dopaminergic tone in type 2 diabetic patients.

Agents acting centrally as well as peripherally (glimins).

## SULFONYLUREAS AND OTHER INSULIN SECRETAGOGUES

Glibenclamide, glipizide, gliclazide, and glimepiride are the four members of SU family available in our country. Besides SU, repaglinide and nateglinide, which have similar mechanism of action but chemically distinct structure, are also available in our country. Both the subgroups together are known as insulin secretagogues. They are rapidly absorbed from the gastrointestinal (GI) tract and transported in blood as protein bound complexes. The free ions, which are gradually released, diffuse in the tissues and reach the site of the action.

## Mechanism of Action

The main action of secretagogues is through acute induction of insulin release from β-cells of islets of Langerhans. When these drugs combine with a SU receptor on adenosine triphosphate (ATP)-sensitive potassium channels in the β-cells, the channels are closed resulting in depolarization of cell membrane, which in turn leads to opening up of calcium channels and internalization of calcium ions in the β-cells. This leads to release of insulin in the circulation. When used for a long term, it is claimed that SUs also act through increasing insulin sensitivity. However, this hypothesis is not yet proved conclusively even though there is some experimental evidence particularly in favor of glimepiride in this regard. These drugs are ineffective in the absence of functional β-cells. Thus, they should not be used in type 1 diabetic patients.

## PROGRESSIVE β-CELL FAILURE IN T2DM

On an average, these agents are effective in controlling blood glucose for about 5–10 years, during this period their effect gradually diminishes and ultimately a stage is reached when they are ineffective in controlling blood glucose even at the highest dose. This stage is popularly described as secondary SU failure. However, it is actually due to failure of β-cells in pancreas to respond. It is estimated that usually at the time of diagnosis of T2DM, only about 50% of the β-cells are functional and these respond to insulin secretagogues. As the time passes, the mass of functionally active β-cells gradually diminishes and in about 5–10 years of time, a stage of secondary failure is reached. The rate at which β-cell mass decreases varies from patient-to-patient. The rate and degree of absorption, degree of protein binding, rate of metabolism, mechanism of excretion, and hypoglycemic properties of individual members of this group vary from each other **(Fig. 2)**.

## Contraindications

All insulin secretagogues are contraindicated in pregnancy and lactation, severe liver disorders, and in type 1 diabetics. The additional contraindications of individual agents are mentioned separately.

*Glibenclamide:* It was introduced in our country about 40 years back. It is a long-acting and potent SU. It should be administered once or twice a day, 30 minutes before meals. Usual daily dose range is 2.5–20 mg. Among all the SUs, it is least expensive thus very suitable for economically average patients. It is contraindicated in renal impairment in addition to common contraindications of the class mentioned above **(Table 1)**.

It does not cross placental barrier in significant quantity. Even though officially contraindicated, it has undergone evaluation in

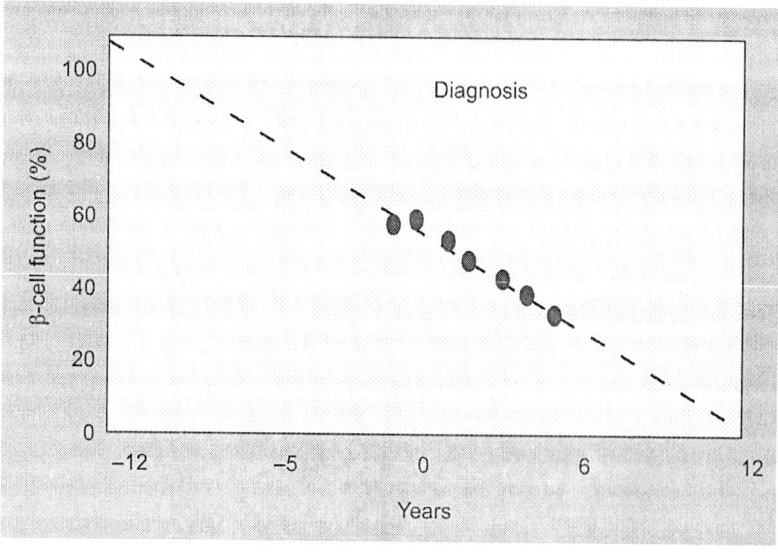

**FIG. 2:** Progressive β-cell failure in type 2 diabetes mellitus.

*Source:* UK prospective diabetes study 16. Overview of 6 years' therapy of type 2 diabetes: a progressive disease. UK Prospective Diabetes Study Group. Diabetes. 1995;44(11):1249-58.

| TABLE 1: Pharmacokinetics of sulfonylurea. | | | |
|---|---|---|---|
| Compound | Half life (hours) | Duration of effect (hours) | Daily dosage range (mg) |
| Glibenclamide | 2–4 | 20–24 | 2.5–20 |
| Glipizide | 1–5 | 12–24 | 2.5–20 |
| Gliclazide | 6–15 | 10–15 | 40–320 |
| Glimepiride | 2–3 | 20–24 | 0.5–6 |

the management of gestational diabetes mellitus (GDM), and some centers have been using it in GDM.

## Indications

1. It can be used as a first-line drug in type 2 diabetic patients who do not tolerate metformin, though with the availability of modern SUs and subsequent introduction of safer agents such as $DPP_4Is$ and $SGLT_2Is$, it is rarely used in this indication nowadays.
2. In patients not controlled on metformin and/or glitazones, $DPP_4Is/SGLT_2Is$, glibenclamide can be added as a first add-on agent or second add-on agent.
3. In those type 2 diabetics who require insulin for blood glucose control but who still have some functional β-cells; glibenclamide can be added to insulin. If β-cells respond to glibenclamide, the dose and frequency of insulin can be reduced. However, very severe and long-standing type 2 diabetics who are in severe hyperglycemia (fasting plasma glucose >200 mg%), in spite of taking four or more tablets of glibenclamide, are unlikely to be benefited from addition of glibenclamide to insulin therapy because they are likely to be in "end stage" failure of β-cells.

*Glipizide:* It is a shorter acting agent as compared to glibenclamide and thus is administered two or three times a day 30 minutes before meals. It is a better SU to control postprandial blood glucose. Modified release once a day preparations are also available. The average daily dose range is 2.5–20 mg%. A few years back, price of glipizide formulations was drastically reduced by a government directive. Thus, like glibenclamide, it is very inexpensive.

Prevalence and severity of hypoglycemia induced by glipizide is a bit lesser than glibenclamide.

*Indications:* In principle, the indications are same as glibenclamide but in those with mild renal impairment, and in those who are prone to hypoglycemia, particularly elderly, it may be preferred to glibenclamide.

*Gliclazide:* It is similar to glipizide and has same indications as glipizide. It is usually administered twice a day 30 minutes before meals. Usual daily dose is 40–320 mg. However, modified release once a day preparations, recently launched in market provide better bioavailability and thus their average daily dose is 30–120 mg taken once a day. It has better safety records than all other SUs, in fact it is as safe as metformin on cardiovascular system. On hypoglycemia front also, it scores over other SUs and is thus safer to use in elderly and patients with renal impairment. International guidelines recommend that gliclazide and glipizide do not require dosage reduction even in severe renal impairment. Its use leads to less weight gain as compared to glibenclamide. Thus, the author feels that gliclazide is an underrated and underutilized SU. It is a bit more expensive than glipizide, which has similar advantages as regards hypoglycemia.

*Glimepiride:* This SU molecule was introduced in our country about two decades back. It has a long duration of action and thus is recommended once a day, however, in some patients it produces a much smoother blood glucose control if administered twice a day. Unlike other SUs, even if administered just before meals, it still gives similar postprandial control as compared to 30 minutes before meals administration. The usual daily dose is 0.5–6 mg. It has a short half-life but still has a long duration of action. It is claimed that stronger extrapancreatic action as compared to other SUs, is responsible for long duration of action in spite of short half-life. Prevalence and severity of hypoglycemia is less as compared to glibenclamide. Sulfonylurea-induced weight gain is also less as compared to glibenclamide. Unlike glibenclamide and glipizide, glimepiride and gliclazide act mainly on receptors on the β-cells in pancreas and have insignificant action on cardiac and vascular receptors. Gliclazide is probably a bit more specific than glimepiride. Theoretically, this property of relative lack of action on SU receptors outside pancreas is an advantage for glimepiride and gliclazide in patients having coronary artery disease. However, practical significance of this is not yet known. As regards gliclazide, in retrospective analysis of data on 9,607 T2DM patients from Netherlands who had started antidiabetic treatment as metformin monotherapy and subsequently who had added various SU and glinide molecules, it was noted that at the end of 9 years, hazards ratio for cardiovascular mortality and morbidity for gliclazide was significantly lower than all other SUs and glinide compounds. The hypothesis behind putative cardiovascular protection of gliclazide is as follows: repeated myocardial ischemia activates coronary dilatation which in turn reduces ischemic burden. For this protective mechanism to remain active, ATP-modulated potassium channels on coronary artery smooth muscle cells should remain in open state. Since first-generation SUs such as glibenclamide are nonspecific SU receptor blockers, if a patient is on glibenclamide during myocardial ischemia, he is unable to activate protective coronary vasodilatation, which is known as ischemic preconditioning, due to closure of ATP modulated potassium channels.

*Indications:* The general indications of glimepiride are same as those of any other SUs. The main indications are:

As first-line drug when metformin is not tolerated or is contraindicated in type 2 diabetic patients.

In type 2 diabetic, patients not controlled on metformin and/or glitazones, $DPP_4Is$ or $SGLT_2Is$.

In type 2 diabetics requiring insulin, it can be coprescribed with insulin. It can be also used as second or occasionally third add-on agent.

Advantages such as once a day dosage, lesser chances of hypoglycemia, lower weight gain, and relative safety in patients with renal impairment and in elderly have made glimepiride a popular SU.

It has no specific contraindication in addition to the group contraindications mentioned above. It can be used in mild to moderate renal insufficiency.

## Side-effects

A number of nonspecific GI symptoms ranging from dyspepsia to diarrhea occur with the SUs in a small number of patients (3–5%). A variety of skin reactions also occur. These are mostly of minor significance and resolve on drug cessation; however, an occasional severe complication may arise such as exfoliative dermatitis or Stevens–Johnson syndrome. A cholestasis type of jaundice and bone marrow depression are very rare complications. Water retention giving rise to dilutional hyponatremia [similar to that seen in the inappropriate antidiuretic hormone (ADH) secretion syndrome] was first described with chlorpropamide but has also been reported with other SUs. Hypoglycemia should be regarded as a consequence of excessive dosage rather than as a side effect, unless due to drug interaction.

## Sulfonylureas and Hypoglycemia

It should be noted that if given indiscriminately, all SUs can lead to dangerous episodes of hypoglycemia, which can be occasionally fatal. In older diabetics, symptoms of sympathetic overactivity, such as palpitations, tremors, sweating, etc. which serve as a warning, are often absent, and hence they could land up straight away in hypoglycemic coma or other types of neurological deficits of acute onset such as hemiplegia or acute delirious state. Renal and hepatic insufficiency, alcohol consumption, infrequent follow-ups, and failure to review the dosage of OADs from time to time are some of the common predisposing factors, and inadequate carbohydrate intake is a common precipitating factor.

Unlike insulin, hypoglycemia induced by SUs could be very prolonged or recurrent, even with drugs like glibenclamide, which has a short biological half-life. Hence, all patients with SU-induced severe hypoglycemia should be hospitalized and maintained on continuous intravenous (IV) 5% glucose drip and observed up to 48–72 hours.

In order to avoid SU-induced hypoglycemia, the following precautions should be taken.

Do not use SUs in patients with hepatic insufficiency. As regards renal insufficiency, avoid glibenclamide and refer to Chapter 17 for the dosage adjustments of other SUs.

Ask the patients to avoid alcohol and take small frequent feeds as per timetable drawn. He/she should not miss the food.

Periodically monitor blood glucose (every 3 months) in laboratory, in addition to home blood glucose monitoring at interval as per individual case (once or twice a week), and if it is well controlled, try to reduce the dosage of SUs.

Stress on diet control and regular exercise so that the dosage of OAD could be kept to the minimum.

If the patients are on a combination of SU plus biguanides, $DPP_4Is$ or incretin mimetics, the upward increment in dosage of SUs and metformin should be more gradual.

In older diabetics (above 70 years), do not insist on a very tight control of blood glucose and avoid glibenclamide.

## Nonsulfonylurea Insulin Secretagogues
### Repaglinide
This is the first insulin secretagogue, which is not a SU derivative but a benzoic acid derivative. Its mechanism of action is same as that of SU. However, the main differences are:
- Its onset of action is much quicker and duration of action much shorter than SUs.
- It can be given in renal impairment.

Repaglinide is a better agent than most SUs to control postprandial hyperglycemia, but at the same time, much weaker agent to control fasting hyperglycemia. It needs to be given before each meal and the usual dose is 0.5–2 mg three times a day. Prevalence of hypoglycemia is much lower than SUs.

#### Indications
The general indications are same as those of SUs, but it can be used as an agent of choice in those who have predominantly postprandial hyperglycemia, tendency for repeated hypoglycemia, irregular lifestyle, elderly diabetics, etc. Multiple doses and higher daily cost are the relative disadvantages.

*Contraindications*: Hepatic impairment.

### Nateglinide
Like repaglinide, it has a quick onset and a short duration of action. Onset, slightly quicker and duration slightly shorter as compared to the former. Thus, it has a slight edge. The usual daily dose is 30 to 120 mg before each meal. Its slot in the management for type 2 diabetic patients and relative advantages and disadvantages over SUs as well as indications and contraindications are same as repaglinide. Of late nateglinide is not freely available in India.

## Future of Sulfonylureas and Glinides
SUs were introduced in clinical practice in 1955 and for around five decades they remained the oral antidiabetic agents of choice. High glycemic efficacy, good GI tolerance and absence of alternatives other than biguanides were factors responsible for exceptional success story of SUs. Severe, persistent or recurrent hypoglycemic

episodes were reported with first-generation SUs. This drawback along with tendency for weight gain was partially taken care of by introduction of modern SUs such as glimepiride and gliclazide in 90s. Till the turn of century, there were hardly any alternatives other than biguanides. Glitazones provide safety from hypoglycemia but they are associated with significantly higher weight gain. Furthermore, due to various issues such as alleged cardiovascular toxicity, tendency to precipitate cardiac failure, alleged carcinogenicity for carcinoma of urinary bladder, their use never really picked up. After the turn of century, successive introduction of $DPP_4Is$, $GLP_1RAs$, and $SGLT_2Is$ have led to the paradigm shift in the management of diabetes. $DPP_4Is$ are safe for heart and kidneys, they do not lead to hypoglycemia and weight gain, while $GLP_1RAs$ provide cardio- and renoprotection in addition, and their use is associated with significant weight loss. $SGLT_2Is$ provide all the advantages of $GLP_1RAs$ and in addition have significant systolic blood pressure reducing action. While $DPP_4Is$ are having moderate glycemic efficacy, the other two groups have moderately strong glycemic efficacy. All the major scientific organizations in the field of diabetology and endocrinology have given expressions to these properties of new antidiabetic agents in their guidelines. New guidelines recommend agents from these three groups as first add on to metformin or as coprescription with metformin in initial combination therapy in most of the situations, relegating SU use to only in those patients who cannot afford these modern agents. Additionally with the availability of generic alternatives to most of these agents, the cost difference has narrowed. Furthermore, in those type 2 diabetic patients with evidence for presence of atherosclerotic cardiovascular disease (ASCVD), heart failure, renal impairment, or high risk for these comorbidities/complications, $GLP_1RAs$ or $SGLT_2Is$ are recommended as first-line agents, along with metformin or even in preference over metformin. All these factors would lead to gradual reduction in use of SUs and glinides, the decline will be faster in urban areas, specialized centers, and affluent areas. Since majority of Indians still live in small towns and villages and are not affluent, the overall decline in prescription will be very gradual.

The sharper reduction in use of glibenclamide and glipizide has additional reasons. In a way, particularly the decline of glibenclamide was beneficial as it is more likely to be associated with episodes of hypoglycemia and cardiovascular adverse events than modern SUs. Very sharp mandatory price reduction of these two molecules ordered by government authorities led to total withdrawal of any marketing and promotional activities by the companies. Some companies shifted their marketing budgets totally to modern SUs, magnified their advantages over first-generation SUs and in the process "killed" these agents. The ultimate looser was poor diabetic patient, because in the hands of experienced and learned doctors who know when and how to use them and when not to use them, these agents are reasonably safe and effective, not only clinically but also economically.

## BIGUANIDES

Metformin is the only biguanide now available in our country as phenformin was banned in December, 2003. However, for historical perspective, some comparative information on phenformin is retained in this book. After absorption from the upper GI tract, phenformin is concentrated predominantly in the liver while metformin in the intestinal mucosa. The former is metabolized in the liver while the latter is excreted unchanged.

Biguanides do not stimulate release of insulin from pancreas; they act at peripheral sites and improve tissue response to available insulin. Thus when given as monotherapy or along with other peripherally acting drugs, they are not liable to cause hypoglycemia. Biguanides mainly act at liver and suppress neoglucogenesis, i.e., formation of glucose from nonglucose sources. In addition, biguanides also have some action on striated muscles where they improve insulin-mediated glucose disposal.

Among the biguanides, metformin is the agent of choice. In fact, phenformin was either banned or voluntarily withdrawn from most of the developed countries between 1978 and 1980. It took exactly quarter of century for Indian regulatory authorities to order its withdrawal from the market.

Metformin is usually administered twice or thrice a day while its slow release preparations can be given once a day. The usual daily dose is 500–2550 mg. It is available in a wide range of formulations to enable the prescriber to titrate the dosage as per the exact requirement of an individual patient (conventional form of metformin is available in four strengths, 250 mg, 500 mg, 850 mg, and 1,000 mg. In addition, extended-release metformin is available in 500 mg and 1,000 mg strengths).

Some patients pass empty shells of extended-release metformin formulations in stool. These shells look like complete extended-release tablets to the naked eye from some distance. Thus, patients feel that their full tablets are coming out from the other end and they are wasting their hard-earned money. These patients should be reassured that they have been prescribed specially formulated tablets having "extended-release technology" and such tablets are coated with special shells from which active medicine is slowly released in their intestine through tiny holes and what they observe in stools is just the empty shell. If their blood glucose is well controlled, it is obvious that they are not wasting their hard-earned money and it is an indirect confirmation that what they saw was just an empty shell. Please remember not to prescribe half tablets (or one and half tablets) of extended-release brands, because in most cases, breaking of tablets in two halves leads to breakdown of the shell and such tablets behave like ordinary tablets releasing the active drug in the circulation rapidly and not in a gradual "controlled release" pattern. There are exceptions to the rule. In some cases, the particular technology used for "controlled release" mechanism is such that even broken tablet works in "slow release" or "controlled release" manner. Such tablet can be differentiated from other tablets by the presence of graduation in the middle on the tablet surface.

## Indications

Metformin is indicated as an agent of first choice in all type 2 diabetic patients, unless it is contraindicated. It should be started along with diet and exercise soon after the diagnosis is confirmed. Universally, metformin is considered as the foundation agent to initiate the treatment of T2DM. Subsequently, if and when required, the agents from other classes of OADs can be added around it. Proved efficacy, safety from hypoglycemia, a track record of more than six decades, absence of cardiovascular side effects, and weight neutrality are some of the main assets of metformin leading to its pivotal status in the management of T2DM. Inexpensiveness is also a big point in its favor. In those type 2 diabetics who do not adequately respond to metformin or who do not tolerate full dose of metformin, it can be combined with glitazones, SUs gliptins, $SGLT_2Is$, or $GLP_1RAs$. Younger patients with severe insulin resistance (clinical markers: central obesity, hypertension, hypertriglyceridemia, etc.) are suitable for metformin—glitazone combination, while others can be prescribed metformin—SU combinations. Affording patients have a choice of metformin—gliptin combination, which has a strong synergy and safety from side effects such as weight gain and hypoglycemia. In those having ASCVD, heart failure, renal impairment or high risk for these comorbidities/complications, $SGLT_2Is$, or $GLP_1RAs$ can be combined with metformin.

In those diabetics on insulin and requiring large doses of insulin due to insulin-resistance overlapping on insulin deficiency, metformin can be added as an adjuvant to insulin.

Metformin has multiple additional indications, such as prevention of diabetes, polycystic ovary syndrome, nonalcoholic hepatic steatosis, and prevention and treatment of certain malignancies. Further details are beyond the scope of this book.

## Role of Metformin in Prevention of Diabetes: DPP Trial

The Diabetes Prevention Program (DPP) was a trial in which people having impaired glucose tolerance (IGT) were divided in following three groups: (1) metformin 850 mg twice a day, (2) intensive lifestyle intervention, (3) placebo. At the end of 2.7 years, compared to placebo, intensive lifestyle intervention and metformin reduced the incidence of diabetes by 58 and 31% respectively. Though intensive lifestyle intervention produced better results, in the day-to-day practice settings, most of the people are unable to comply with such intensive interventions over a long term. In this context, 31% relative reduction of incidence of diabetes with metformin is quite impressive [Diabetes Prevention Program (DPP) Research Group. The Diabetes Prevention Program (DPP): description of lifestyle intervention. Diabetes Care. 2002;25(12):2165-71].

In India, Ramachandran from Chennai has done similar study with lower dosages of metformin and documented comparable reduction in incidence rates of diabetes with metformin [Ramachandran A, Snehalatha C, Mary S, Mukesh B, Bhaskar AD, Vijay V, et al. The Indian Diabetes Prevention Programme shows that lifestyle modification and metformin prevent T2DM in Asian Indian subjects with impaired glucose tolerance (IDPP). Diabetologia. 2006;49(2):289-97].

## Contraindications

Metformin is contraindicated in severe hepatic insufficiency and renal insufficiency [estimated glomerular filtration rate (eGFR) <30 mL/min/1.73 m$^2$]. Please refer to Chapter 17 for details regarding use of metformin in milder renal impairment. It is also contraindicated in conditions such as severe cardiac failure, severe bronchospastic conditions such as bronchial asthma and severe chronic obstructive pulmonary disease (COPD) and in patients in shock. This precaution is taken to avoid metformin-induced lactic acidosis, which is more likely to develop in hypoxic environment. It is also contraindicated in diabetic ketoacidosis, pregnancy, and lactation and in T1DM. Theoretically, all noninsulin drugs are contraindicated in pregnancy, including metformin. However, based on its safety demonstrated in several clinical trials, it is routinely used in many pregnant diabetic women, particularly in those with gestational diabetes.

## Biguanides and Lactic Acidosis

Between the two biguanides, metformin is now universally considered as the drug of choice because of its relative safety as regards occurrence of lactic acidosis, which is extremely rare but a life-threatening complication of biguanide therapy having 50% mortality rate even after prompt diagnosis and treatment in well-equipped intensive care unit (ICU) with dialysis facilities. This is precisely the reason for withdrawing phenformin from the most of the advanced countries in 1978-1980 and continuing with metformin.

Most of the patients who developed biguanide-associated lactic acidosis had hepatic, renal, or circulatory impairment, and in fact, they should never have received a biguanide. However, there are a few case reports of lactic acidosis in patients who did not have any contraindications for use of phenformin, which was prescribed in correct dose. A noteworthy feature about metformin-induced lactic acidosis is that in all patients, metformin was consumed in spite of a contraindication or in very large doses, hence, lactic acidosis was avoidable. The lesser incidence of metformin-associated lactic acidosis can be explained by the fact that metformin is less lipophilic than phenformin, and it is not concentrated and metabolized in the liver thus hepatic insufficiency does not increase the probability of metformin-induced lactic acidosis.

It was generally believed by Indian diabetologists that lactic acidosis is rare in our patients as compared to western countries. Our patients consume complex carbohydrates containing higher amounts of fiber content in large amounts. Alcohol consumption is also less as compared to western countries and possibly, because of these reasons our patients are controlled with comparatively smaller doses of biguanides leading to lesser incidence of lactic acidosis.

However, considering the lack of laboratory facilities required for estimation of blood lactic acid and blood pH and lack of awareness about lactic acidosis in some clinicians, one can assume that lactic acidosis is not as rare as it appears and possibly many cases are missed. A few cases of biguanide-associated lactic acidosis have already been reported from our country.

In order to avoid biguanide-induced lactic acidosis, the following precautions should be taken:
- Do not use biguanides in hepatic or renal insufficiency (eGFR <30 mL/min/1.73 m$^2$) and in patients with severely impaired left ventricular function and severe bronchial asthma or COPD or any condition, which can lead to severe hypoxia.
- Advise the patients not to consume alcohol
- Use minimal effective doses of biguanides and try to reduce it from time to time
- Keep the possibility of biguanide-induced lactic acidosis in mind whenever you come across a diabetic on biguanides having symptoms suggestive of lactic acidosis, such as deep, rapid breathing, dyspnea, upper abdominal discomfort, drowsiness, unexpected deterioration in health, etc. when

other common causes are excluded. Under such circumstances, promptly withdraw biguanides and hospitalize the patient for further management.

## THIAZOLIDINEDIONES

### Pioglitazone, Rosiglitazone, and Lobeglitazone

Thiazolidinediones also known as glitazones work as insulin sensitizers. They act only on peripheral tissues, mainly muscle and fat cells, and increase their sensitivity to insulin. They do not directly increase pancreatic insulin secretion but they act through increasing sensitivity of tissues to insulin, thus, like metformin, they require presence of insulin and in an environment devoid of insulin, as in T1DM, they are ineffective. When given alone or in combination with any antidiabetic medication other than insulin or insulin secretagogue (SUs and repaglinide), they rarely cause hypoglycemia. Glitazones are potent and highly selective agonists of peroxisome proliferator-activated receptor gamma (PPAR-$\gamma$), which are intranuclear receptors. The cellular site of action is predominantly adipocytes and muscle cells with some action on hepatocytes. Glitazones sensitize tissues toward insulin and reduce circulating free fatty acid levels. The action on hepatocytes is responsible for beneficial effects seen in management of nonalcoholic steatohepatitis (NASH) with pioglitazone. NASH is an important but grossly underestimated, underdiagnosed, and undertreated complication/associated condition with significant mortality and morbidity through progressive deterioration in hepatic pathology as well as acceleration of cardiovascular complications.

Because of some misconceptions in minds of clinicians, pioglitazone is somewhat underused in our country. It is a potent insulin sensitizer and even in today's scenario, with availability of several new antidiabetic medications, if used judiciously, it has a definite role to play in the management of a subset of type 2 diabetic patients with significant insulin resistance. So let us study how and when to use pioglitazone and when not to use it. Recently, another TZD, lobeglitazone has been introduced in India.

## Indications

Thiazolidinediones are classified among high potency antidiabetic agents with ability to reduce glycated hemoglobin (HbA1c) up to 1.5%. They are indicated in the following situations:
- In predominantly insulin resistant type 2 diabetic patients, pioglitazone is used as an alternative to metformin particularly if the latter is not tolerated or contraindicated. It can also be combined with metformin when monotherapy with metformin fails to achieve glycemic targets.
- In dual or triple drug combination along with any one or two from metformin, $DPP_4Is$, $SGLT_2Is$, SUs/repaglinide, and $GLP_1$ agonists when monotherapy or two-drug therapy fails to meet glycemic targets and the patient is still some distance away from end-stage β-cell failure, particularly in those who have features of significant insulin resistance. Experienced clinicians can make such a judgment. Presence of features of insulin resistance (central obesity, raised triglycerides, acanthosis nigricans, hypertension, fatty liver, etc.).
- Though no agent is officially recommended for nonalcoholic fatty liver disease (NAFLD), among all the agents being used and studied in trails, pioglitazone has given best results in biopsy proved cases.

## Contraindications

Pioglitazone is contraindicated in severe hepatic insufficiency, NYHA class II and III cardiac failure, and pregnancy. It is ineffective in type 1 diabetic patients.

## Precautions

- Water retention leading to increased volume of fluid in intravascular compartment is liable to occur with pioglitazone. Precipitation of incipient cardiac failure has occurred with the use of pioglitazone particularly when used along with other fluid retaining agents such as insulin.
- By now, pioglitazone is in clinical practice for about two decades. During this period, cases developing hepatotoxicity were very rare and thus formal guidelines about pretreatment

and subsequent periodic monitoring of serum glutamic-oxaloacetic transaminase (SGOT) and serum glutamic-pyruvic transaminase (SGPT) have been relaxed and the prescriber should use his discretion to advise liver function tests depending upon individual case. Those with SGOT, SGPT values more than twice the upper limit of normal should not use pioglitazone or discontinue if already on therapy. Physicians should use their discretion for those with values in between higher limit of normal and two times normal.

- A small increase in risk for carcinoma of urinary bladder has been observed in patients on pioglitazone. However, cause and effect relationship was not proved.

  In 2011, in response to observation of higher incidence of carcinoma of bladder in patients on pioglitazone in clinical studies, French authorities banned pioglitazone and German authorities applied restrictions to its use, while the USA and UK allowed unrestricted use of pioglitazone. In the same year, the Drugs Controller of India temporarily suspended the sales of pioglitazone but within few weeks revoked suspension order. Since then pioglitazone is uninterruptedly available in India. Subsequently in August, 2014, the dark clouds over pioglitazone were permanently cleared when 10-year study involving 200,000 patients to examine potential association between pioglitazone and urinary bladder cancer concluded that pioglitazone was not associated with statistically significant increased risk of bladder cancer [Lewis JD, Habel LA, Quesenberry CP, Strom BL, Peng T, Hedderson MM, et al. Pioglitazone Use and Risk of Bladder Cancer and Other Common Cancers in Persons with Diabetes. JAMA. 2015;314(3):265-77].

  To be on safer side, pioglitazone should not be prescribed in those with history of carcinoma of urinary bladder. Before starting pioglitazone, routine urine examination should be performed and those with unexplained hematuria should be subjected to cystoscopy to rule out carcinoma of urinary bladder. Patients on pioglitazone should be subjected to periodic urine examination.

- Glitazones are associated with a small increase in incidence of fractures of lower ends of long bones, particularly in lower extremities and in women. As regards rosiglitazone, it was observed in DREAM study on prevention of diabetes and ADOPT study on durability of glycemic effects in T2DM, and as regards pioglitazone, it was seen in PROactive trial done to study cardiovascular protection offered by pioglitazone. Thus, glitazones should be used with caution.

## Dosage

The usual daily dose of pioglitazone is 15–45 mg. in a single dose. Most of the Indian doctors do not prescribe it beyond 30 mg/day. Many experienced diabetologist in India use 7.5 mg. of pioglitazone per day and they have observed reasonable efficacy and reduced side effects with this dose. Patients on pioglitazone usually gain some weight, which can be as much as 10 kg in some patients. The weight gain is mainly due to water retention with some contributions from subcutaneous adipogenesis and weight regain due to better metabolic control. In those with significant edema or weight gain, glitazones need to be discontinued.

## Glitazones in Prevention of Diabetes

**DREAM** *(Diabetes Reduction Assessment with ramipril and rosiglitazone Medication) trial* has demonstrated that use of rosiglitazone in the dose of 16 mg daily by those having IGT led to 60% relative risk reduction as regards conversion to diabetes [DREAM (Diabetes REduction Assessment with ramipril and rosiglitazone Medication) Trial Investigators; Gerstein HC, Yusuf S, Bosch J, Pogue J, Sheridan P, et al. Effect of rosiglitazone on the frequency of diabetes in patients with impaired glucose tolerance or impaired fasting glucose: a randomised controlled trial. Lancet. 2006;368(9541):1096-105].

**ACT NOW** *(Actos Now for the prevention of diabetes) trial:* In this prevention trial, administration of 45 mg of pioglitazone led to 72% relative risk reduction of diabetes as compared to placebo in those with impaired glucose tolerance. However, there was significant weight gain in patients on pioglitazone [DeFronzo RA, Tripathy D, Schwenke DC, Banerji M, Bray GA, Buchanan TA, et al. Pioglitazone for diabetes prevention in impaired glucose tolerance. N Engl J Med. 2011;364(12):1104-15].

**TABLE 2: Relative efficacy of various oral antidiabetic drugs for prevention of T2DM.**

| OADs/lifestyle intervention | Risk reduction % | Trial |
|---|---|---|
| Pioglitazone | 72 | ACT NOW |
| Rosiglitazone | 60 | DREAM |
| Metformin | 33 | DPP |
| Acarbose | 25 | STOP NIDDM |
| Aggressive diet + exercise | 56 | DPP |

(T2DM: type 2 diabetes mellitus; ACT NOW: Actos Now for the prevention of diabetes; DPP: Diabetes Prevention Program; DREAM: Diabetes Reduction Assessment with ramipril and rosiglitazone Medication; OADs: oral antidiabetic drugs; STOP NIDDM: STOP-noninsulin-dependent diabetes mellitus)

Table 2 gives relative efficacy of various OADs and lifestyle measures in prevention of diabetes in those having IGT.

Please note that in spite of excellent efficacy in prevention of diabetes, due to tendency of weight gain, pioglitazone is not recommended for this indication. Rosiglitazone is not available. Table 2 can be referred for comparing efficacies of different agents used in diabetic prevention studies.

### Some Important Studies on Glitazones

**PROactive study:** [Erdmann E, Dormandy J, Wilcox R, Massi-Benedetti M, Charbonnel B. PROactive 07: pioglitazone in the treatment of T2DM: results of the PROactive study. Vasc Health Risk Manag. 2007;3(4):355-70].

PROactive was a prospective comparative controlled study in 5,238 patients to find out whether pioglitazone can prevent cardiovascular events in type 2 diabetic patients. It proved that pioglitazone was successful in reducing the risk of secondary macrovascular events such as nonfatal myocardial infarction and nonfatal stroke in statistically significant manner in high-risk type 2 diabetic patients with established macrovascular disease. [In primary end point of the main study, a composite of 10 different events including intervention in lower limbs for management of peripheral vascular disease were included and the difference between pioglitazone and placebo was nonsignificant. This had created initial negative impression about the study, however subsequent subanalysis focusing on different end points brought out the encouraging positive findings and true value of the study].

**IRIS Study:** [Vascoli CM, et al. Am Heart J. 2014;168:823-9].

Iris was a 5-year prospective placebo controlled study in non-diabetic insulin resistant patients with history of transient ischemic attack (TIA) or completed stroke. It proved that pioglitazone in the dose of 15–45 mg daily was able to reduce the risk of major cardiovascular events and new onset diabetes in statistically significant manner as compared to placebo.

Since macrovascular disease is very common in T2DM and it is responsible for death in two-thirds of the patients, the macrovascular protective property of pioglitazone increases its value in the management of T2DM.

**ADOPT Study:** [Kahn SE, Haffner SM, Heise MA, Herman WH, Holman RR, Jones NP, et al. Glycemic durability of rosiglitazone, metformin, or glyburide monotherapy. N Engl J Med. 2006;355(23): 2427-43].

This comparative study was done with rosiglitazone, metformin, and glibenclamide to study and compare the glycemic durability at the end of 5 years of monotherapy with these agents. It was found out that cumulative incidence of monotherapy failure at 5 years was 15% for rosiglitazone, 21% for metformin, and 34% for glibenclamide. This represents a risk reduction of 32% for rosiglitazone as compared to metformin and 63% as compared to glibenclamide. Though similar comparative studies are not available with pioglitazone, high durability of rosiglitazone is likely to be a class effect and thus, shared by pioglitazone.

## Rosiglitazone: A Roller-coaster Journey and Current Status

In 2007, a meta-analysis[†] published in New England Journal of Medicine by Steven Nissen from Cleveland Clinic, USA, (NEJM. 2007;356:2457-71) suggested higher incidence of myocardial infarction and increased cardiovascular mortality in patient on rosiglitazone as compared to other antidiabetic agents including pioglitazone. It was thought that though both carry out their insulin-sensitizing action through PPAR-γ agonism, their additional actions on other PPAR receptors such as PPAR-α and PPAR δ/β differ. Thus, while pioglitazone is associated with reduction of low-density lipoprotein (LDL) cholesterol levels, rosiglitazone is associated with increase in LDL cholesterol levels.

**RECORD Trial** [Home PD, et al. Lancet. 2009;373:2025-35].

In June 2009, results of RECORD trial were published. It included 4,447 patients and was designed to study cardiovascular side effects of SUs, metformin, and rosiglitazone. Patients not controlled on SUs or metformin monotherapy were divided in three groups and treated with SUs plus rosiglitazone, metformin plus rosiglitazone, or SUs plus metformin. Rosiglitazone was not associated with increased cardiovascular mortality or morbidity but the data was inconclusive regarding increased risk of myocardial infarction. However, as expected, use of rosiglitazone was associated with increased risk of cardiac failure and limb fractures. Since rosiglitazone was significantly more expensive than SUs and metformin, particularly in western countries, the regulatory authorities as well as media viewed the findings of the trial in negative manner and saw no reason to continue it. Record was a large scale prospective comparative study with hard end points and not merely a meta-analysis† and its findings refuted many of the fears about cardiovascular side effects of rosiglitazone raised by meta-analysis published in 2007. However, based on

---

†What is meta-analysis?

Let us understand meta-analysis. It is a retrospective analysis of research work. In the clinical trials on drugs, whenever studies having a large number of patients are not available to get a reliable insight into efficacy or safety of a particular drug, meta-analysis of several smaller studies already completed is done. Studies having similar design are added up and the data are analyzed. The strength of meta-analysis is inclusion of a large number of patients thus data is more reliable. The weaknesses include retrospective nature of study, design of individual studies may differ significantly, each individual study may be too small or of a short-term nature and the aim of meta-analysis may differ from the main aim of the original study. Network meta-analysis is done when direct comparative studies are not available, e.g., if there are no comparative studies between hypothetical drug A and C, but there are studies comparing A with B and B with C, in network meta-analysis A is indirectly compared with C based on the results of comparative studies between A and B and B and C.

abovementioned meta-analysis, European countries including UK banned rosiglitazone and in September, 2010, the USA imposed severe restrictions on its use including requirements such as a need for obtaining special permission from authorities to use it only in those patients where other antidiabetic medications were ineffective. Following the actions taken by western countries, the Drugs Controller of India banned use of rosiglitazone in November, 2010.

The roller-coaster journey of rosiglitazone was far from over. On November 25, 2013, 3 years after awarding virtual death sentence, the FDA of USA reviewed the findings of RECORD trial and removed the restrictions on prescriptions and free availability of rosiglitazone in the USA. Till date, the authorities in other countries and territories including the European Union and India have not reviewed their decision and rosiglitazone remains unavailable in these countries. The 2013 The United States Food and Drug Administration (US FDA) decision threw the ball into prescribes court who were free to use it in the USA. However, because of many reasons including lack of enthusiasm from the originator of rosiglitazone, its use in the USA never picked up and though it is still available there it is rarely prescribed.

## Lobeglitazone

Lobeglitazone is a recently introduced TZDs in our country. It originated in South Korea and is available in few Asian countries. Its mechanism of action is same as that of pioglitazone. In placebo controlled monotherapy study, lobeglitazone reduced HbA1c by 0.44% at the end of 24 weeks, while in comparative trial versus pioglitazone as add on to metformin, both the molecules reduced HbA1c by 0.74% at the end of 24 weeks. In a comparative phase III Indian study on 180 patients, both lobeglitazone and pioglitazone reduced HbA1c by 1.0% at the end of 16 weeks, when used on top of stable dose of metformin. 0.5 mg of lobeglitazone once a day was compared to 15 mg of pioglitazone in this study. The side effects profile (edema, weight gain) was similar.' Unlike pioglitazone, lobeglitazone has not undergone any cardiovascular outcome studies. Its glycemic efficacy studies are essentially short-term studies and done in smaller number of patients restricted to East Asia.

### *Indications of Lobeglitazone*

Lobeglitazone shares exactly same indications with pioglitazone and till now, no clear advantage over later has emerged. Larger glycemic efficacy studies in wider indications and cardiovascular and renal outcome studies are eagerly awaited. Its usual dose is 0.5 mg once a day. Its contraindications and limitations are same as those of pioglitazone.

## ALPHA-GLUCOSIDASE INHIBITORS

Acarbose and voglibose are available in India. They act locally on the surface of small intestine. By inhibiting $\alpha$-glucosidase enzymes which convert complex carbohydrates into monosaccharides, they delay digestion of carbohydrates and convert them into glucose gradually thus their absorption in circulation is slowed down and postprandial peaks are blunted. They have moderate glycemic efficacy. These agents are not very effective in controlling fasting blood glucose and thus are usually used as an adjuvant to other antidiabetic agents for improving postprandial glycemic control. They tend to produce abdominal distention, borborygmi, and diarrhea in some patients, particularly when given in higher doses. These side effects are more common in Indians as compared with western people because we take a lot of fiber in our diet. However, since an average Indian derives 65% of calories through carbohydrates, we have higher postprandial glucose values for the same level of HbA1c as compared to westerners. Hence, AGIs are more suitable for Indians, they are hardly prescribed in the west. Usual dose is 1–2 tablets with meals, the pill to be taken with first bite of food (acarbose 25–50 mg with meals, voglibose 0.2–0.3 mg with meals). The frequency of administration can be individualized (e.g., if postbreakfast and postdinner glucose values need improvement, but postlunch values are under control, AGIs can be given with breakfast and dinner, or if a particular patient takes very heavy dinner, but light breakfast and lunch, and among postprandial glucose values, only postdinner value is high, AGIs can be administered only with dinner).

## Indications

It is indicated as a monotherapy in patients with mild and predominantly postprandial hyperglycemia, if metformin is contraindicated or not tolerated. This is an uncommon "niche indication".

As an adjuvant to insulin, metformin, glitazones, insulin secretagogues as well as modern agents such as $DPP_4Is$, $SGLT_2Is$, and $GLP_1$ agonists for improvement in postprandial glucose control. By themselves, they have moderate efficacy and are usually used as adjuvants to mainline agents in the management of T2DM. They can be used as first, second, third, and occasionally even forth add-on therapy. Whenever mainline agents have established reasonable glycemic control and fasting glucose is controlled but mild postprandial hyperglycemia is coming in the way of reaching A1c target, one can think of AGIs.

### Role of Acarbose in Prevention of Diabetes: STOP-NIDDM Trial

People with IGT who received 50 mg of acarbose three times a day had 25% relative risk reduction from new onset diabetes as compared to placebo. In addition, they had significant risk reductions as regards acute myocardial infarction and new onset hypertension during the trial period. However, though it was able to reduce the risk of abovementioned cardiovascular end points in those with prediabetes, in other trials done in established diabetes, acarbose was unable to significantly reduce the risk of hard cardiovascular end points. Acarbose is used as an alternative to metformin in those with IGT who are unable to implement required lifestyle measures [Chiasson JL, Josse RG, Gomis R, Hanefeld M, Karasik A, Laakso M, et al. Acarbose for prevention of T2DM: the STOP-NIDDM randomised trial. Lancet. 2002;359(9323):2072-7].

## Contraindications

Alpha-glucosidase inhibitors are contraindicated in inflammatory bowel disorders, obstructive disorders of the GI tract, and in pregnancy and lactation.

## Precautions

If a patient develops hypoglycemia, he should be treated by administering glucose, even if hypoglycemia is mild because, in patients on these agents, carbohydrates including disaccharides such as sucrose take longer time for conversion to glucose.

## INCRETIN-BASED THERAPY

Two new classes of antidiabetic agents with novel and totally different mechanisms of action, as compared to insulin and traditional OADs, have been introduced in clinical practice. Incretin-based agents along with $SGLT_2Is$ have made paradigm shift in the way T2DM is managed. Incretin-based agents are:
- *Glucagon-like peptide-1 receptor agonists* are injectable agents, with the exception of semaglutide, which is available in injectable as well as oral form (injectable semaglutide is not available in India).
- *Dipeptidyl peptidase-4 inhibitors or gliptins* are oral agents. Their mechanisms of action partially overlap each other. Before looking into these agents, let us review incretin physiology.
  - *Incretin physiology:* Incretins are hormones secreted by small intestine in response to food intake. The two important incretins are: (1) $GLP_1$ and (2) GIP (glucose-dependent insulinotropic peptide). Circulating levels of these hormones, particularly $GLP_1$ are reduced in type 2 diabetics. They respond to IV infusion of $GLP_1$ but are resistant to action of GIP, thus it has no therapeutic value.

Thus, let us now concentrate on $GLP_1$. Its four important physiological actions are:
1. Glucose-dependent enhancement of insulin secretion by β-cells in pancreas
2. Glucose-dependent suppression of postprandial glucagon secretion by α-cells in pancreas
3. Delaying gastric emptying
4. Stimulation of satiety center in hypothalamus, leading to reduction in appetite

All these actions lead to control of blood glucose in normal persons. In type 2 diabetic patients, reduced levels of $GLP_1$ are one of the contributing pathophysiological factors responsible for hyperglycemia. $GLP_1$ has very short biological half-life because immediately after its formation and secretion in ileum. It is degraded by $DPP_4$ enzyme, which is locally secreted in small intestine. Thus, in order to be therapeutically effective, it has to be given in continuous IV infusion, which is not practicable.

## $GLP_1RAs$

Glucagon-like peptide-1 receptor agonists are large molecular weight proteins with significant homology (structural similarity with $GLP_1$ as regards amino acids and their sequence). When injected subcutaneously or given orally in specially designed formulation (oral semaglutide), they share physiological actions of $GLP_1$ and since they are resistant to the action of $DPP_4Is$, they have therapeutic value in the management of T2DM. Information on agents available in India is given here in chronological order as per their introduction in our country.

*Exenatide*, which is a synthetic derivative of exendin found in saliva of Gila monster has a biological half-life of 2 hours and remains effective for about 12 hours after subcutaneous (SC) administration in human beings. It is available in our country as Byetta since 2007. It shares all the physiological actions of $GLP_1$ and is not degraded by $DPP_4$ enzymes. Its administration in the dosage of 5–10 μg in SC injection twice a day 30–60 minutes before meals in type 2 diabetics with viable β-cells leads to significant reduction in postprandial blood glucose, about 1% reduction in HbA1c, and some reduction in fasting plasma glucose. Its main advantages over SU are weight reduction and absence of hypoglycemic episodes since it acts only in presence of hyperglycemia. These two properties have led to its vast popularity of $GLP_1RAs$ in western countries. It is a good alternative to SUs in the management of T2DM, particularly those who are overweight and affording. The main side effects seen in about 10% patients are nausea and vomiting. Starting with the dose of 5 μg for 4 weeks and then increasing to 10 μg, if required helps to reduce GI side effects. With introduction of liraglutide, which has clear advantages, its use of exenatide has become negligible.

*Liraglutide:* It is a GLP$_1$ agonist having longer biological half-life and needs to be given once a day subcutaneously thus is more patient-friendly. As compared to exenatide, its other subtle differences are:
- Less pronounced effect on gastric emptying leading to lesser reduction of postprandial blood glucose and also lesser GI side effects
- It reduces fasting blood glucose as well as HbA1c by a greater extent
- It has greater homology with glucagon-like polypeptide-1. Liraglutide was introduced in India in 2010. Its dose is 1.2–1.8 mg SC once a day. The starting dose is 0.6 mg and if well tolerated, the dose should be stepped up to 1.2 mg after 1 week. It is available in India as Victoza. Unlike exenatide and lixisenatide, liraglutide is cardioprotective.

*Lixisenatide:* It is once daily short-acting GLP$_1$RA based on exendin platform. Its glycemic efficacy is a bit inferior to liraglutide and it does not offer protection from ASCVD and renal impairment. Its combination product with glargine in single pen assembly for once a day administration is available in west and is more popular. The combination product is convenient, user friendly but at the same time moderately effective and pragmatic option when one wants a trade-off between ease of administration and aggressive control. Needless to say that such products offer convenience at the cost of very limited flexibility. It can be considered in elderly patients with moderate, nonaggressive HbA1c targets needing GLP$_1$RAs as well as logistic simplicity of dosage administration. Plain lixisenatide is available in India.

*Dulaglutide:* It is a long-acting GLP$_1$RA based on human GLP platform and needs only once a week administration, thus is more convenient. The starting dose is 0.75 mg subcutaneously once a week to be stepped up if well tolerated and if required to 1.5 mg once a week. It is only once a week, GLP$_1$RA available in India and marketed as Trulicity. Obviously, many patients have shifted from liraglutide to dulaglutide. It also offers protection against ASCVD.

*Semaglutide*: It is a long-acting $GLP_1RA$ based on human $GLP_1$ platform, initially introduced in west as once a week injection and subsequently as once a day oral tablet, only tablets are available in India. Injectable semaglutide offers all the advantages of dulaglutide, in addition offers more weight reduction.

Introduction of a high molecular weight protein such as semaglutide in oral formulation is considered as one of the greatest achievement of pharmaceutical science. In oral formulation, semaglutide is coformulated with a chemical called sodium N-[8-(2 hydroxybenzoyl)amino]caprylate (SNAC). SNAC protects semaglutide from enzymatic digestion in stomach and facilitates its absorption across the gastric mucosa. Semaglutide is available as Rybelsus tablets in 3 mg/7 mg/14 mg strengths. Semaglutide needs to be taken once a day on empty stomach, first thing in morning with up to 120 mL of water. Patient should not eat or drink for 30 minutes after taking semaglutide. The starting dose is 3 mg daily and if well tolerated it should be up titrated to 7 mg once daily at the end of 4 weeks and subsequently if required, to 14 mg daily at the end of another 4 weeks.

## Advantages of $GLP_1RA$

Glucagon-like peptide-1 receptor agonists offer following benefits:
- Moderately strong glycemic efficacy
- Freedom from hypoglycemia
- Significant weight reducing action
- Cardiovascular protection, particularly against ASCVD and renoprotection (liraglutide, dulaglutide, and semaglutide)

*Side effects and precautions*: The main side effects are GI and are seen in initial period of therapy. Nausea, vomiting, diarrhea, and abdominal distension are not uncommon. Introduction of the drug in small doses and gradually stepping up the dose every 4 weeks takes care of the problem in many patients. Taking the medicine with light nonfatty breakfast and use of symptomatic therapy with antivomiting agents and proton pump inhibitors is another solution. Temporary worsening of diabetic retinopathy and macular edema has been reported in some studies on injectable semaglutide and is probably due to rapid improvement in glycemic control.

## Cardiovascular Outcome Studies on GLP$_1$RA

Cardiovascular protective effect of liraglutide, dulaglutide, and injectable semaglutide has been conclusively demonstrated. Study on oral semaglutide is ongoing. The protection develops more slowly as compared to that offered by SGLT$_2$I because mechanism works through slowing down the process of atherosclerosis. These agents also offer renoprotection. No significant protection was seen against hospitalization for heart failure. The molecules based on exendin platform (lixisenatide and exenatide) offer cardiovascular safety but no cardiovascular protection. **Table 3** gives salient features of CVOTs done on GLP$_1$RAs.

## Indications of GLP$_1$RA

Based on the findings of CVOT studies, most guidelines across the globe are now recommending GLP$_1$RAs with proven cardiovascular and renal protection (liraglutide, dulaglutide, injectable semaglutide) for use as first-line agents (as an alternate option to SGLT$_2$I) in patients with ASCVD and renal impairment and in those having high risk for these comorbidities. In other patients, any one agent from the entire GLP$_1$RA family can be added as first or second add on in combinations with metformin, SUs, and pioglitazone (with one or two of these agents per the individual situation), particularly in those where freedom from hypoglycemia and weight reduction is a priority. They can be combined with insulin for better glycemic control, lesser hypoglycemic episodes, and lesser weight gain as compared with insulin monotherapy. This indication is rapidly getting acceptance in western countries. There is no point in combining these agents with DPP$_4$I because when GLP$_1$RA is on board, DPP$_4$Is are redundant.

Cost of therapy (around ₹9,000/month) and GI side effects are the limiting factors for widespread use of these agents in a day-to-day practice particularly in our country.

**Table 4** gives comparative pharmacokinetic profiles of GLP$_1$RAs and their dosage schedules.

## DPP$_4$Is/Gliptins

As mentioned above, DPP$_4$ is an enzyme secreted by small intestinal mucosa in areas next to incretin secreting cells.

## TABLE 3: GLP$_1$ RA CVOTs: Design and primary safety/efficacy outcomes.

| | ELIXA | LEADER | SUSTAIN-6† | EXSCEL | HARMONY | REWIND | PIONEER 6† | AMPLITUDE-O | FREEDOM CVO |
|---|---|---|---|---|---|---|---|---|---|
| Study intervention | Lixisenatide | Liraglutide | Injection semaglutide | Exenatide ER | Albiglutide | Dulaglutide | Oral semaglutide | Efpeglenatide | Exenatide continuous SC infusion |
| Number of patients | 6,068 | 9,340 | 3,297 | 14,752 | 9,463 | 9,901 | 3,183 | 4,076 | 4,156 |
| Patient population | T2DM + ACS | T2DM + CVD or CV risk | T2DM + CVD and/or CKD stage 3 or higher or CV risk | T2DM with/without CV event | T2DM + established CVD | T2DM + CVD or CV risk | T2DM + CVD and/or CKD stage 3 or CV risk | T2DM + CVD or CV risk | T2DM + CVD or CV risk |
| Primary outcome | 4P-MACE | 3P-MACE | 3P-MACE | 3P-MACE | 3P-MACE | 3P-MACE | 3P-MACE | 3P-MACE | 4P-MACE |
| Median follow-up (years) | 2.1 | 3.8 | 2.1 | 3.2 | ~1.6 | 5.4 | 1.3 | 1.81 | 1.3 |

*Continued*

*Continued*

|  | ELIXA | LEADER | SUSTAIN-6[†] | EXSCEL | HARMONY | REWIND | PIONEER 6[†] | AMPLI-TUDE-O | FREEDOM CVO |
|---|---|---|---|---|---|---|---|---|---|
| Number of events for primary MACE outcome | 805 | 1,302 | 254 | 1,744 | 766 | 1,257 | 137 | 314 | 174 |
| Primary MACE outcome result[§] | HR 1.02 (95% CI 0.89, 1.17); $p = 0.81$ | HR 0.87 (95% CI 0.78, 0.97); $p < 0.01$ | HR 0.74 (95% CI 0.58, 0.95); $p < 0.02$[¶*] | HR 0.91 (95% CI 0.83, 1.00); $p = 0.06$ | HR 0.78 (95% CI 0.68, 0.90); $p = 0.0006$ | HR 0.88 (95% CI 0.79, 0.99); $p = 0.026$ | HR 0.79 (95% CI 0.57, 1.11); $p = 0.17$ | HR 0.73 (95% CI 0.58, 0.92); $p = 0.007$ | HR 1.21 (95% CI 0.90, 1.63); $p = 0.004$[^] |

(ACS: acute coronary syndrome; CI: confidence interval; CKD: chronic kidney disease; CVD: cardiovascular disease; CVOTs: cardiovascular outcome trials; ER: extended-release; GLP₁RA: glucagon-like peptide-1 receptor agonist; HR: hazard ratio; MACE: major adverse cardiovascular events; SC: subcutaneous; T2DM: type 2 diabetes mellitus)

Comparison of trials should be interpreted with caution due to differences in study design, populations and methodology.

\* All trials used placebo as a comparator.

[†] Noninferiority margin for upper bound of 95% CI: <1.8; superiority testing for MACE was prespecified in PIONEER 6 but not in SUSTAIN-6.

[§] *p*-value for superiority (except for FREEDOM CVO); all trials demonstrated noninferiority versus comparator.

[^] Higher CV risk outcomes estimated from meta-analysis of studies for this formulation, in patients aged ≥65 years and a trend for higher CV risk in patients with worse renal function.

[¶] Nominal *p*-value; @Doses pooled for analysis.

**TABLE 4: Pharmacokinetics and pharmacodynamics of available $GLP_1$ agonists.**

| Duration of action | Name | Base | Homology to native $GLP_1$ | Dose/Range | Route |
|---|---|---|---|---|---|
| Short acting | Exenatide | Exendin | 53% | 5–10 µg twice daily | SC |
| Short acting | Lixisenatide | Exendin | 50% | 10–20 µg once daily | SC |
| Long acting | Liraglutide | Human GLP | 97% | 1.2–1.8 mg once daily | SC |
| Long acting | Dulaglutide | Human GLP | 90% | 0.75–1.5 mg once weekly | SC |
| Long acting | Oral semaglutide | Human GLP | 94% | 7–14 mg once daily | Oral |

($GLP_1$: glucagon-like peptide-1; SC: subcutaneous)

It degrades incretins including $GLP_1$ immediately after formation. In normal persons, a small amounts of GLP and GIP which escape degradation by $DPP_4I$ circulate and carry their physiological functions. In diabetes, the circulating levels of these hormones are low and in addition GIP is ineffective. $DPP_4Is$ are orally active agents, which inhibit $DPP_4$ enzyme. This action leads to sustained availability of physiological amounts of incretins including $GLP_1$. If given to diabetic patients, these agents effectively reduce blood glucose level by working through $GLP_1$ axis. **Figure 3** explains the mechanism of action of incretin-based therapies.

*Sitagliptin (Januvia)* is the first agent from this class, to be introduced in clinical practice in our country. It is given in once a day in 100 mg dosage by mouth, just before breakfast. It is a bit less potent than $GLP_1RAs$ because it does not have equally potent actions on gastric motility and satiety center. Unlike $GLP_1RAs$, its use does not lead to significant weight reduction. It is weight neutral. When used alone or in combination with insulin sensitizers, it does not lead to significant hypoglycemia because of its glucose-dependent action (action is triggered only in hyperglycemic state) on β-cells. Availability in oral form and relative cost-effectiveness are its main advantages over $GLP_1RAs$.

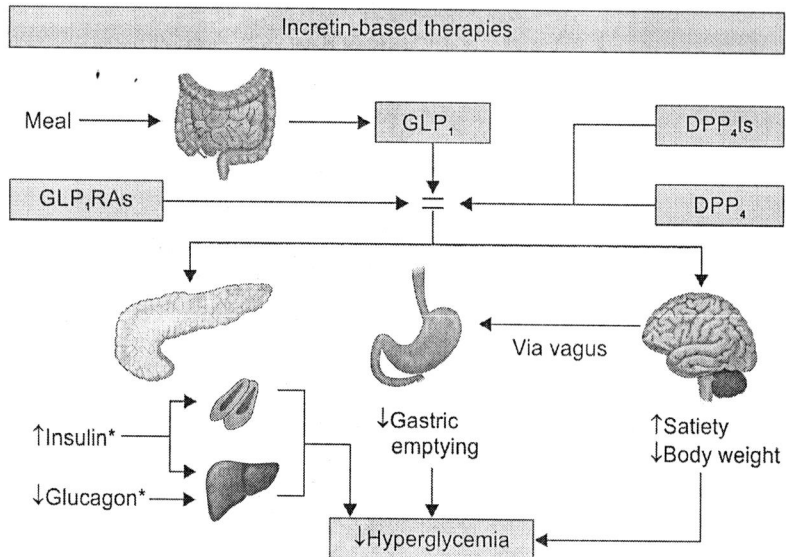

*Glucose-dependent effects.

**FIG. 3:** Mechanism of action of $DPP_4Is$ and $GLP_1RAs$. *(For color version, see Plate 3)*

($DPP_4Is$: dipeptidyl peptidase-4 inhibitors; $GLP_1$ RAs: glucagon-like peptide-1 receptor agonists)

*Source:* Drucker DJ, Nauck MA. The incretin system: glucagon-like peptide-1 receptor agonists and dipeptidyl peptidase-4 inhibitors in type 2 diabetes. Lancet. 2006;368(9548):1696-705; Tahrani AA, Bailey CJ, Del Prato S, Barnett AH. Management of type 2 diabetes: new and future developments in treatment. Lancet. 2011;378(9786):182-97.

Furthermore, its GI tolerance is excellent and it does not require dose titration. With the introduction of several branded generics, the cost of sitagliptin has substantially reduced.

It can be a good alternative to SUs both as monotherapy if metformin is unsuitable and in combination with metformin and/or glitazones. Though a bit less potent than SUs it scores over them in terms of safety (safety from hypoglycemia and weight gain) and cardiovascular safety. In mild renal impairment, the dose need not be changed. In moderate and severe renal impairment, the dose is 50 mg and 25 mg once a day, respectively. Tablets in 50/25 mg strengths are available, but the cost of both is same as 100 mg tablets. Its safety in those with ASCVD and heart failure and also renal impairment has been proved in a dedicated cardiovascular outcome trial (CVOT), named TECOS.

*Vildagliptin (Galvus)* is another agent from this class, which was introduced soon after sitagliptin in India. Its usual dose is 50 mg twice a day and has a profile similar to that of sitagliptin. Recently, slow release once a day preparations containing 100 mg. of vildagliptin have been introduced by many companies. Both sitagliptin and vildagliptin are available in fixed dose combinations with metformin in our country. Vildagliptin is widely available globally except in the USA. Unlike other gliptins of western origin (sitagliptin, saxagliptin, linagliptin, and alogliptin), vildagliptin has not undergone CVOT to prove its safety in those with ASCVD and heart failure. It has been generally accepted that it is safe to use it in those with abovementioned comorbidity. The acceptance is based on reasonable proof of cardiovascular safety obtained during studies to prove glycemic efficacy, which, unlike usual glycemic efficacy studies, included some elderly patients with abovementioned comorbidities (usually glycemic efficacy studies are done in young patients devoid of any comorbidity). In addition, some mechanistic studies to prove cardiovascular safety have also been performed on vildagliptin. Thus, though CVOT data is not available, vildagliptin has more data on safety as compared to teneligliptin and evogliptin, two other gliptins from East Asian origin, which are available in India and which lack significant safety data. Please note that for any antidiabetic agent introduced in the USA after 2009, and to be introduced in future, it is mandatory to prove cardiovascular safety of the agent through successful completion of specifically designed cardiovascular outcome studies. Since vildagliptin is not marketed in the USA, it was not mandatory and Novartis, the company which invented not only vildagliptin, but also the entire concept of $DPP_4Is$ for the first time, has opted out of doing such elaborate time consuming and expensive study.

## *Verify Study [Lancet. 2019;394:1519-29]*

This study, published in Lancet, is a feather in cap for vildagliptin. VERIFY included recently diagnosed T2DM patients and divided them in two groups. One group received metformin monotherapy while the other received 100 mg of vildagliptin plus metformin. At the end of 6 months both the groups received metformin vildagliptin combination and were followed up at 13 weeks interval. Failure to maintain HbA1c at or below 7.0% at two successive follow-ups was considered as treatment failure and insulin was added. On an average patients were followed up for 5 years. It was observed that in spite of both the groups receiving identical treatment from 6 months after initiation of treatment, those with initial combination therapy fared better in statistically significant manner as compared to those who started treatment on metformin monotherapy, as regards ability to maintain HbA1c at or below target for longer duration. The study strongly supports initial or primary combination therapy with two OADs in management of T2DM and since, as on today, vildagliptin-metformin is the only combination with published reports based on long-term comparative blinded study in respected journal such as the Lancet, this combination gets a head start in initial combination therapy. Based on our experience, gut feeling and common sense, we, Indians, have been using initial combination therapy with SU + metformin for decades, now our pragmatic manner of treating T2DM has been authenticated by VERIFY study. When we started using SU/metformin combination, vildagliptin was nonexistent. VERIFY study is one more reason why SUs will be gradually replaced by gliptins and other agents in future. Recently cost of the vildagliptin formulations has significantly come down due to introduction of branded generics.

*Saxagliptin (Onglyza)* is available in India for more than a decade. It is available as a formulation containing 5 mg tablet and is administered once daily. Its indications are same as those of other $DPP_4$ Is. Though it proved cardiovascular safety against ASCVD and renal safety, in dedicated CVOT study, patients on saxagliptin had statistically significant chances of requiring hospitalization for heart failure as compared to those on placebo. Thus, it is contraindicated in those with history of cardiac failure or current cardiac failure.

*Linagliptin (Trajenta)* the 4th in series of gliptins, was launched in India in 2012. It has a long biological half-life as well as ability to maintain raised $GLP_1$ level for about 24 hours. Thus, it is true once a day agent. It is safe in all grades of renal insufficiency and is administered in same full therapeutic dose as in those with normal renal functions, thus frequent monitoring of renal functions is not required for those on linagliptin. Thus, it is more convenient to prescribe in those with renal impairment, though all gliptins are equally safe in renal impairment. Some require dosage adjustments while others do not. Linagliptin is the only antidiabetic medication which has undergone two separate CVOT studies, including CAROLINA, which was done against active comparator, glimepiride. Linagliptin can be prescribed in all grades of hepatic insufficiency. Recently cost of the linagliptin formulations has significantly come down due to introduction of branded generics.

*Alogliptin:* It is 5th in the series of western well tested multinational gliptins to be introduced in India. Being a product of the USA origin, it has undergone CVOT study in which its cardiovascular safety against ASCVD was proved. Patients on alogliptin had slightly higher but statistically nonsignificant chance of requiring hospitalization for heart failure as compared to placebo. Like linagliptin, it has to be administered once a day and no dosage changes are required in renal impairment. Alogliptin was introduced very late in India and by the time several $DPP_4I$ molecules and brands were already established.

*Teneligliptin* is once a day gliptin which does not require dosage adjustments in any degree of renal impairment. Like all the other gliptins, it has moderate glycemic efficacy. It is a product of Korean research and was introduced by a large number of companies almost simultaneously at considerably cheaper rates as compared to multinational gliptins. Though, it does not have a backing of large glycemic efficacy studies and CVOT studies, it appears to be as effective as any gliptin on glycemic front and probably as safe on cardiovascular and renal front. That is the gut feeling of majority of Indian doctors. It has reached record sales figures in India. Some feel that teneligliptin has opened the doors of gliptin therapy for average Indians.

*Evogliptin:* It is the last of the gliptins introduced in India and has a very similar profile like teneligliptin (once a day dosage schedule), no adjustment in renal impairment, lack of extensive safety and efficacy data; and moderate glycemic efficacy as estimated through small studies and gut feeling.

The main advantages of gliptins over SUs are lack of weight gain, and absence of GI side effects and hypoglycemic episodes.

Proof of cardiovascular and renal safety against increased chances of cardiovascular disease with SUs is another point favoring $DPP_4Is$. **Table 5** gives salient features of CVOTs on $DPP_4Is$. In addition, in experimental animals, long-term exposure of these agents has led to some degree of β-cell preservation. Beta cell regeneration, replication as well as reduced apoptosis have been postulated. Sulfonylureas do not have this property. The practical advantage of this property is durability of glycemic effect, which is better as compared to SUs. Furthermore, cost difference between these two groups has significantly come down. Thus, in urban India, these agents are expected to slowly replace SUs. However, in rural India, based on economic necessity and also based on the fact that rural Indian doctors get very few opportunities to upgrade their scientific knowledge, hence changeover from SUs to newer and safer antidiabetic agents would be very slow. Thus, it is a bit early to write obituary of SUs.

## SODIUM-GLUCOSE COTRANSPORTER-2 INHIBITORS

The introduction of $SGLT_2Is$ in a short period after the agents acting on incretin axis and subsequent discovery of their excellent cardio and renoprotective properties has further accelerated the paradigm shift in the management of T2DM from previous glucocentric approach to the dual approach involving end-organ protection along with glycemic control. This approach has brought $SGLT_2Is$ in the center court of pharmacological management of T2DM. Though the kidney is involved in glucose homeostasis through multiple mechanisms, the main mechanism involves glucose filtration, reabsorption and excretion. In normal persons under euglycemic conditions, kidneys filter about 180 g of glucose into the renal tubules, around 99% of filtered glucose is reabsorbed in the circulation. SGLT group of enzymes are responsible for this physiological action. $SGLT_1$ reabsorbs 10% of filtered glucose and $SGLT_2$ reabsorbs remaining 90%. While the former is mainly present in the intestinal mucosa, the latter is exclusively present in the brush borders of renal tubular epithelium. $SGLT_2Is$ are orally acting agents which inhibit $SGLT_2$ and block around 50% of filtered glucose reabsorption into the circulation. The loss of glucose through urine results in blood glucose reduction. These medications essentially lower the renal threshold for glucose

**TABLE 5: DPP$_4$I CVOTs: Design and primary safety/efficacy outcomes.**

| | SAVOR-TIMI 53 | EXAMINE | TECOS | CARMELINA | CAROLINA |
|---|---|---|---|---|---|
| Study intervention | Saxagliptin | Alogliptin | Sitagliptin | Linagliptin | Linagliptin (vs. glimepiride) |
| Number of patients | 16,492 | 5,380 | 14,671 | 6,979 | 6,603 |
| Patient population | Established CV disease or CV risk factors | History of ACS | Established CV disease | Established CV disease and/or prevalent CKD | Established CV disease or CV risk factors |
| Primary outcome (first event of primary composite endpoint) | 3P-MACE | 3P-MACE | 4P-MACE | 3P-MACE | 3P-MACE |
| Median follow-up (years) | 2.1 | 1.5 | 3.0 | 2.2 | 6.3 |
| Number of events for primary MACE outcome | 1,222 | 621 | 1,390 | 854 | 718 |
| Primary MACE outcome result$^§$ | HR 1.00 (95% CI 0.89, 1.12) $p = 0.99$ | HR 0.96 (upper CI 1.16)$^@$ $p = 0.32$ | HR 0.98 (95% CI 0.89, 1.08) $p = 0.65$ | HR 1.02 (95% CI 0.89, 1.17) $p = 0.74$ | HR 0.98 (95.47% CI 0.84, 1.14)* $p = 0.76$ |

(ACS: acute coronary syndrome; CI: confidence interval; CKD: chronic kidney disease; CV: cardiovascular; CVOTs: cardiovascular outcome trials; DPP$_4$I: dipeptidyl peptidase-4 inhibitor; HR: hazard ratio; MACE: major adverse cardiovascular events)

Comparison of trials should be interpreted with caution due to differences in study design, populations and methodology.

*95.47% bound for CI reflects an O'Brien–Fleming alpha-spending adjustment for the two interim analyses of the primary outcome, in addition to Bonferroni adjustment for change from 4P-MACE to 3P-MACE.
$^§$ $p$-value for superiority; all trials demonstrated noninferiority versus comparator.
$^@$ Upper boundary of one-sided repeated CI.

excretion. The loss of energy in the form of glucose results in weight loss. Use of $SGLT_2I$ is also associated with significant reduction of systolic and some reduction of diastolic blood pressure. The other metabolic effects include reduction in serum uric acid levels and a small reduction in serum potassium levels without causing hypokalemia.

Four agents namely (1) canagliflozin, (2) dapagliflozin, (3) empagliflozin, and (4) remogliflozin are available in India, all have similar glycemic efficacy, they reduce HbA1c by 0.7-1.0% on an average. Out of these 4 agents, first three have been extensively studied in phase 3 trials for glycemic efficacy, CVOT for cardiovascular protective properties, renal outcome studies for renoprotective properties, and various studies on heart failure with reduced as well as preserved ejection fraction.

Now let us have brief discussion of these agents.

## Canagliflozin (Invokana)

It is available in 100 mg as well as 300 mg strength tablets and the dosage is one tablet of either strength daily. The higher strength is recommended in obese patients seeking significant weight reduction, while 100 mg. Strength is more commonly used in routine practice. It is claimed that 300 mg of canagliflozin matches the glycemic as well as weight reducing efficacy of $GLP_1RAs$ at significantly lesser cost and with oral route of administration, which is preferred by the patients. It is claimed that it has slightly higher glycemic efficacy than other agents from this class and this is attributed to additional $SGLT_1$ blocking action in the intestinal wall and in renal tubules. Other $SGLT_2Is$ are pure $SGLT_2Is$ without having any $SGLT_1$ inhibitory action. CVOT done on canagliflozin proved its cardioprotective action, while renal outcome study proved its renoprotective properties. It has not undergone dedicated heart failure study.

## Dapagliflozin (Forxiga)

It is available in 5 and 10 mg strength and the later strength is usually used in a day-to-day practice as it has better glycemic efficacy. It is administered once a day. Besides its glycemic properties, CVOT trial has proved its safety on cardiovascular system.

Unlike canagliflozin and empagliflozin, it could not prove its cardioprotective effect, probably because two-thirds of the patients included in the study had only risk factors for cardiovascular disease but had not suffered from any cardiovascular episodes in past while CVOT studies on other two agents had more patients with cardiovascular disease (100% in case of empagliflozin). The renal outcome study on dapagliflozin clearly established its renoprotective properties both in diabetic as well as nondiabetic patients while studies on heart failure in patients with reduced as well as preserved ejection fraction in diabetic as well as nondiabetic patients proved its efficacy.

## Empagliflozin (Jardiance)

It is available in 10 and 25 mg. Strength and glycemic efficacy of lower strength is only marginally lower. It is administered once a day. CVOT proved cardioprotective properties; studies on diabetic as well as nondiabetic patients with heart failure were successful. Empagliflozin has recently completed dedicated renoprotective study, wherein its renoprotective properties ere conclusively proved. A notable feature of EMPA-REG, a CVOT study done on empagliflozin was far higher (38%), relative risk reduction for cardiovascular death as compared to CVOT studies done across all antidiabetic drug classes.

### Remogliflozin (Remo)

It is available in 100 mg tablet strength and its dosage is 100 mg twice a day. It has not undergone any cardiovascular and reno protective studies and is not available in advanced western countries. After the introduction of generic versions of well studied $SGLT_2Is$ in India relative cost advantage of remogliflozin has been nullified.

*Advantages of $SGLT_2Is$*: Good glycemic efficacy combined with cardio- and renoprotective properties and protection from heart failure; which is very common in diabetic patients, ability to reduce systolic BP; which is also very common in diabetics; and weight reducing properties catapulted $SGLT_2Is$ in the forefront of diabetes management. **Table 6** shows salient features of CVOTs on $SGLT_2Is$.

TABLE 6: SGLT$_2$I CVOTs: Design and primary safety/efficacy outcomes.

| | EMPA-REG OUTCOME | CANVAS program* | DECLARE-TIMI 58 | VERTIS CV | CREDENCE (Cardio-renal Outcome Trial) |
|---|---|---|---|---|---|
| Study intervention | Empagliflozin | Canagliflozin | Dapagliflozin | Ertugliflozin | Canagliflozin |
| Number of patients | 7,020 | 10,142‡ | 17,160 | 8,246 | 4,401 |
| Patient population | T2DM + ASCVD | T2DM + ASCVD or ≥2 CV risk factors | T2DM + established ASCVD or multiple risk factors | T2DM + established ASCVD | T2DM + Stage 2 or 3 CKD + macroalbuminuria |
| Primary outcome (first event of primary composite endpoint) | 3P-MACE | 3P-MACE | 3P-MACE, CV death + HHF§^ | 3P-MACE | ESKD + doubling of SCr + death from kidney disease + CV death |
| Median follow-up (years) | 3.1 | 2.4¶ | 4.2 | 3.0 | 2.6 |
| Number of events for primary MACE outcome | 772 | 1,011 | 1,559 | 1,103 | 486# |
| Primary MACE outcome result§ | HR 0.86 (95% CI 0.74, 0.99) p = 0.04 | HR 0.86 (95% CI 0.75, 0.97) p = 0.02 | HR 0.93 (95% CI 0.84, 1.03) p = 0.17 | HR 0.97 (95% CI 0.85, 1.11)@ p = Not available | HR 0.80# (95% CI 0.67, 0.95) p = 0.01 |

(ASCVD: atherosclerotic cardiovascular disease; CI: confidence interval; CKD: chronic kidney disease; CV: cardiovascular; CVOTs: cardiovascular outcome trials; ESKD: end-stage kidney disease; HHF: hospitalization for heart failure; HR: hazard ratio; MACE: major adverse cardiovascular events; SGLT$_2$I: sodium-glucose transport protein 2 inhibitor; T2DM: type 2 diabetes mellitus)

Comparison of trials should be interpreted with caution due to differences in study design, populations, and methodology.

*Data in CANVAS Program based on pooled data from CANVAS and CANVAS-R.
‡4330 patients in CANVAS and 5812 patients in CANVAS-R.
¶5.7 years in CANVAS and 2.1 years in CANVAS-R.
^Primary safety outcome of 3P-MACE and coprimary efficacy outcomes of 3P-MACE and CV death + HHF.
§p-value for superiority; all trials demonstrated noninferiority vs. comparator.
@95.6% CI.
#MACE was not the primary outcome in CREDENCE; the data is shown for first event of 3P-MACE in CREDENCE.

*Precautions*: SGLT$_2$Is should be used with care in elderly patients, those on diuretics and volume contracted patients. Volume depletion should be corrected before starting these agents to prevent postural hypotension and resultant falls and fractures. Occasionally, acute kidney injury can occur when these agents are prescribed in patients having abovementioned conditions and in those on nonsteroidal anti-inflammatory drugs (NSAIDs) and diuretics. In acutely ill and in those with vomiting or irregular oral intake, these agents should not be used. When used along with insulin, one should not reduce the dose of insulin rapidly and in postoperative state after major surgery, one should not hastily withdraw insulin. In these situations, rapid withdrawal of insulin can lead to ketoacidosis. This is a rare complication of SGLT$_2$I therapy but likely to be diagnosed late because of unawareness about the condition at first-line clinician's level and also because peculiarity of having blood glucose in near normal range in spite of ketoacidosis leading to noninclusion of ketoacidosis in the list of differential diagnosis. Prevalence of urinary tract infections and fungal genital infections is more common, the later particularly in women. Improvement in personal hygiene can reduce the prevalence. An encouraging news is that coprescription of DPP$_4$Is with SGLT$_2$Is reduces the prevalence of fungal genital infection. In clinical practice, these two agents are commonly coprescribed. As regards urinary tract infections, in most cases, patients develop lower urinary tract infections which are amenable to treatment with oral antimicrobial agents. Generally, these agents are not recommended in those with eGFR <45–30 mL/min/1.73 m$^2$, as glycemic efficacy goes down with the reduction of eGFR. However, the exact level of eGFR beyond which these agents are proscribed keeps on varying from country-to-country, even for same agent from the same manufacturer. The trend is towards reducing eGFR level. Based on findings of DAPA CKD trial, it is prescribed by nephrologists as a pure renoprotective agent in diabetic as well as nondiabetics even in those with eGFR of 25 mL/min/1.73 m$^2$, while canagliflozin, based on CREDENCE trial is being prescribed as nephroprotective agent in diabetic nephropathy up to eGFR of 30 mL/min/1.73 m$^2$. Some loss of glycemic efficacy should be accepted in such situations and should be managed through other antidiabetic agents. All SGLT$_2$Is are contraindicated in pregnancy and lactation.

*Specific precautions for those on canagliflozin:* Fractures of lower limbs are a bit more common with this agent as compared to other $SGLT_2Is$. Higher number of lower limb amputations, mostly small part amputations such as toe amputations were reported in early studies on canagliflozin but CREDENCE trial did not report this adverse findings. Exact cause is not known and could be due to difference in recording and reporting of the event. Hyperkalemia is occasionally reported in those on canagliflozin, while generally slightly lower levels of potassium are reported with $SGLT_2Is$.

## Quick-release Bromocriptine Tablets

Conventional bromocriptine has been in clinical practice for more than two decades for the management of Parkinsonism and galactorrhea. Quick-release preparation of bromocriptine has been introduced in India in mid-2010 and in the USA in November, 2010. It is indicated in the management of T2DM.

In T2DM, dopaminergic tone in hypothalamic area is reduced. This is associated with increased secretion of noradrenaline in hypothalamic-hypophysial axis, which in turn leads to insulin resistance, obesity, and hyperglycemia. Bromocriptine is dopamine agonist. Administration of quick-release version leads to rapid build-up of its blood levels and resetting of dopaminergic tone. This is associated with reduction in insulin resistance and improvement in glycemic status, particularly postprandial hyperglycemia.

Quick-release bromocriptine has better bioavailability than its conventional version. It is available in tablet form; each tablet contains 0.8 mg of bromocriptine in special quick-release formulation. The therapeutic dosage is 1.6–4.8 mg once daily 2 hours after getting up in morning, preferably after food. In order to avoid GI side effects, treatment should be started with 0.8 mg and dosage should be stepped up at weakly interval.

Quick-release bromocriptine is the first antidiabetic medication, which has successfully undergone elaborate premarketing cardiovascular safety studies in the USA. After the publication of report of excess cardiovascular mortality with rosiglitazone in the New England Journal of Medicine in June 2007, the US FDA has made these tests mandatory for any new antidiabetic agent before its introduction in the market.

Quick-release bromocriptine can be used as one of the add-on agents, particularly in those with manifestations of insulin resistance.

## Glimins

These agents belong to a new class of antidiabetics which have dual action. They act on β-cells in pancreas and increase insulin secretion and release through glucose-dependent mechanism using a pathway which is different from the one used by SUs and glinides. Glimins improve mitochondrial function thereby reducing the rate of apoptosis of β-cells and improving cellular energy metabolism. Peripherally, glimins enhance insulin action in liver and muscles.

Mechanisms of action of glimins are complementary to other antidiabetic agents with which they can be combined.

Unlike SUs and glinides, glimins are not liable to produce hypoglycemia, and unlike metformin, they are not associated with lactic acidosis.

*Imeglimin*, the first in class agent from glimin family, was introduced in India toward the end of 2022. It is available as 500 and 1,000 mg tablets and the usual dosage is 500–1,000 mg twice a day. It has good gastrointestinal tolerability and is not contraindicated in renal impairment. Unlike $SGLT_2Is$ and $GLP_1RAs$, it does not have a special niche for use as preferred agent. Prevalence of GI intolerance including diarrhea is significantly lower than that of metformin, thus imeglimin can be used in place of metformin in case of metformin intolerance.

## Clinical Applications of OADs

Oral antidiabetic drugs are indicated in T2DM patients when diet fails to control hyperglycemia. Stressful conditions such as severe infections, pregnancy, major surgery, and severe renal and hepatic insufficiency are contraindications to the use of OADs. There are exceptions, as regards use in renal insufficiency. Refer to Chapter 17 for use of OAD in renal insufficiency. Linagliptin is an exception as regards contraindication in hepatic impairment. OADs with exception of $SGLT_2Is$ and AGIs do not work in the absence of insulin, hence should not be used alone in T1DM. OADs should be avoided in pregnancy. **Table 7** shows comparative pharmacological features and **Figure 4** shows comparative glycemic efficacies. Also refer **Flowchart 1** for selecting appropriate pharmacological agent depending upon individual needs.

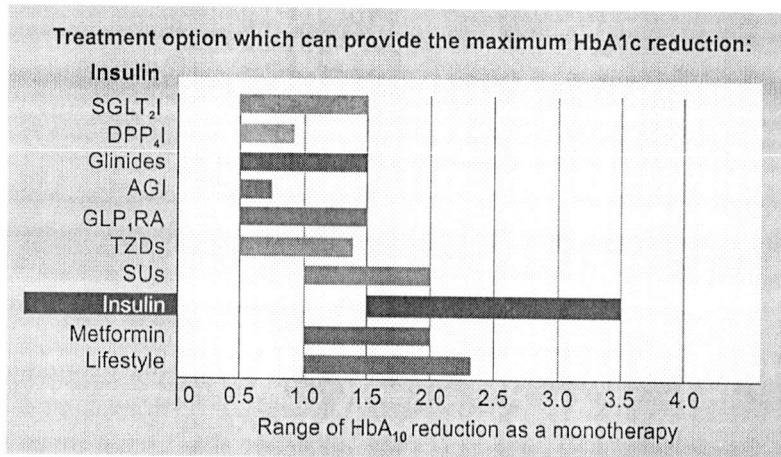

**FIG. 4:** Comparative glycemic efficacies of antidiabetic agents. *(For color version, see Plate 3)*

**TABLE 7:** Comparative pharmacological features of antidiabetic agents used in T2DM.

|  | Metformin | SU | TZD | SGLT$_2$I | GLP$_1$RA | Insulin |
|---|---|---|---|---|---|---|
| Efficacy | High | High | High | Intermediate | High | Highest |
| Risk of hypoglycemia | Low | Moderate | Low | Low | Low | High |
| Weight | Loss | Gain | Gain | Loss | Loss | Gain |
| Side-effects | GI | Hypo | Edema, HF, fractures | Genital infections | GI | Hypo |

(GI: gastrointestinal; GLP$_1$RA: glucagon-like peptide-1 receptor agonist; HF: heart failure; SGLT$_2$I: Sodium-glucose cotransporter-2 inhibitor; SU: sulfonylurea; TZD: thiazolidinedione)

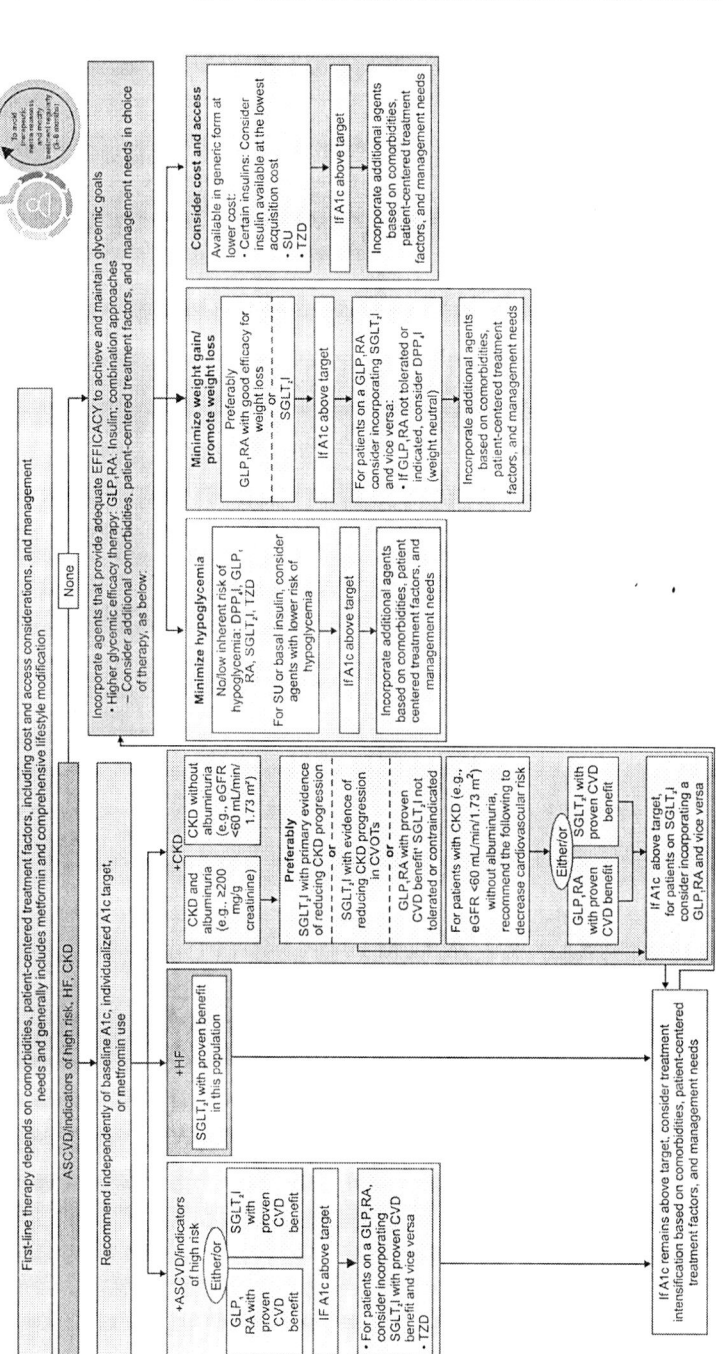

**FLOWCHART 1:** Pharmacologic treatment of hyperglycemia in adults with type 2 diabetes mellitus.

*Source:* American Diabetes Association. Standards of Medical Care in Diabetes-2022 Abridged for Primary Care Providers. Clin Diabetes. 2022;40(1):10-38.

## CRITERIA FOR CONTROL

One should aim at steady near normal blood glucose. **Table 8** gives conventional glycemic criteria for control and **Figure 5** gives time in range (TIR) targets calculated from CGM data, depending upon presence of comorbidities and special situations. General HbA1c goal should be <7%. After achieving this goal, one should carefully and gradually try to reach lower goal such as near 6.0% in pregnant women and 6–6.5% in young without any comorbidities. In middle aged, one should try to be nearer to 6.5%. While on the road to lower HbA1c levels, if there are hypoglycemic episodes particularly when there were no blunders committed by the patients, one should settle for slightly higher level. In elderly patients, particularly in those with cardiovascular disease, renal impairment, impaired cognitive function, in those with lack of manpower help at home for emergency handling, one should target 7.5% and in those bedridden or with limited life expectancy, one should plan to keep it around 8.0% or at level to block osmotic symptoms.

Of late continuous glucose monitoring (CGM) is easily available and should be used in type 1 diabetics, those with T2DM on insulin, particularly on large dosages, those difficult to control including brittle diabetics, where severe hypoglycemia needs to be avoided at all costs, pregnancy, those reluctant to increase dosage of antidiabetics due to fear of hypoglycemia, etc. The data generated should be analyzed, particularly metrics such as TIR. The desired values are as follows: (TIR 70–180 mg%, around 70% or 16 hours 40 minutes out of 24 hours), time below range (TBR, <5% or <30 minutes out of 24 hours), and time above range (TAR, 25% or <6 hours). CGM throws light on current glycemic control **(Fig. 5)** and is more useful to get clues for adjustment of antidiabetic

**TABLE 8:** Criteria for metabolic control.

| Time | Good | Fair | Poor |
|---|---|---|---|
| Fasting* | <110 mg% | 110–130 mg% | >130 mg% |
| Two hours postmeal* | <140 mg% | 140–180 mg% | >180 mg% |
| Glycated hemoglobin (HbA1c) | 6.5–7% | 7–7.5% | >7.5% |

*Venous plasma true glucose values.

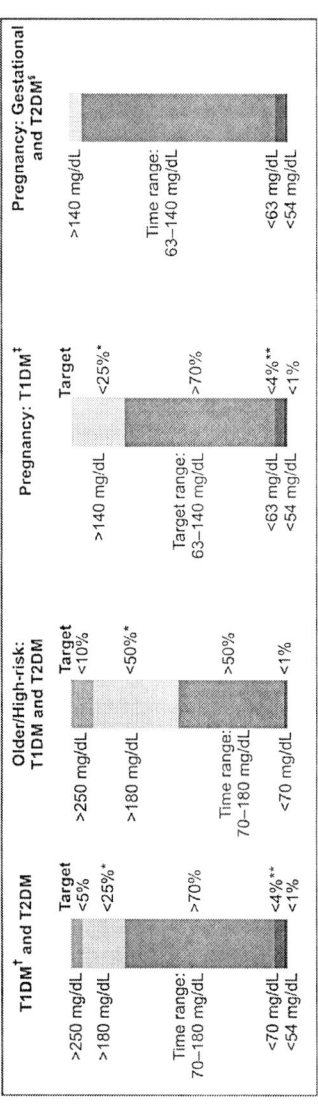

**FIG. 5:** CGM-based targets for different diabetes populations. *(For color version, see Plate 4)*

(CGM: continuous glucose monitoring; TIR: time-in-range; T1DM: type 1 diabetes mellitus; T2DM: type 2 diabetes mellitus)

*Source:* Battelino T, Danne T, Bergenstal R, et al. Clinical Targets for Continous glucose monitoring data interpretation: Recommendations from the international consensus on time in range. Diabetes Care. 2019;42(8):593-1603.

□ For age <25 year, if the A1c goal is 7.5, then set TIR target to approximately 60%.
† Percentages of time-in-ranges are based on limited evidence. More research is needed.
§ Percentages of time-in-ranges have not been included because there is very limited evidence in this area. More research is needed.
*Includes percentage of values >250 mg/dL (13.9).
**Includes percentage of values <54 mg/dL (3.0).

medication dosages and fine tune therapy, while HbA1c give historical data of past 3 months. In other words, HbA1c is helpful to analyze past performances while CGM derived data including TIR is helpful to plan future therapy.

## FAILURE OF CONTROL

A common cause of failure is inadequate lifestyle adjustments. Some diabetics are under the wrong impression that since they are taking OAD, they are at liberty to eat anything and they need not make any effort to burn the extra calories. In addition to review of lifestyle in patients failing to respond to OAD, a systematic search for occult infection (e.g., tuberculosis, urinary tract infection, etc.) should be made. It is also advisable to thoroughly analyze all the medicines he/she is taking. In addition to medicines prescribed by you, he/she may be taking, say for example, steroids for asthma (some powders dispensed by quacks for "asthma" and "jaundice" contain steroids), strong potassium wasting diuretics like furosemide; and diphenylhydantoin can also interfere with the action of OAD. If a failure occurs even after proper lifestyle regulations and maximal dose of one OAD, drugs from other groups (i.e., $DPP_4I$ or $SGLT_2I$ or SU in those taking metformin and vice versa) should be added and the dosage gradually increased in case of SU. In those not responding to two agents, if the pressing demands for insulin therapy are not present (severe osmotic symptoms, weight loss, presence of major infection, very unstable cardiovascular or renal status), one can try third agent with complementary action, always keeping in mind that with every additional oral medication or up-titrating the dosages of traditional medications such as metformin, SU, pioglitazone, the glycemic yield will be lesser and lesser. In order to reach glycemic targets quickly, start with two-drug therapy if baseline HbA1c is > 7.5% or if you prefer a less aggressive approach, start with two-drug therapy if the gap between current and target HbA1c is 1.5% or more. If one starts with monotherpay, which would be metformin in most cases, the up-titration if required, should be completed by 12 weeks and then if required, second agent should be added. By the end of 24 weeks, third OAD, or insulin should be on board if required. The reason for progressive need for additional agents is not the drug failure but progressive failure of β-cells and

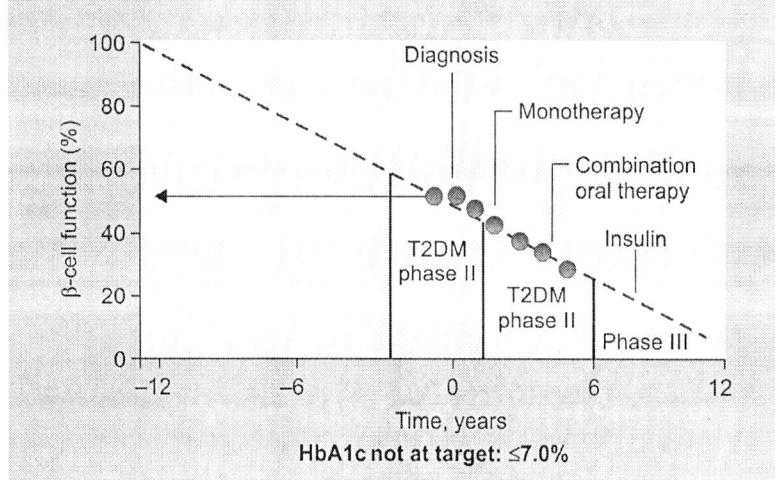

**FIG. 6:** Progressive β-cell failure. *(For color version, see Plate 5)*
(HbA1c: glycated hemoglobin; T2DM: type 2 diabetes mellitus)
*Source:* Based on data from U.K. prospective diabetes study 16. Overview of 6 years' therapy of type 2 diabetes: a progressive disease. U.K. Prospective Diabetes Study Group. Diabetes. 1995;44(11):1249-58; Kendall DM, Cuddihy RM, Bergenstal RM. Clinical application of incretin-based therapy: therapeutic potential, patient selection and clinical use. Am J Med. 2009;122 (6 Suppl): S37-50; Kendall DM, Bergenstal RM. Comprehensive management of patients with type 2 diabetes: establishing priorities of care. Am J Manag Care. 2001;7(10 Suppl):S327-43; quiz S344-8.

thus progressively lesser insulin secretion in response to treatment **(Fig. 6)**. The only agents which are effective in absence of insulin are $SGLT_2Is$ and AGIs and on an average their capacity to reduce HbA1c is 0.8–1% and 0.5%, respectively. Agents such as metformin and pioglitazone having extra pancreatic action also require presence of insulin to reduce blood glucose; they do not secrete extra insulin but act by increasing sensitivity of tissues to insulin. Thus, in absence of insulin, they are ineffective.

## DRUG INTERACTIONS

These occur mainly with SUs. Alcohol intolerance occurs in a number of patients particularly those on chlorpropamide. Many drugs potentiate hypoglycemic effects of SUs. These include clofibrate, dicumarol, large doses of salicylates, β-blockers, NSAIDs, and biguanides. In those taking biguanides, the risk of lactic acidosis increases if they consume alcohol **(Table 9)**.

**TABLE 9: Synopsis of actions of antidiabetic agents.**

| | Insulin | SU and glinides | Metformin | Alpha-glucosidase inhibitors | Glitazones | DPP$_4$ Is | Incretin mimetics |
|---|---|---|---|---|---|---|---|
| Fasting glucose | ↓↓ | ↓ | ↓ | - or ↓ | ↓ | ↓ | ↓ |
| Postprandial glucose | ↓↓ | ↓ | ↓ | ↓ | ↓ | ↓↓ | ↓↓ |
| Insulin concentration | ↑↑↑ | ↑ | - or ↓ | - or ↓ | ↑ | ↑ | ↑ |
| Body weight | ↑ | ↑ | - or ↓ | - | ↑ | - | ↓↓ |
| Free fatty acid | ↓ | - or ↓ | - or ↓ | - | ↓ | - | ↑ |
| Triglycerides | - | - | - or ↓ | - | - or ↓ | - | - |
| Total cholesterol | - | - | - or ↓ | - | - or ↑ | - | - |
| Safety | Hypoglycemia | Hypoglycemia | Lactic acidosis | - | ? | - | - |
| Tolerability | Inject | - | GI disturb | GI disturb | - | - | GI disturb |
| Exclude/caution | - | Liver/kidney impairment | Liver kidney impairment, hypoxia | Inflammatory bowel disease | Liver impairment | - | |
| Monitor | - | Creatinine | Creatinine | LFT | LFT cardiac function | - | - |

(DPP$_4$Is: dipeptidyl peptidase-4 inhibitors; GI: gastrointestinal; LFT: liver function test; SU: sulfonylurea)

## ACKNOWLEDGMENTS

The preparation of content (tables) on summary of cardiovascular outcome trials, included in this chapter, has been facilitated by Dr Jignesh Ved. He is an employee of Boehringer Ingelheim. India; his contribution to this chapter has been in his individual scientific capacity, and does not represent or endorse the views of Boehringer Ingelheim.

## SUGGESTED READINGS

### DPP$_4$I CVOTs

1. Scirica BM, Bhatt DL, Braunwald E, Steg PG, Davidson JM, Hirshberg B, et al. Saxagliptin and cardiovascular outcomes in patients with type 2 diabetes mellitus. N Engl J Med. 2013;369(14):1317-26.
2. White WB, Cannon CP, Heller SR, Nissen SE, Bergenstal RM, Bakris GL, et al. Alogliptin after acute coronary syndrome in patients with type 2 diabetes. N Engl J Med. 2013;369(14):1327-35.
3. Green JB, Bethel MA, Armstrong PW, Buse JB, Egnel SE, Garg J, et al. Effect of Sitagliptin on Cardiovascular Outcomes in Type 2 Diabetes. N Engl J Med. 2015;373(3):232-42.
4. Rosenstock J, Perkovic V, Johansen OE, Cooper ME, Kahn SE, Marx N, et al. Effect of Linagliptin vs Placebo on Major Cardiovascular Events in Adults with Type 2 Diabetes and High Cardiovascular and Renal Risk: The CARMELINA Randomized Clinical Trial. JAMA. 2019;321(1):69-79.
5. Rosenstock J, Kahn SE, Johansen OE, Zinman B, Espeland MA, Woerle HJ, et al. Effect of Linagliptin vs Glimepiride on Major Adverse Cardiovascular Outcomes in Patients with Type 2 Diabetes: The CAROLINA Randomized Clinical Trial. JAMA. 2019;322(12):1155-66.

### SGLT$_2$I CVOTs

6. Zinman B, Wanner C, Lachin JM, Fitchett D, Bluhmki E, Hantel S, et al. Empagliflozin, Cardiovascular Outcomes, and Mortality in Type 2 Diabetes. N Engl J Med. 2015;373(22):2117-28.
7. Wanner C, Inzucchi SE, Lachin JM, Fitchett D, von Eynatten M, Mattheus M, et al. Empagliflozin and Progression of Kidney Disease in Type 2 Diabetes. N Engl J Med. 2016;375(4):323-34.
8. Neal B, Perkovic V, Mahaffey KW, de Zeeuw D, Fulcher G, Erondu N, et al. Canagliflozin and Cardiovascular and Renal Events in Type 2 Diabetes. N Engl J Med. 2017;377(7):644-57.
9. Radholm K, Figtree G, Perkovic V, Solomon SD, Mahaffey KW, de Zeeuw D, et al. Canagliflozin and Heart Failure in Type 2 Diabetes Mellitus: Results from the CANVAS Program. Circulation. 2018;138(5):458-68.

10. Mahaffey KW, Neal B, Perkovic V, de Zeeuw D, Fulcher G, Erondu N, et al. Canagliflozin for Primary and Secondary Prevention of Cardiovascular Events: Results from the CANVAS Program (Canagliflozin Cardiovascular Assessment Study). Circulation. 2018;137(4):323-34.
11. Wiviott S, Raz I, Bonaca MP, Mosenzon O, kato ET, Cahn A, et al. Dapagliflozin and Cardiovascular Outcomes in Type 2 Diabetes. N Engl J Med. 2019;380(4):347-57.
12. Cannon CP, Pratley R, Dagogo-Jack S, Mancuso J, Huyck S, Masiukiewicz U, et al. Cardiovascular Outcomes with Ertugliflozin in Type 2 Diabetes. N Engl J Med. 2020;383(15):1425-35.
13. Cosentino F, Cannon CP, Cherney DZI, Masiukiewicz U, Pratley R, Dagogo-Jack S, et al. Efficacy of Ertugliflozin on Heart Failure-related Events in Patients with Type 2 Diabetes Mellitus and Established Atherosclerotic Cardiovascular Disease: Results of the VERTIS CV Trial. Circulation. 2020;142(23):2205-15.
14. Cherney DZI, Charbonnel B, Cosentino F, Dagogo-Jack S, McGuire DK, Pratley R, et al. Effects of ertugliflozin on kidney composite outcomes, renal function and albuminuria in patients with type 2 diabetes mellitus: an analysis from the randomised VERTIS CV trial. Diabetologia. 2021;64(6):1256-67.
15. Perkovic V, Jardine MJ, Neal B, Bompoint S, Heerspink HJL, Charytan DM, et al. Canagliflozin and Renal Outcomes in Type 2 Diabetes and Nephropathy. N Engl J Med. 2019;380(24):2295-306.

**GLP$_1$RA CVOTs**

16. Pfeffer MA, Claggett B, Diaz R, Dickstein K, Gerstein HC, Kober LV, et al. Lixisenatide in Patients with Type 2 Diabetes and Acute Coronary Syndrome. N Engl J Med. 2015;373(23):2247-57.
17. Marso SP, Daniels GH, Brown-Frandsen K, Kristensen P, Mann JFE, Nauck MA, et al. Liraglutide and Cardiovascular Outcomes in Type 2 Diabetes. N Engl J Med. 2016;375(4):311-22.
18. Marso SP, Bain SC, Consoli A, Eliaschewitz FG, Jodar E, Leiter LA, et al. Semaglutide and Cardiovascular Outcomes in Patients with Type 2 Diabetes. N Engl J Med. 2016;375(19):1834-44.
19. Holman RR, Bethel MA, Mentz RJ, Thompson VP, Lokhnygina Y, Buse JB, et al. Effects of Once-weekly Exenatide on Cardiovascular Outcomes in Type 2 Diabetes. N Engl J Med. 2017;377(13):1228-39.
20. Hernandez AF, Green JB, Janmohamed S, D'Agostino Sr RB, Granger CB, Jones NP, et al. Albiglutide and cardiovascular outcomes in patients with type 2 diabetes and cardiovascular disease (Harmony Outcomes): a double-blind, randomised placebo-controlled trial. Lancet. 2018;392(10157):1519-29.
21. Gerstein HC, Colhoun HM, Dagenais GR, Diaz R, Lakshmanan M, Pais P, et al. Dulaglutide and cardiovascular outcomes in type 2 diabetes (REWIND): a double-blind, randomised placebo-controlled trial. Lancet. 2019;394(10193):121-30.

22. Husain M, Birkenfeld AL, Donsmark M, Dungan K, Eliaschewitz FG, Franco DR, et al. Oral Semaglutide and Cardiovascular Outcomes in Patients with Type 2 Diabetes. N Engl J Med. 2019;381(9):841-51.
23. Gerstein HC, Sattar N, Rosenstock J, Ramasundarahettige C, Pratley R, Lopes RD, et al. Cardiovascular and Renal Outcomes with Efpeglenatide in Type 2 Diabetes. N Engl J Med. 2021;385(10):896-907.
24. Ruff CT, Baron M, Im K, O'Donoghue ML, Fiedorek FT, Sabatine MS. Subcutaneous infusion of exenatide and cardiovascular outcomes in type 2 diabetes: a non-inferiority randomized controlled trial. Nat Med. 2022;28(1):89-95.

# CHAPTER 14

# Role of Insulin in Management of Diabetes

## INTRODUCTION

Diabetes is a lifelong disease with high mortality and morbidity, mainly through macrovascular and microvascular complications. The only way to prevent, postpone, or slow down the rate of progression of microvascular complications is to achieve persistent tight control of blood glucose levels. Major clinical trials [Diabetes Control and Complications Trial (DCCT) in type 1 diabetes mellitus (T1DM) and United Kingdom Prospective Diabetes Study (UKPDS) in type 2 diabetes mellitus (T2DM)] have proved the importance of appropriately aggressive treatment. In T1DM, intensive therapy can reduce the incidence of microvascular complications by up to 60% while reduction is less impressive in T2DM only because in some patients, by the time diagnosis of diabetes is established, complications have already set in. In our pursuit to achieve the glycemic and other targets, we must aggressively manage diabetes by judiciously utilizing all the modalities of management namely, diet, exercise and medications including insulin in coordinated manner. Insulin is a must in all type 1 diabetic patients and at any point in a busy diabetic clinic; about 33% of type 2 diabetic patients would require insulin if they are to achieve the goal of tight blood glucose control. Aggressive management and tight blood glucose control are also associated with higher prevalence of hypoglycemic episodes. Thus, insulin and other antidiabetic agents should be used judiciously.

Till 80s, we had only bovine insulin and practically only one brand of insulin. Moreover, it was available in only one strength, 40 units/mL. New developments have taken place in the field of insulin therapy over last four decades at a rapid rate. Bovine insulin and subsequently introduced porcine insulin has virtually become extinct and totally replaced by human insulin. Human insulin is manufactured by the genetic engineering technology, which has virtually eliminated raw material shortages. We also have ready-made insulin mixtures in different proportions. We now have a choice of two different strengths of insulin and also have a choice regarding insulin administration devices due to availability of patient-friendly insulin pens. We also have several designer insulin analogs such as lispro insulin, insulin aspart, glargine, detemir, degludec and glargine 300. Thus, besides deciding when to use insulin and in what dosage schedules, a practitioner now has to take several decisions such as which strength? Which device? When to use rapid-acting and long-acting insulin analog? How to achieve good metabolic control without significantly increasing hypoglycemic episodes? Thus, he needs to update his knowledge.

## INSULIN PHYSIOLOGY AND PATHOPHYSIOLOGY IN DIABETES

Insulin is secreted by β-cells of the islets of Langerhans in pancreas. Islets are scattered throughout the pancreas. Typically, each islet contains about 1,000 cells, 80% of which are β-cells. Insulin is secreted by the β-cells in response to changes in glucose concentrations. Insulin is released directly in portal vein from where 50% of it is extracted for local action during first pass through the liver. Insulin is an important anabolic hormone with profound control over carbohydrate, protein as well as fat metabolism. In T1DM, β-cells are completely destroyed thus there is hardly any endogenous insulin secretion. These patients are dependent on externally administered insulin for their survival. In such patients, discontinuation of insulin will lead to severe metabolic disturbances, terminating into diabetic ketoacidosis and coma, and ultimately death. In T2DM, there is β-cell dysfunction leading to insufficient first phase insulin secretion and gradually diminishing overall insulin secretion. In addition to the insulin secretory β-cell defects, about 85% of type 2 diabetic patients also have varying degrees of insulin resistance. In these patients, peripheral tissue response to available insulin is less than normal. In addition, there is an α-cell defect due to which there is inappropriately high secretion of glucagon (in normal persons glucagon secretion is controlled by blood glucose level: it is increased during hypoglycemia and suppressed during hyperglycemia). Most of the type 2 diabetic patients have varying degrees of these defects; however, till they reach 'end-stage β-cell failure', they retain capacity to produce varying amounts of endogenous insulin which, even though not sufficient to control blood glucose, is sufficient to prevent diabetic ketoacidosis. Type 2 diabetic patients are not dependent on insulin for survival, thus they were classified as noninsulin-dependent diabetics in past. However, over the years, the capacity of their β-cells gradually diminishes and a time comes when they cannot be controlled on oral pills, even if all the major classes are combined together. At this stage, they require insulin for achieving blood glucose control.

## INSULIN PHARMACOLOGY

On the basis of onset of action and duration of action, the insulin preparations available in the market are divided in following categories:

### Short-acting Insulin

Short-acting insulin is also called regular, clear, or crystalline insulin and was previously available in bovine, porcine as well as human forms in our country; however, human insulin has virtually replaced both the varieties of animal insulin. It is used for control of postprandial rise in blood glucose level. Regular human insulin has onset of action in 30–60 minutes, peak action between 2 and 3 hours, and duration of effective action for 3–6 hours. However, there are many variations from patient to patient. Short-acting insulin is usually used in combination with intermediate- or long-acting insulin. In many type 1 diabetic patients and other diabetics after having reached the stage of β-cell failure, short-acting insulin is required before each meal to control postprandial hyperglycemia. However, short-acting insulin administered before dinner is unlikely to control next morning's fasting blood glucose (FBG), while the shot administered before lunch is unlikely to be effective till dinner. Intermediate- or long-acting insulin administered concurrently along with short-acting insulin takes over at these times by providing basal insulinization. Short-acting insulin should be injected 30 minutes before meals. Often, in a day-to-day practice either this instruction is not conveyed to the patient or he does not understand it or ignores it and injects insulin just before meals. Such action can lead to poor postprandial control and in pursuit of improving postprandial glucose; insulin dose is often increased without paying attention to timing of insulin injection. This can lead to late postprandial hypoglycemia.

### Rapid-acting Insulin Analogs

Insulin analogs are especially designed insulin in which amino acid sequence of native human insulin is altered to get a favorable pharmacokinetic profile, without altering biological activity of insulin. The rapid-acting insulin analogs available in India are lispro insulin, insulin aspart, and glulisine. Lispro insulin happens to be the first marketed insulin analog. In lispro insulin, amino acids at positions B28 and B29 are interchanged. It has onset of action in 15–30 minutes, peak action between 30 and 90 minutes after administration, and effective duration of action of 3–4 hours. In insulin aspart, proline at B28 is replaced by aspartic acid. This alters the pharmacokinetic profile which is similar to that of lispro. Glulisine is manufactured by replacing asparagine with lysine at B3 position and lysine with glutamic acid at B26 position. Its pharmacokinetic profile is similar to that of lispro and aspart insulin. Lispro, aspart, or glulisine insulin should be used in place of short-acting insulin in those patients in whom short-acting insulin is unable to control postprandial blood glucose peaks or its use leads to late postprandial hypoglycemia. Another advantage of rapid-acting insulin over short-acting insulin is flexibility as regards time of administration. Short-acting insulin is relatively slowly absorbed from subcutaneous tissue and thus is required to be injected 30 minutes before meals for optimizing postprandial blood glucose levels. Unpredictable delivery of food, change of decision regarding amount and time of food, vomiting can lead to poor postprandial control. In pursuit of minimizing abovementioned controllable variables, the patient loses his flexibility. Rapid-acting insulin is more rapidly absorbed and eliminated than short-acting insulin. Thus, postprandial blood glucose control is a bit better and also chances of late postprandial hypoglycemia are a bit lesser than in those using rapid-acting insulin as compared to short-acting insulin. Because of quicker absorption, rapid-acting insulin is injected just 10 minutes before the meals and in case of unpredictability, even if it is administered just before food, rise in postprandial blood glucose is not very significant.

## Ultrarapid-acting insulin (Fiasp)

In Fiasp, niacinamide, which facilitates absorption from subcutaneous tissues at slightly faster rate than rapid-acting insulin; and an amino acid arginine, which stabilizes it, are added to aspart. It has two advantages over rapid-acting insulin. When time or amount of food consumed or retained is unpredictable, it can be given just before, with or up to 20 minutes after food. Comparative studies have shown that 1 hour postprandial blood glucose levels are better with Fiasp than aspart. In short, it is one step ahead of the three rapid-acting insulins.

## Intermediate-acting Insulin

Two intermediate-acting insulins are available, viz., neutral protamine hagedorn (NPH) insulin and lente insulin. In former, protamine is added to prolong the duration of action of insulin while in latter, zinc is used for the same purpose. Onset of action of NPH insulin is 2–4 hours after administration, peak action occurs between 6 and 10 hours after administration, while effective duration of action is for 10–16 hours. The corresponding pharmacokinetics for lente insulin is 3–4 hours, 6–12 hours, and 12–18 hours, respectively. Combination of NPH with short-acting insulin is more stable than that of lente insulin. However, if injected immediately after mixing, lente insulin can be combined with short-acting insulin. Of late, lente insulin has disappeared from the market. As compared to long-acting insulin, intermediate-acting insulin has following disadvantages: (1) shorter duration of action, thus not covering 24 hours span and (2) peak effect around 8 hours, thus higher chances of hypoglycemia around 6–10 hours after injection, particularly when dose is increased to improve FBG control. NPH insulin is still very commonly used in a day-to-day practice as a substitute to long-acting insulin because it is inexpensive as compared to long-acting insulin. The disadvantages described above can be partly overcome by administering it twice a day, or at late night (postdinner, around 10–11 PM) in once a day dosage in those with small to moderate insulin requirements. The idea is to maintain adequate blood and liver insulin levels from dawn to prebreakfast time. When intermediate insulin is injected before dinner particularly in early diners such as Jains, its levels start dwindling by dawn and early morning, when counterregulatory hormones are at their peak. The combined effect can lead to a sharp rise in blood glucose level at morning. If the reason behind this phenomenon is misunderstood and predinner dose is increased, there is too much insulin in circulation at around 3 AM, leading to hypoglycemia at that time. This can be avoided by shifting the time of injection of intermediate-acting insulin to around 10–11 PM. This action helps to avoid reactive morning hyperglycemia by avoiding 3 AM hypoglycemia (Somogyi effect).

## Long-acting Insulin

Ultralente insulin was the only long-acting insulin available in India in past. It had onset of action 6–10 hours after administration, peak at 10–14 hours, and duration of action of 18–20 hours. Ultralente insulin was used to provide basal insulin requirement. It was administered as a solo treatment or was combined with oral antidiabetic drugs (OADs) or premeal short-acting insulin as per patient's requirement based on his functional capacity of β-cells. It had much higher tendency for hypoglycemia. The research and development on long-acting insulin analogs having smoother, truly round the clock action without significant episodes of hypoglycemia started simultaneously with that of rapid-acting analogs and all the current long-acting insulin preparations in the market are examples of insulin analogs.

*Peakless insulin—insulin glargine:* This long-acting analog of insulin has been introduced in India about 15 years back, within 1 year after its international launch. Following structural changes have been incorporated in glargine to get improved pharmacokinetic profile: (1) in position 21 in A chain, asparagine is replaced by glycine and (2) at the end of B chain two arginine residues are added. It is "peakless" insulin with 22–24 hours action. The currently available traditional intermediate-acting insulin like NPH or lente insulin do not have round the clock action and thus need to be given twice a day to avoid wide blood glucose fluctuations. Moreover, they peak around 8 hours after administration. This may lead to hypoglycemic episodes during the peak action. Glargine has following advantages as compared to conventional intermediate-acting insulin:

- It can be taken any time of the day as per patient's convenience (of course it should be taken at the same time every day).
- In most of the patients, it needs to be taken only once a day.
- Episodes of hypoglycemia are less as compared to conventional insulin.
- It is ideal insulin to be used along with OADs for a tight blood glucose control in type 2 diabetic patients who do not respond adequately to OADs but still have some residual β-cell function. When FBG crosses 150 mg%, in spite of taking two or three different OADs in submaximal to maximal doses, one may continue the pills and add glargine 10 units daily and gradually increase if required. It will lead to better blood glucose control.
- It can also be used as an ideal basal insulin component in any intensive insulin therapy, which is usually required in type 1 diabetic patients and severe type 2 diabetic patients with secondary failure to oral agents. In this plan, glargine is given once a day and short- or rapid-acting insulin is separately given before each meal.
- Usual starting dose of glargine is 10 units once a day. It may be noted that glargine should not be mixed with any other insulin in the same syringe.

*Concentrated (U/300) glargine*: Its formulation in three times concentrated form and resultant smaller size of deposited mass in subcutaneous tissue after injection is one of the reasons leading to slower release of insulin crystals as compared to glargine 100, with which it shares exactly same amino acid structure. As compared to conventional glargine (U/100), concentrated (U/300) form of glargine has a flatter pharmacokinetic profile and slightly longer duration of action. It is true once a day insulin. In some patients who have difficulty in controlling their FBG with glargine, one may consider using glargine (300 units).

*Detemir insulin*: It was the first long-acting insulin analog to be marketed anywhere. Following structural changes have been incorporated in detemir: (1) Amino acid at position B30 has been removed and (2) Myristic acid side chain has been attached to amino acid 29 in B chain. These changes are responsible for long duration of action. Like glargine, detemir is a long-acting insulin analog with generally similar pharmacokinetics and indications. It has a slightly shorter duration of action than glargine. Thus, even though it works on once a day basis in many type 2 diabetic patients, some patients, particularly those having T1DM, are better-off with twice a day dosing of detemir. In fact, in European countries it is mandatory to prescribe it twice a day. Weight gain in patients on detemir is a bit less than those on equal doses of other insulin preparations. With the availability of 24 hours acting peakless insulin such as glargine 300 and degludec, use of detemir has come down considerably. In some countries, it has received official clearance for use in pregnancy, no other long-acting insulin analog has been officially cleared for this indication.

*Degludec*: This long-acting basal insulin analog was introduced in India in September, 2013. It has truly 24 hours long action span, as its biological half-life is 42 hours. Following structural changes are responsible for its long action: (1) Removal of amino acid from position 30, (2) attachment of a fatty acid, hexadecanedioic acid through a spacer at B29. Its other advantages over traditional long-acting insulin are: (i) flexibility as regards timing of insulin injection, since it has a long biological half-life, unlike other basal insulin preparations, the patient is not likely to lose glycemic control even if he delays his insulin injection by a few hours. Thus, in case patient forgets to take insulin injection at scheduled time or is unable to take it due to logistic reasons, he can take it as soon as he remembers or as soon as he can take it. Subsequently, he should continue his 24 hourly schedules. At least 8 hours must elapse between two injections. This is a big plus point; (ii) hypoglycemia—the frequency and severity of hypoglycemia, particularly nocturnal hypoglycemia is less with insulin degludec as compared with insulin glargine. Glargine 300 nearly matches pharmacokinetic profile of degludec and shares most of the advantages including flexibility as regards time of injection. Though far more flexible as compared to glargine and detemir, as regards time of injection, it is less flexible than degludec (3 hours extension vs. 8 hours extension).

Degludec is ideal basal insulin and can be combined with short or rapid-acting insulin preparations in basal-bolus insulin therapy for type 1 diabetic patients and some of the type 2 diabetic patients. It can be also used along with metformin or other oral antidiabetic agents in type 2 diabetic patients with some β-cell activity. However, degludec is costlier than glargine (**Table 1** for pharmacokinetic profiles of insulin preparations).

*Insulin mixtures:* Ready-made insulin mixtures of short-acting insulin and intermediate-acting NPH insulin are available in 25/75, 30/70, and 50/50 proportions. These are called premix

**TABLE 1:** Summary of insulin pharmacokinetics.

| Generic name | Brand names | Time of onset of action (h) | Time to peak action (h) | Duration of action (h) |
|---|---|---|---|---|
| Regular human | Actrapid | 0.5 | 1.5–2.5 | 8 |
| Aspart | Novorapid | Within 0.25 | 0.5–1.5 | 4–6 |
| Fast-acting aspart | Fiasp | Within 0.25 | 1 | 2–4 |
| Lispro | Humalog | Within 0.25 | 0.5–1.5 | 4–6 |
| Glulisine | Apidra | Within 0.25 | 0.5–1.5 | 4–6 |
| NPH | Insulatard | 2–4 | 4–10 | 12–18 |
| Detemir | Levemir | 2–4 | Flat | 14–24 |
| Glargine 100 | Lantus | 2–4 | Flat | 20–24 |
| Glargine 300 | Toujeo | 6 | Flat | Up to 36 |
| Degludec | Tresiba | 1 | Flat | >42 |

*Source:* Medications for the treatment of diabetes mellitus, 2022–2023, ADA.

insulin. Mixtures of rapid-acting analogs, lispro, and aspart are also available in 30/70 and 50/50 proportions with NPH insulin. Some patients have difficulty in mixing insulin. For such patients, these mixtures are useful. Depending upon individual need, a particular mixture can be selected. However, one must note that the flexibility of independently altering either short-acting or intermediate-acting component of insulin is lost with ready-made mixtures. When one increases or decreases the dose of such mixtures, both the components are proportionately altered. In other words, insulin mixtures are like ready-made garments, they do not suit everybody ("one size does not necessarily fit all"). The convenience of ready mixture comes with the limitations regarding flexibility of dosages. If a given mixture can provide both the short-acting and intermediate-acting components in exact units as per the individual need, then mixtures are suitable. This is as far as theoretical limitation of insulin mixtures. However, in real-life situation, if a patient ideally requiring individual insulin preparations to be mixed manually, just cannot master the process of mixing insulin or does not have any intention of learning the same—it is far better to prescribe ready premix insulin if he can manage to take it. After all, theoretical limitations apart, glycated hemoglobin (HbA1c) of 8% is far better than 10%. Many frontline doctors are also not very confident of prescribing full basal bolus insulin therapy to their patients. Because of all these reasons, premixed insulin is very commonly prescribed in India and developing countries. For your information, Mixtard is number one prescribed medicine in India. Its sales are more than any other medicine in India, across all the categories of medicines. Premixed insulin with 30 or 25% short-acting components are used as staple premixed insulin. Patients on these insulin with difficulty in achieving postprandial glucose control can be shifted to 50/50 premixed concentration. But keep the possibility of spoiling control 7–8 hours down the line due to automatic reduction in intermediate-acting insulin concentration from 70 to 50%. Remember famous English proverb *"You can't always have a cake and eat it too."*

*Coformulated insulin*: Coformulation of aspart with degludec is available under trade name Ryzodeg. Differences between coformulation and premix insulin are: (1) In former, both the components retain separate identities and their individual pharmacokinetic properties. (2) The longer acting component in Ryzodeg is degludec, the true 24 hours acting insulin, whereas in premixed insulin, it is NPH insulin, which is an intermediate-acting insulin. The resultant clinical benefits are (i) lower chances of late postprandial hypoglycemia due to absence of 'shoulder effect' or prolongation of action span of shorter acting insulin and (ii) better FBG control due to superiority of degludec over intermediate-acting insulin.

**Which Patients need Insulin?**
T1DM patients should be put on insulin immediately after the diagnosis as their life is dependent on it and they would develop diabetic ketoacidosis leading to coma, if insulin is withheld. However, it should be remembered that true T1DM is very uncommon in our country (2%).

Many young diabetics in their 20s and 30s are poorly controlled in spite of taking large dosages of insulin, but they are glutamic acid decarboxylase (GAD) negative and do not develop ketoacidosis if insulin is withdrawn, unless there are severe associated disorders such as infections. Thus they are not type 1 diabetic patients but need large doses of insulin.

**Insulin in Type 2 Diabetes Mellitus (Fig. 1)**
About 95-96% of diabetics in our country have T2DM. More than 60% of them can be controlled on diet and OADs. However, in the following circumstances, insulin should be used:
- During severe stressful situations, e.g., septicemia, tuberculosis, other severe infections, myocardial infarction, etc. During such situations, there is increase in counterregulatory hormone secretion in response to stressful situations. Under such conditions, lifestyle changes and OADs are not sufficient to establish and maintain glycemic control.
- During perioperative period in patients undergoing major surgery
- During pregnancy and lactation
- In those patients in whom highest dosage of OADs from two/three different groups fails to bring down blood glucose levels to normal
- When OADs are contraindicated (e.g., severe hepatic and renal failure)

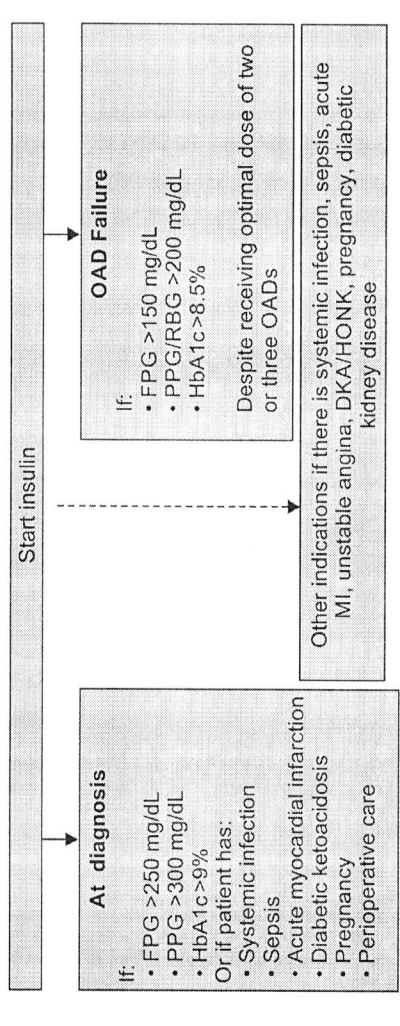

**FIG. 1:** Indian guidelines on initiation and intensification of insulin therapy.

(DKA: diabetic ketoacidosis; FPG: fasting plasma glucose; HbA1c: glycated hemoglobin; HONK: hyperosmolar nonketotic coma; MI: myocardial infarction; OAD: oral antidiabetic drug; PPG: postprandial plasma glucose; RBS: random blood sugar)

*Source:* Das AK, Sahay BK, Seshiah V, Mohan V, Muruganathan A, Kumar A, et al. Indian National Consensus Group: national guidelines on initiation and intensification of insulin therapy with premixed insulin analogs. Med Update. 2013;2013:227.

- When patients present with very high glucose levels [FBS >300 mg%; postprandial blood sugar (PPBS) >400 mg%; HbA1c >10.5%] associated with severe symptoms such as polyuria, polydipsia and weight loss.

## Initiation of Insulin Treatment

Acutely ill patients requiring changeover to insulin, or all newly diagnosed T1DM patients requiring insulin, should be preferably admitted for a few days for initiation, dosage adjustment and training regarding insulin injection techniques, for method of monitoring and also for training regarding prevention/detection and self-treatment of hypoglycemia. The opportunity should also be utilized for patient education program on various other aspects of diabetes.

Now, let us see how to handle insulin initiation in outpatient family practice.

Let us first understand the action spans of different insulin formulations. The prebreakfast, short-acting, and rapid-acting insulin control blood glucose rise following breakfast and to some extent following lunch, while intermediate-insulin controls blood glucose levels mainly from afternoon period up to dinner time when injected in morning and the overnight period when injected in evening. In other words, when the effect of short-acting insulin starts wearing off, intermediate-acting insulin takes over. Similarly, predinner short-acting insulin controls blood glucose rise following dinner, while predinner intermediate-insulin takes care of blood glucose control during the late night and early morning period up to breakfast time. Long-acting insulin provides basal needs for 24 hours **(Table 1)**.

### Insulin Initiation

The starting dose depends on several factors including blood glucose level, associated complications and infections, capacity of $\beta$-cells to synthesize and release insulin (about 50% of the $\beta$-cells are functional at the time of onset of T2DM and as the times passes, the % of the $\beta$-cells which are functional, gradually reduces), insulin resistance (judged by weight of the patient and other signs), etc. The dose is 0.2–0.5 U/kg body weight. Usual starting dose is 0.2 U/kg body weight. In those with predominantly fasting hyperglycemia, and in whom insulin is being introduced fairly early and at appropriate time, entire daily dose can be given at bedtime in the form of intermediate- or long-acting insulin. In others with more severe hyperglycemia and/or associated complications, the daily dose is divided into two equal portions and administered before breakfast and dinner. At each time, one-third to half the number of units are given as short-acting insulin and the remaining as intermediate-acting insulin.

## Insulin Regimens in T2DM

- *Basal-only regimen*: Ambulatory patients who are having diabetes for around 5 years but not responding to 2–3 oral agents and having HbA1c <8.5% and FBS and PPBS values around 150–160 and 220–270 respectively can respond to once a day intermediate- or long-acting insulin plus OADs. The decision between intermediate- or long-acting insulin will depend upon the affordability and need for higher insulin. The starting dose is usually 10 units once a day. Intermediate-acting insulin to be given around 10 PM while true long-acting insulin can be given any time of the day.
- *Basal-plus regimen*: Those already on once a day insulin as above and having reasonable fasting glucose control but one of the postprandial sugars are above 200 mg%, add a short-acting insulin before a meal which produces highest postprandial glucose level.
- *Basal-bolus regimen:* Those patients having very high fasting and postprandial glucose with A1c at or above 9% need a combination of short- or rapid-acting insulin and intermediate- or long-acting insulin. Total daily dose (TDD) to be calculated as above. 50% of TDD to be given as intermediate- or long-acting insulin and remaining 50% to be divided in three equal doses and given before each meal. Long-acting insulin can be given any time of the day while short- or rapid-acting insulin to be given before each major meal. If from affordability point of view one is using intermediate-acting insulin, one can start with full dose at 10 PM and subsequently split it in two doses if required.

## Examples.

- A 45-year-old male weighing 70 kg has T2DM for 5 years. In last few months, he has been gradually losing control over his blood glucose. His last two fasting and postlunch blood glucose readings were around 150–160 mg% and 210–220 mg%, respectively, and his HbA1c is 8.4%. He is on 4 mg of glimepiride and 2 g of metformin. This patient can be put on 12–14 units of NPH/glargine/detemir at bedtime and his metformin continued while glimepiride to be discontinued or dose reduced by 50%.
- A 50-year-old female patient weighing 60 kg, a known diabetic for 8 years, has been in poor metabolic control for over last 1 year. Her recent laboratory values are: fasting plasma glucose 217 mg%, postlunch plasma glucose 342 mg%, and HbA1c 10.2%. She is currently on 6 mg of glimepiride and 2 g of metformin daily. She has been recently diagnosed to have severe urinary tract infection. Her total daily insulin dose is 60 × 0.4 = 24 units; 12 units before breakfast and dinner (4 units of short-acting insulin plus 8 units of NPH insulin at each time). Her current metformin dose can be continued after ruling out contraindications to its use, while glimepiride can be discontinued or continued in half the dose.

## Dose Adjustment

If FBG is high, increase predinner dose of intermediate/long-acting insulin by 2–4 units while if FBG is low, decrease the same by 2–4 units. The usual FBS target is 80–120 mg%. Adjust the dosage of morning's short-acting insulin for controlling postbreakfast and postlunch blood glucose levels. If postbreakfast blood glucose is at goal but postlunch is not coming down or increase in prebreakfast short-acting insulin leads to prelunch hypoglycemia, then instead of increasing prebreakfast short-acting insulin, add a small dose such as 4 units of short-acting insulin before lunch. To adjust the dosage of prebreakfast, intermediate-acting insulin, since one usually does not order predinner blood glucose levels (actually, one should, from time to time), use the indirect method, i.e., if there are symptoms of hypoglycemia in the evening (please resort to direct questioning, if the patient does not mention them, or ask the patient to monitor his capillary blood glucose by glucometer at a particular frequency, which will depend upon individual situation and bring the logbook during consultation). Suggestion for more accurate evaluation of control at this particular time is as follows.

Since all the clinicians are in their clinics in the evening, you can do random capillary blood glucose at your clinic with glucometer and use the information obtained for dosage adjustment of prebreakfast, intermediate-acting insulin.

As regards adjustment of dosage of predinner, short-acting insulin, please teach the patient to do self-monitoring of blood glucose by using glucometer, 2 hours after dinner. If blood glucose is high at postdinner time, increase predinner short-acting insulin, while low blood glucose or symptoms of hypoglycemia at late night are signals for reducing the dose of predinner, short-acting insulin. While adjusting insulin dosage observe the following rules:
- Handle one insulin at a time, starting with intermediate-acting predinner insulin
- Do not increase the dosage by >4 units at a time, unless blood glucose is extremely high.
- Do not increase the dosage more frequently than every third day. Before increasing the dosage, verify other variants such as missing previous insulin dose, eating an unusually large meal, etc.

Many of the T2DM patients retain at least minimal β-cell function even when they fail to show adequate response to OAD. They secrete insulin which is inadequate for metabolic control but which can be judiciously utilized in combination with externally administered insulin so that dosage and frequency of external insulin can be minimized. This is the reason why some of the T2DM patients can be well controlled with only one shot of intermediate-acting insulin or short-plus intermediate-acting combination of insulin.

In those diabetics, where FBG is persistently normal, one can attempt withdrawing evening insulin and use a dipeptidyl peptidase-4 inhibitor ($DPP_4I$), sodium-glucose cotransporter-2 inhibitor ($SGLT_2I$), or a sulfonylurea (SU) instead. An alternate method is to use intermediate-/long-acting insulin in the evening and OAD in the daytime. This method results in better control of FBG in some patients.

## TRICKS OF THE TRADE IN DIFFICULT SITUATIONS

In some patients, it is difficult to control fasting plasma glucose in spite of high dosages of predinner, intermediate-acting insulin. Under such circumstances, giving intermediate-acting insulin at around 10–11 PM will serve the purpose. If the patient is also taking short-acting insulin before dinner, either it should be given separately before dinner, or in T2DM patients, an attempt could be made to replace it by SU/DPP$_4$I/AGI (α-glucosidase inhibitor).

This strategy is used when patients require more than 20 units of intermediate-acting insulin in the evening. Increasing its dosage beyond 20 units and persisting with predinner time may lead to late night or early morning hypoglycemia with rebound hyperglycemia during prebreakfast hours. This hyperglycemia is liable to be wrongly interpreted, resulting in further increase in predinner, intermediate-acting insulin dosage.

Another approach in such a situation (i.e., high FBG in spite of >20 units of intermediate-acting insulin in the evening) is to do random blood glucose around 3 AM (by asking the patient or his relatives to do it at home with glucometer). If it is more than 150 mg%, increase the intermediate-acting insulin, but if it is 70 mg% or lower, reduce the intermediate-acting insulin, and you would have better control of FBG in spite of reducing the insulin. Replacing NPH insulin with one of the peakless analogs is an excellent but expensive alternative.

What to do about OADs when initiating or intensifying insulin regimen?

If there are no contraindications to use of oral agent which you want to use, continue metformin, DPP$_4$Is, SGLT$_2$Is, and AGIs.

Long-acting SUs to be avoided and modern SUs can be continued, usually in reduced dosages. In Western countries SUs are used only with basal-only insulin but avoided in basal-bolus therapy, the reason being overlapping actions of externally administered insulin and endogenous insulin secreted in response to SUs. In some Western countries again coprescription of insulin and pioglitazone is avoided, the reason being since both can retain sodium, and chances of cardiac failure are higher. In patients having very poor glycemic control in spite of a large dose of insulin, some diabetologists in India are using this combination while very carefully monitoring the patient. Under such situations, insulin sensitizing action of pioglitazone occasionally works wonders.

## MISTAKES WHILE TAKING/PRESCRIBING INSULIN

*Mistakes due to mismatch between insulin vials and syringes—Some real-life "comic mistakes" leading to tragic implications*: Today, the most common mode of administration of insulin is through subcutaneous route by using insulin syringes. Looking at rapid economic development of our country, very aggressive strategies of insulin marketing companies to encourage shift from syringes to pens (margins are higher in cartridges and regulated by government for vials), and rapid conversion rate in last few years, this situation will change sooner than later but clinicians have to be alert. After having prescribed insulin injections, it is prescribing doctor's duty to ensure that the prescription bears all the details such as units and type of insulin, its frequency, the time gap between injection and food intake, vial strength, and specifications of insulin syringe. Insulin vials are available in two strengths: U/40 and U/100, containing 40 units and 100 units, respectively, per each milliliter. Insulin syringes are also available in two types: U/40 and U/100, each made specifically to suit specific insulin vial. Besides teaching proper insulin injection techniques, it is advisable that the treating doctor also briefs them about different vial strengths and syringe types. He should advise them to always verify the vial strength whenever a new vial is to be used and to draw insulin in matching syringes. However, in a day-to-day practice, occasionally, major mistakes occur, either due to lack of time available at doctor's disposal or because of carelessness of the patient. These mistakes in insulin injection technique lead to hypoglycemia or hyperglycemia as per individual mistake. Sometimes, life-threatening emergencies are created. Some of the actual mistakes the author has come across have been described below:
- A patient was on injection Huminsulin (30/70) (U/40 vial) 40 units twice a day and his blood glucose was poorly controlled, thus he was advised injection Huminsulin (30/70) 50 units twice a day. Since capacity of U/40 syringe is only 40 units, he was advised to use U/100 syringe so that *"you can take up to 50 units*

*mark and avoid two pricks"*. Patient followed the advice and his blood glucose further worsened. At this point he consulted us. The reason for worsening of blood glucose was obvious. If one takes U/40 insulin up to 50 units mark in U/100 syringe, he actually takes only 20 units. So, instead of increasing insulin from 40 to 50 units, he ended reducing it to 20 units.

*Take-home message*: In such situations instruct the patient to change over to U/100 vial as well as U/100 insulin syringe, or to change over to insulin pens.

- An uneducated patient taking injection Mixtard (30/70) 48 units, before breakfast and 34 units before dinner came to outpatient department alone. His blood sugars were high. His compliance with insulin injections was apparently good, so was his diet control. He was investigated for the lack of blood glucose control in spite of apparent high dose of insulin. He could not answer questions regarding the type of insulin syringe. However, when asked about the cost of insulin vial, he could answer the question correctly and from this information, we derived that he was taking U/40 insulin. When asked, "How long the bottle lasts"? We found that his bottle was lasting 2.5 times the expected period. From this data, we concluded that he was taking U/40 insulin with U/100 syringe, thus actually taking only 40% of the prescribed dose. We asked him to come back with vial and syringe and confirmed the same. When he changed over to U/40 syringe, his blood glucose was controlled.

*Take-home message:* If your patient's blood glucose is not well controlled in spite of good compliance, always find out from him how many days the vial lasts. If vial is lasting for much longer time than expected (around 2.5 times), suspect the mismatch between insulin vial and syringe (specifically, suspect that patient is injecting insulin from U/40 vial with U/100 syringe. For example, if your patient is prescribed 20 units of insulin twice a day, he would finish the vial in exactly 10 days. Each vial contains 400 units of insulin: 40 units/mL in 10 mL vial). However, if uses U/100 syringe and draws insulin up to 20 units mark, he will end up using only 8 units of insulin at a time, or 16 units per day, thus vial will last for 25 days.

Many of the patients have at least one relative in the USA. Whenever these nonresident Indian relatives know that their India-based kin is on insulin injections, they send a large carton containing disposable insulin syringes. These are invariably U/100 syringes, which are made to inject U/100 insulin, the only strength of insulin available for common use in the entire developed world. However, in India, even though both the strengths of insulin are available, 99 out of 100 times the patient is on U/40 strength. Thus, if insulin from U/40 vials is drawn up in U/100 syringes, patients end up injecting only 40% of the prescribed dose, unless they draw 2.5 times the prescribed dose in the syringe. Thus, it is better to avoid using U/100 syringe for U/40 insulin injection. However, in emergency, one may multiply the prescribed dose 2.5 times and use U/100 syringe for U/40 insulin. For example, if one is prescribed 20 units of insulin and is usually using U/40 vials and U/40 syringes, if he has to use U/100 syringe, he should withdraw insulin from U/40 vial up to 50 units mark in U/100 syringe.

On the other hand, in case of an extremely rare situation of needing to inject U/100 insulin with U/40 syringe, one has to multiply by a factor of 0.4. For example, if one is prescribed 20 units of insulin and is usually using U/100 vials with U/100 syringes, if he has to use U/40 syringe, he should draw insulin from U/100 vial up to 8 unit mark on U/40 syringe (U/40 syringes have red top and are marked up to 40 in red, while U/100 syringes have orange top and are marked up to 100 in black. In order to find out the strength of insulin vial, ask the questions regarding the cost of vials to get the information. U/40 vial costs between ₹125 and ₹150, while U/100 vial obviously costs more than ₹300.

- A patient was taking 40 units of Huminsulin (30/70) in morning and 20 units in evening. His FBG was well controlled but postlunch blood glucose was high, thus his morning dose was increased to 44 units while no change was made in evening dose. Since one can only take up to 40 units of insulin in U/40 syringe, he was rightly advised to change over to U/100 insulin vial and inject it with U/100 insulin syringe. However, he continued to take evening dose of 20 units from U/40 vial and with U/40 syringe and ordered fresh stocks of U/40 vial and syringes even after the vial in use was finished. He did not make any technical mistake but after using all the remaining insulin from U/40 vial for the evening dose, he could have taken 20 units in evening from the U/I00 vial which he was using for morning. There was no need to keep inventory of two vials and two types of syringes.

*Take-home message:* You can use U/100 insulin vials and syringes for small as well as large doses, but you cannot inject >40 units of U/40 insulin with U/40 syringe.

Thus, always match insulin vial strength with insulin syringe.

- A 45-year-old female patient, whose blood glucose was not controlled in spite of triple drug oral combination, was put on Mixtard (30/70) 8 units before breakfast and dinner. She was a resident of a village on the mainland about 50 km across Mumbai island, and was in hurry to catch the last launch, thus skipped training session for insulin injections, which we hold for all patients requiring insulin for first time. On reaching the shore, around dinner time, she approached a "trainee nurse" in a private nursing home in her village and literally forced her to give her insulin, even though the nurse was reluctant. Under pressure, the "nurse" accepted the proposal and injected entire vial containing 10 mL or 400 units through 10 mL conventional multipurpose syringe. Patient walked 1.5 km to reach home and subsequently developed typical symptoms of hypoglycemia. Her husband immediately contacted me and narrated the incidence. She was advised to be shifted to a nursing home immediately. She was kept in the nursing home for 48 hours under constant intravenous (IV) glucose infusion and dire life-threatening emergency was avoided. Faulty technique leading to partial injection and poor absorption from a large subcutaneous deposit could have contributed to some extent. Availability of mobile phone saved the life. This was my first experience with emergency lifesaving teleconsultation about 20 years back.

*Take-home message:* Such things can happen in India. It is prescribing doctor's duty to ensure safe administration of insulin to his patients and nothing should be taken for granted.

- A patient was prescribed 10 units of Huminsulin (30/70) (U/40) before dinner. She was well controlled with appropriate syringes and vials purchased from the market, till she received a vial of Huminsulin (30/70) (U/100) free of cost from her employer's medical services department. Nobody briefed her about the difference between U/40 and U/100 vials and the need to use appropriate syringes. For a few days, she used U/40 syringe to inject insulin from U/100 vials. One fine day, the family doctor, who used to come to visit her daily for injecting insulin, noticed that he was drawing U/100 insulin in U/40 syringe. He decided to draw up to 25 units mark to account for the difference (he should have drawn up to 4 units mark). Thus, he injected 62.5 units subcutaneously. In other words, he magnified the mistake 2.5 times. Patient developed severe hypoglycemia.

*Take-home message:* All patients on insulin, their relatives who are involved in their care and their primary care medical and paramedical personnel, all should receive intensive education on availability of insulin vials and syringes in different strengths. As far as possible, do not use inappropriate syringes to avoid calculation mistakes. Use of insulin pens, which eliminate this problem, should be encouraged.

- A 43-year-old female patient was put on injection Mixtard (pen) (30/70) 20 units before breakfast and dinner, and was having stable blood glucose control till she decided to do cost-cutting by purchasing Mixtard (30/70) U/40 vial from the market and by refilling empty Mixtard cartridges via syringe filled with insulin drawn from Mixtard U/40 vial. Soon her blood glucose rose significantly. The reason is obvious. While Mixtard cartridge contains 100 units/mL, Mixtard U/40 from vial contains 40 units/mL. Thus, the patient ended up taking only 8 units of insulin twice a day instead of 20 units twice a day.

  **Figure 2** depicts how the patient improvised by refilling insulin cartridge from its rear end by injecting Mixtard drawn from U/40 vial.

- A 66-year-old female patient was prescribed 15 units of Mixtard (30/70) before breakfast. She went to a small chemist shop in the bylanes of Mumbai for purchasing insulin vial and syringes. Chemist gave her U/l00 vial and U/40 syringes. She was regularly taking "15 units of insulin" daily before breakfast

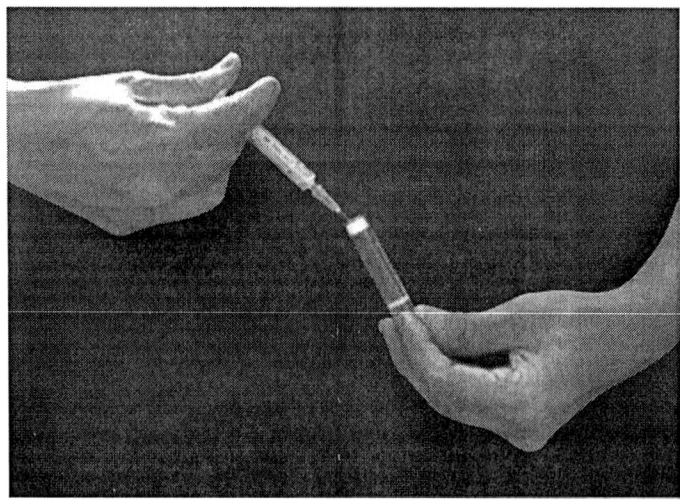

**FIG. 2:** Faulty improvization: Patient filling empty Mixtard cartridge by injecting Mixtard, drawn from U/40 vial, through rear end of cartridge.

and was occasionally experiencing hypoglycemic episodes. At this stage, she came to us for second opinion. We asked her to come back with her insulin vial and syringe for verification and identified her mistake.

Her mistake was explained in details and she was trained to change over to U/40 vials and draw 15 units of insulin in U/40 syringe for injection. An elaborate prescription with highlighting of relevant portion was handed over to her. Her young daughter was also briefed in details.

*Take-home message:* Do not take anything for granted. Do not rely on patient. Verify each step. In case of doubt, physically inspect the vials and syringes.

- *A mistake which luckily turned out to be beneficial*: A 43-year-old male, a known diabetic for 3 years, was hospitalized for anterior wall infarction. He was on IV insulin infusion for 48 hours and was subsequently discharged on 10 units of Mixtard before breakfast and dinner. He was prescribed U/40 insulin with U/40 insulin syringes. When he came for follow-up after 6 weeks, his fasting and post-lunch plasma glucose values were 100 mg% and 132 mg%, respectively.

Everything was apparently fine. However, on routine verification drive, it was found out that the vials of insulin were lasting much longer than expected. On further investigations, it was found out that he was using U/100 syringe for injection of U/40 strength insulin, thus effectively, he was taking only four units of premixed (30/70) insulin twice a day and still his blood glucose was well controlled. Subsequently, his insulin was discontinued and he was kept on aggressive lifestyle measures and when he came for follow-up after 4 weeks, his fasting and post-lunch plasma glucose values were 96 mg% and 130 mg%, respectively. Thus, in his case, if he had taken insulin correctly as advised, he would have landed into hypoglycemia. His insulin requirement probably went down faster than anticipated due to disappearance of transient insulin resistance associated with acute myocardial infarction.

*Take-home message:* Even in those patients apparently doing very well, do not take things for granted and verify compatibility between insulin vials and syringes.

- *Double mistakes also happen:* A 65-year-old woman, having T2DM for 10 years with grossly uncontrolled blood glucose in spite of three OADs, was prescribed injection Huminsulin (30/70) 10 units before breakfast and dinner. The most reputed chemist of the area having a few practicing diabetologists and several consultant physicians in his drainage area filled the prescription by supplying U/40 huminsulin vial and U/100 insulin syringe. The vial and syringe were carried to her family doctor who administered the insulin injection twice a day for 10 days with syringes carried by the patient. Thus, the patient ended up taking only four units of insulin twice a day, which was 40% of the prescribed dose. Thus, after 10 days, when she repeated her blood glucose levels, they were only marginally better than baseline. The mistake was identified at first follow-up. The problem was overlooked at two stages: (1) the chemist and (2) the family doctor.

*Take-home message:* Do not take anybody for granted. Specifically mention vial strength and syringe subtype as a suffix after insulin and syringe prescription, respectively.

All the cases described earlier are 100% real cases, none of them are imaginary. However, the very encouraging news is that of late I am not getting such cases, indicating that there is a vast improvement in insulin administration-related knowledge among patients, caregivers and medical and paramedical staff. Additionally, a larger percentage of patients shifting to insulin pens has helped.

**When to Use Insulin Vials and When to Use Insulin Pens**
The traditional method of injecting insulin consists of using disposable plastic insulin syringes, which are used to draw insulin from the glass vials as well as to inject insulin in patient's body. This is the least expensive way of injecting insulin but a bit more time-consuming and cumbersome as compared to injecting insulin through insulin pens. The patients opting for economy should be advised to continue injecting insulin in this manner. Patients requiring > 40 units of insulin at a time should be prescribed U/100 insulin vials and syringes in order to avoid extra prick (the capacity of U/40 syringe is 40 units). The additional advantage of using insulin from U/100 vial is reduced volume of injected insulin which is less painful.

Injecting insulin through pens is less time-consuming and more convenient. In addition, the dosing is precise. The upper portion of pen is rotated in clockwise manner till the numerical figure of insulin dose appears in a window at its upper end. This is known as "dialing of dose". In short, insulin pens are smarter and convenient option. Disposable pens are preloaded with insulin cartridge inside the sealed compartment. They are in "ready to use" form, but once all the insulin (300 units) is used up, pens cannot be refilled. In reusable pens one needs to replace insulin cartridge, just like one replaces the ball pen refills. When one is expected to use insulin for short-term or if one wants to try out suitability of pens, he should be advised to use disposable pens. Long-term insulin users are advised to use reusable pens, as it is less expensive to use them as compared to disposable pens. The maximum one-time cost of reusable pen is approximately ₹1,000. The insulin analogs are usually available only in pen forms, with the exception of Lantus, (glargine 100) and Novorapid, which are also available in conventional vial form (U/100 only). With little bargaining, reusable insulin pens can be obtained free of cost (insulin in cartridge form has better margin thus companies can afford to give free reusable pens if the user is expected to use them, and thus their insulin cartridges for a long-term).

## SUMMARY

Since its introduction exactly a century ago, insulin has remained on the centerstage of diabetes management. Prior to the availability of exogenous insulin, diagnosis of T1DM was essentially a death certificate. While insulin products and delivery systems have dramatically improved over a period of 100 years, insulin still remains a medical necessity in all type 1 diabetic patients and is also required in many type 2 diabetic patients to reach the glycemic targets. Improvement in insulin quality and delivery systems is an ongoing process and thus every clinician who treats diabetic patients requires to acquire working knowledge on use of insulin and constantly update it.

# CHAPTER 15

# Combination Therapy in Diabetes

## INTRODUCTION

When one discusses combination therapy in diabetes, he is usually referring to various combinations of blood glucose-lowering medications only, even though technically one can include various antihypertensive medications as well as lipid-lowering medications, which are often used in combination in a diabetic patient. Even among the blood glucose-lowering agents, regimens containing combinations of insulin are not included under the title of antidiabetic drug combinations. Thus, conventionally antidiabetic combination therapy includes: (1) combination of two or more oral antidiabetic drugs (OADs) given in separate dosage form or fixed-dosage form, (2) combination of OADs with insulin, and (3) combinations of glucagon-like peptide-1 receptor agonists ($GLP_1RAs$) with insulin/OADs.

## COMBINATIONS OF ORAL ANTIDIABETIC MEDICATIONS

For almost four decades after OADs were introduced, there were only two classes of drugs, sulfonylureas, and biguanides (coincidentally in the same era, Indian's choice for automobiles was restricted between only two cars, Ambassador and Fiat!). In the olden days, pharmacological treatment with OADs always started with monotherapy, sulfonylurea for thin or average weight diabetic patients, and biguanide for overweight diabetic patients.

The concept of primary combination therapy, albeit, with two separate tablets was nonexistent. Fixed-dose combinations were rarely available, that too in very few countries. When a domestic pharmaceutical company introduced a combination of glibenclamide and metformin in India in late 80s, an average clinician was confused about its exact slot and a section of senior diabetologists just did not accept the concept. They considered this combination as irrational because it was not available in the USA. Incidentally, some of these doctors avoided metformin like one would avoid a person suspected of coronavirus infection, again because during that era, the US Food and Drug Administration (US FDA) had declined permission to introduce metformin in the USA, though across Europe, it was available and very commonly prescribed. Pragmatic clinicians accepted the concept of fixed-dose combinations as the need of the day, because anyway, after initial years with monotherapy, most of the patients were on both sulfonylureas and biguanides combinations in separate tablets and gradually the acceptance for the concept of fixed-dose combination grew and many more formulations were launched. The concept grew in leaps and bounds after a major pharmaceutical company in the USA launched the same combination of glyburide, (official name for glibenclamide in the USA), and metformin in the year 2000. Earlier, metformin was ultimately accepted by the US FDA in 1995 and within 1 year after its introduction, had become the USA's most widely prescribed OAD and third most widely prescribed drug. Over last two decades, the scenario has changed drastically due to several reasons such as:
- Introduction of agents belonging to totally new classes of OADs, such as glitazones, alpha-glucosidase inhibitors (AGIs), dipeptidyl peptidase-4 inhibitors (DPP$_4$Is), GLP$_1$RAs, and sodium-glucose cotransporter-2 inhibitors (SGLT$_2$Is), whose mechanism of action is different from that of older agents and having synergistic effect with the older drugs.
- Availability of new information on pathophysiology of type 2 diabetes mellitus (T2DM) particularly as regards role played by insulin resistance and incretin deficiency and hypersecretion of glucagon and realization that one needs to tackle multiple pathophysiological defects simultaneously and obviously with different antidiabetic agents in polytherapy. Thus from

pragmatic point of view, fixed-dose combination concept received gradual acceptance.
- Aggressive promotion of fixed-dose combinations by pharmaceutical companies.

In primary combination therapy, two antidiabetic agents are prescribed together at the beginning of pharmacological treatment bypassing monotherapy. While traditionally, OAD treatment starts with monotherapy and second agent is added if blood glucose remains uncontrolled in spite of taking maximum dosage of one agent.

*Last but not the least.* Recent studies showing that establishment of good metabolic control in the initial years after the diagnosis of diabetes helps to reduce macrovascular complications several years later and also the proof obtained through VERIFY study on long-term glycemic benefits of metformin vildagliptin combination versus metformin monotherapy in initial 6 months, though after 6 months both the groups received combination therapy.

*Now let us have a look at some commonly used combinations and their niche in today's settings.*

## A Combination of Sulfonylurea with Metformin

Central action of sulfonylurea is complemented by peripheral action of metformin.

Thus, this combination has a strong rationale. Since most type 2 diabetic patients have a combination of β-cell defect, which is addressed by sulfonylurea, with insulin resistance, which is addressed by metformin; nowadays, many diabetologists start the pharmacological therapy of T2DM with sulfonylurea plus metformin combination (primary combination therapy). The advantage of this therapy is that the dosage and thus side effects of each agent are lower than in monotherapy.

Metformin-sulfonylurea combination can be used as initial combination therapy or when monotherapy with one of the agents fails. The selection of particular combination will depend upon the sulfonylurea component of the fixed-dose combination (refer to the Chapter 13 for selection of sulfonylurea depending on the underlying specific situation in an individual patient). All the four sulfonylureas available in our country are also available in fixed-dose combination with metformin.

## Combination of Sulfonylurea plus Pioglitazone

Any sulfonylurea can be combined with pioglitazone. As regards fixed-dose combinations, several combinations containing glimepiride and pioglitazone are available. Peripheral action of pioglitazone is complementary to central action of sulfonylurea and a rationale for use of such a combination is same as that for sulfonylurea plus metformin combination. What is the place of such a combination in therapy? In type 2 diabetic patients not responding to sulfonylurea alone, one can use such a combination. Predominantly insulin-resistant type 2 diabetic patients, who started drug treatment with pioglitazone but subsequently failed to reach glycemic targets with monotherapy, can be considered for sulfonylurea plus pioglitazone combinations. Moreover, since most type 2 diabetic patients have both β-cell defect as well as insulin resistance, some diabetologists use a combination of a secretagogue and insulin sensitizer from the beginning of drug therapy, in such a situation, this combination can be used. However, it should be noted that in these indications preference may be given to sulfonylurea plus metformin combination and if metformin is not tolerated or is contraindicated, sulfonylurea plus pioglitazone can be used.

## Limitations of Sulfonylurea plus Metformin/Pioglitazone Combinations

The combinations are unsuccessful if there is no viable β-cell mass as in very long-standing type 2 diabetic patients. The clinical pointer is poor blood glucose control in spite of a large dose of sulfonylurea. Metformin and pioglitazone work only in presence of insulin, either endogenous insulin secreted in response to sulfonylurea, or exogenous administered insulin. Hence, in such conditions, addition of metformin or pioglitazone is superfluous.

## Combination of Metformin plus Pioglitazone

Both these agents are insulin sensitizers. They act peripherally and increase sensitivity of tissues to insulin. While metformin acts predominantly on liver with some action at muscles; pioglitazone acts predominantly on muscles and fat tissues with some action on liver. Thus, they have synergistic effect when given together. Since they do not stimulate β-cells in pancreas to release insulin, the combination will not work in patients who have significant β-cell defect, unless insulin is separately given in addition to the combination. The main place for this combination is predominantly insulin resistant type 2 diabetic patients with reasonable residual β-cell function. In such patients, β-cells produce some amount of endogenous insulin, which is insufficient to control blood glucose level due to severe insulin resistance, leading to very high demand on β-cells. Many of these patients would not tolerate full dose of metformin if it is used as monotherapy, or would still be uncontrolled after full dose. Under such circumstances, a combination of metformin plus pioglitazone would be useful. Other alternative in such circumstances is to use monotherapy with pioglitazone. However, monotherapy may not be sufficient to bring down blood glucose to normal or may increase weight and pedal edema to an unacceptable level.

## Combinations of Repaglinide

The broad mechanism of action of repaglinide is same as that of sulfonylureas. Thus, repaglinide can be combined with metformin, pioglitazone, and acarbose or any of the new OADs. The broad indications are same as those for combinations of sulfonylureas with respective agents. Repaglinide-based combinations are preferred over similar sulfonylurea-based combinations if patients have renal impairment, predominantly postprandial hyperglycemia, in elderly patients and in patients prone for hypoglycemia.

## Metformin plus $DPP_4Is$ Combinations

The use of safer/organ protective, weight neutral/weight reducing agents which also offer safety from hypoglycemia is gradually increasing and $DPP_4Is$, $SGLT_2Is$, and $GLP_1RAs$ are gradually occupying the center stage in management of T2DM at the cost of SUs. Many doctors are not fully comfortable with the use of pioglitazone. Thus abovementioned modern antidiabetic agents are now increasingly available in combinations with metformin and with each other. Let us study them.

Main mechanism of action of metformin is reduction of hepatic glucose production, while main mechanisms of action of $DPP_4Is$ are increasing glucose-mediated insulin secretion and suppressing excessive rise of glucagon in postprandial period. These actions are mediated by increasing levels of $GLP_1$. Recently, it has been demonstrated that metformin also works through incretin axis. In patients on metformin, $GLP_1$ levels are elevated. It probably works through several mechanisms such as increase in production of $GLP_1$ as well as slowing down its metabolism. Additionally, it is also postulated that use of metformin is associated with increased effect of $GLP_1$ at the tissue level.

Thus, the actions of metformin and $DPP_4Is$ are complementary to each other. Metformin (500/850/1,000 mg) can be combined with 50 mg of sitagliptin or vildagliptin for twice a day administration or can be combined with 2.5/5 mg of linagliptin or saxagliptin for once/twice a day administration. Teneligliptin—metformin combination are also commonly used. Fixed-dose combinations are also available. Such combinations can be used at the beginning of OAD therapy as well as in those patients where metformin monotherapy has failed.

## Combinations of $SGLT_2Is$ with Metformin, $DPP_4Is$, and Triple Drug Combinations Containing these Three Agents

Sodium-glucose cotransporter-2 inhibitors have moderate to strong glycemic efficacy, offer protection from atherosclerotic cardiovascular disease (ASCVD), heart failure, and progression of renal impairment. These agents are recommended as joint first choice medications along with metformin in those with abovementioned comorbidities or very high risk for them. Additionally, even in those who do not have abovementioned comorbidities or high risk for them. These agents are preferred whenever weight reduction or hypoglycemia prevention is a priority. The mechanism of glycemic action is complimentary to metformin as well as $DPP_4Is$ and thus they are increasingly used in combinations with these agents as per individual needs of patients. Of late their fixed-dose combinations with metformin, $DPP_4Is$ as well as triple drug combinations containing all these three agents have become very popular.

## Combinations of Alpha-glucosidase Inhibitors

Acarbose and voglibose act locally on the small intestinal mucosa. This action is distinct from and complementary to any other OAD. Thus, AGIs can be combined with any other OADs. They can be used as an adjuvant along with sulfonylurea, metformin, or pioglitazone or a combination therapy containing two of these agents whenever postprandial blood glucose control needs improvement. Fixed-dose combinations of acarbose and voglibose with metformin are available for some years. During mid-2013, when pioglitazone was temporarily banned in India, it was replaced by voglibose in triple drug combinations (metformin plus glimepiride plus voglibose). Even after reintroduction of pioglitazone, triple drug combinations containing voglibose continued to be available in the market and receive acceptance of clinicians.

## Fixed-dose Drug Combinations

Since the combination therapy has come to stay, many pharmaceutical companies have marketed branded combinations of two or three OADs in tablet form.

Combinations of various sulfonylureas with metformin, pioglitazone with metformin, glimepiride with pioglitazone, as well as combinations of sulfonylureas plus metformin plus voglibose/pioglitazone are available in the market. Many $DPP_4Is$ are available in fixed-dose combinations with metformin, $SGLT_2Is$ as well as metformin plus $SGLT_2Is$ in triple drug combinations. The range of combinations, the number of brands and availability of each brand in multiple stock-keeping units (SKUs) is mind boggling and sometimes confusing. A company is marketing glimepiride-metformin combination in 10 different SKUs or strengths. Convenience and thus better compliance is the obvious advantage of fixed-dose combinations over separate dosage forms.

*However, one must observe following precautions while prescribing fixed-dose combinations.*
- Study patient's needs based on individual pathophysiological factors, associated comorbidities, history of tolerance, affordability, and then decide which OAD or combination of OAD is required and in what individual doses. After deciding

these variables, choose a brand exactly providing the individual patient's requirement.
- Verify whether any contraindication exists for each ingredient of combination therapy.
- Prescribe the fixed-dose combination if all the individualized requirements can be fulfilled by a fixed-dose combination available in the market.

In other words, do not select a brand and then prescribe it to a patient in anticipation of him adjusting to the contents and strengths of a brand, it should be other way round.

## Examples of Irrational Combinations

- *Combination of two sulfonylureas or a nonsulfonylurea secretagogues (repaglinide) with sulfonylurea*: All these act through the same mechanism; hence, there is no point in combining them. If one is unsuccessful, others are unlikely to succeed in the same situation.
- *Combination of four different OADs*: If three different OADs are unable to control blood glucose, it indicates that patient has developed β-cell failure and he needs insulin. Furthermore, more the number of agents in a combination, more are dosage flexibility issues, even three in one is often problematic in this regard.
- Combination of metformin with glitazones in thin, lean, long-standing diabetic who is likely to have significant β-cell defect as a major contributor toward hyperglycemia.
- *Combination of $DPP_4Is$ with $GLP_1RAs$*: These two groups of agents have common mechanism of action.
- *Combinations of OADs with a statin and aspirin*: It amounts to stretching a combination concept beyond the limits.

## COMBINATIONS OF INSULIN WITH ORAL ANTIDIABETIC DRUGS

About 33% of type 2 diabetic patients require insulin for achieving good glycemic control. In some of these patients, OADs can be judiciously added to achieve better blood glucose control with lesser insulin dose and/or lesser frequency of insulin administration.

Similarly, in type 1 diabetic patients with associated acquired insulin resistance, leading to further worsening of blood glucose or requiring higher insulin dosage, addition of metformin or pioglitazone to insulin leads to better blood glucose control and reduction in insulin dosage.

## Insulin plus Sulfonylurea or Repaglinide Combinations

Insulin plus sulfonylurea are the most commonly used insulin plus OAD combinations. To be successful, patient selection is important. Such a combination will not provide any additional benefits if used in patients with advanced β-cell failure for obvious reasons. If one does not wait till end-stage failure, but adds insulin when fasting plasma glucose crosses 150 mg% persistently; better blood glucose control can be obtained and dosage of insulin or frequency of insulin administration can be reduced. The most common example of such a therapy is to give once a day basal insulin [neutral protamine hagedorn (NPH) insulin/glargine preferably at 10 PM and give sulfonylureas during the daytime]. Adequate hepatic insulinization at night achieved through bedtime basal insulin administration leads to better control over fasting blood glucose. One of the sulfonylureas is administered in the daytime to stimulate β-cells to release endogenous insulin formed by the surviving β-cells. In affording patients glargine/glargine 300/degludec can be used in place of NPH insulin. In those patients who do not respond adequately to this therapy but still are likely to have some β-cell function left in them, OADs can be combined with twice daily insulin, usually given before breakfast and dinner in a combination of short- and intermediate-acting forms. In conditions better suited for repaglinide, instead of sulfonylureas, a combination of insulin with repaglinide can be administered.

## Insulin plus Metformin Combination

This combination is used in type 2 diabetic patients and in type 1 diabetic patients associated acquired insulin resistance.

Addition of metformin will help through its insulin sensitizing action in achieving better blood glucose control with lesser dosage of insulin.

## Insulin plus Pioglitazone Combination

The rationale and indications are essentially same as those for insulin plus metformin combination; pioglitazone can be used instead of metformin if the latter is not tolerated or contraindicated. However, such a combination is contraindicated in Europe as a precautionary measure to prevent exacerbation of cardiac failure.

## Insulin plus Alpha-glucosidase Inhibitor Combination

Administration of one of the AGIs added to basal insulin therapy helps in achieving better postprandial blood glucose control. It also helps to reduce dosage and frequency of insulin. This combination is suitable for those patients on insulin therapy who need a small improvement in postprandial blood glucose control. Under such circumstances, addition of one of the AGIs is a good alternative to additional dosage and/or frequency of insulin. Viability of β-cells is not an issue for insulin plus AGI combination.

## Insulin plus $DPP_4I$/$SGLT_2I$ Combinations

Several members of these two classes of agents have successfully undergone clinical trials in combination with insulin and for the obvious reasons discussed above, will gradually replace SUs for this indication.

## $GLP_1RAS$ COMBINATIONS WITH INSULIN/ METFORMIN/PIOGLITAZONE/SULFONYLUREA

The rationale behind the combinations of $GLP_1RAs$ with metformin/ pioglitazone/sulfonylurea/insulin is same as the combinations of $DPP_4Is$ with these agents. $GLP_1RAs$ have following two advantages over $DPP_4Is$: (1) they are more potent, (2) their use leads to significant weight reduction while $DPP_4Is$ are generally weight neutral. Both share the advantage of freedom from hypoglycemia. However, with the exception of oral semaglutide, $GLP_1RAs$ are injectable and several times costlier than $DPP_4Is$. The combination therapy with $GLP_1RAs$ plus OADs (other than $DPP_4Is$), and with insulin is rapidly becoming popular in the west and lixisenatide in combination with glargine in a single pen assembly, with facilities to adjust glargine dose and release both the agents in single prick, is available. A similar combination of liraglutide with degludec is available. Addition of $GLP_1RA$ to insulin helps to reduce insulin dose and thus reduce side effects such as weight gain and hypoglycemia.

Diabetes is often associated with comorbidities such as hypertension, hyperlipidemia, macrovascular disease, etc. Often, each of these comorbidities requires multidrug therapy. As the time passes, pill burden of antihyperglycemic agents keeps on increasing. Under such circumstances, use of a rationally formulated fixed-drug combination is pragmatic.

# 16
## CHAPTER

# Management of Diabetes in Elderly

## INTRODUCTION

Diabetic patients above the age of 65 years are classified as elderly diabetics. Several factors, such as reduction in mortality from infectious diseases leading to longer life expectancy, have led to an ever-increasing proportion of individuals to survive long enough to get afflicted with chronic degenerative diseases such as diabetes mellitus (DM). An increasing number of diabetic people reach old age by virtue of better understanding of the disease and availability of treatment, including the treatment for complications such as end-stage renal failure and coronary artery disease. At the same time, more and more nondiabetic individuals reach old age and subsequently develop diabetes, resulting from long-standing exposure to the endogenous and environmental risk factors such as obesity, inadequate physical activity, stress associated with rapid urbanization, etc. As a result prevalence of diabetes increases with age. In studies done in South India where overall prevalence of type 2 diabetes mellitus (T2DM) is approximately 14% in urban population, its prevalence was found to be 21% in population above the age of 40 years, and 41% in the age group of 55–64 years. At this rate the problem of elderly people with diabetes will soon become unmanageable.

While planning management of diabetes in elderly, some of the important factors needing consideration are as follows:
- Elderly diabetics are more likely to be unaware of hypoglycemia, thus exposing them to significantly higher mortality

and morbidity associated with drug-induced hypoglycemia. Moreover, elderly long-standing diabetics are more likely to have significant cardiovascular diseases. Under such circumstances, sudden hypoglycemia could be life-threatening. Hence, metabolic goals should be especially set for them. Fasting plasma glucose of 120–150 mg%, postprandial plasma glucose 150–200 mg%, and HbA1c of 7.5–8.0% should be aimed at.

- Elderly diabetics are more likely to have renal impairment, thus renal functions need to be monitored frequently. Long-acting sulfonylureas such as glibenclamide should be avoided and agents such as gliclazide and glimepiride should be preferred.
- Elderly diabetics are more likely to have multiple comorbidities and receiving multiple medications simultaneously, thus before prescribing any medication, the likely drug interactions should be studied.

All said and done, elderly diabetics is a group of heterogeneous people with age >65 years and presence of diabetes as common features shared by all but having very significant variability as regards various degrees of physical disabilities, cognitive impairments, associated comorbidities and age. A 66-year-old fully fit diabetic, though elderly diabetic by definition, will not require any special care and should be handled like any other diabetic, while a 90-year-old bedridden diabetic with dementia will need a very high degree of special care.

## PREVENTION OF DIABETES IN THE ELDERLY

The only cost-effective way to handle this enormous problem is to reduce the incidence of diabetes and its complications. Primary prevention of diabetes in elderly, by preventing obesity with prudent meal planning and proper physical activity, is an effective and inexpensive approach; however, it is difficult to make changes in lifestyle at late stage in life; moreover, other medical conditions such as osteoarthritis and cardiovascular disease may come in the way of physical exercise. Thus, the strategies for primary prevention of diabetes should be implemented early in life. Secondary prevention aims to reduce chronic complications and sustain quality of life in diabetic patients. To accomplish this, therapeutic goals should be clearly and specifically set for elderly diabetics after duly considering associated comorbidities. In elderly patients, emphasis should be on control of symptoms and prevention of acute complications, including diabetic foot problems rather than achieving strict glycemic control with the intention of preventing long-term complications, unlike in younger patients.

## MANAGEMENT OF DIABETES

### Patient and Family Education

Absorbing capacity and memory deteriorate with age. Associated vascular and metabolic complications further deteriorate cognitive functions. Thus, while imparting education to elderly diabetics, the educator should be very patient. He should adapt a speed with which the patient is comfortable. It is advisable to impart training in several short sessions tackling one important aspect at a time. Simple patient-friendly language should be used and the educator should assess the impact of his talk from time to time before moving ahead. For the patients staying in a joint family, training should be simultaneously imparted to spouse and a younger member of family along with the patient. The emphasis of training should be on: (1) the need for constant metabolic control and importance of periodic assessment; (2) diagnosis, prevention, and treatment of hypoglycemia; (3) sick day schedule; and (4) foot care.

### Diet

Considerable effort is required to change the eating habits of elderly patients. It is unrealistic to expect a drastic change in diet. Emphasis should be on restriction of calories in overweight patients, increasing complex carbohydrate and fiber content, avoidance of sugar and jaggery, restriction of oils and fats, and last but not the least, taking small and frequent meals. Many elderly patients are depressed and sudden decision to reduce or totally skip a meal is not uncommon. In order to avoid hypoglycemic episodes, detailed and repeated talks should be given to them about importance of maintaining the timing and amount of food intake and its interrelation with antidiabetic medications.

## Exercise

Physical exercise prescriptions have little value for many elderly patients because of osteoarthritis, cardiovascular, and foot problems. If physical condition permits, short daily walk should be encouraged. Patients should be thoroughly assessed as regards their cardiovascular fitness, foot problems if any, and screening for presence of severe proliferative retinopathy, before giving them exercise prescriptions.

## Drug Treatment

The principles of treatment in elderly diabetics do not differ from those in other diabetic population, and will not be discussed in details. Only specific aspects will be discussed. It is to be noted that elderly diabetics form a heterogeneous group. Even though, most of them have T2DM, there are gross differences as regards functional capacity of β-cells, degree of insulin resistance, presence and extent of vascular complications, etc. Hence, therapy will have to be tailor-made. Relatively young and active elderly diabetics are to be treated like any other diabetic with usual metabolic goals.

### *Oral Antidiabetic Drugs*

*Sulfonylureas*: In elderly patients with T2DM, sulfonylureas are indicated in those who cannot be controlled on diet plus metformin and who have not yet reached significant β-cell failure.

Gliclazide or glimepiride should be preferred. The incidence of hypoglycemia, particularly severe, prolonged, and recurrent hypoglycemia is comparatively lesser with these agents as compared to glibenclamide. Gliclazide and glimepiride may be continued with utmost care in renal impairment. However, when estimated glomerular filtration rate (eGFR) is reduced to <45 mL/min/1.73 m$^2$, the dose of glimepiride should be reduced by 50%. Six monthly estimation of serum creatinine should be done. Sulfonylureas are contraindicated in severe hepatic insufficiency.

About two decades back, nonsulfonylurea insulin secretagogues were introduced in the market. Repaglinide is still available in our country. These agents are suitable for use in elderly diabetics.

One should start with a low dose (half tablet of standard strength), and gradually increase if required. Sulfonylureas are usually very well tolerated by the gastrointestinal (GI) tract. The most important side effect is hypoglycemia, which is more common in elderly diabetics.

*Drug interactions with sulfonylureas:* Gatifloxacin, aspirin, nonsteroidal anti-inflammatory agents, sulfonamides, oral anticoagulants, tricyclic antidepressants, and alcohol are some of the agents which enhance the effect of sulfonylureas, while thiazide diuretic and steroids reduce their effect. Beta blockers, particularly nonselective agents such as propranolol block adrenergic symptoms of hypoglycemia, thus leading to late diagnosis and treatment which could increase mortality and morbidity associated with hypoglycemia.

*Metformin:* In elderly diabetics with normal renal functions and stable cardiovascular and respiratory status, metformin can be used with care if diet alone is not sufficient to control symptoms. It can be also used as add-on therapy to sulfonylureas if required. When used alone, it is unlikely to produce hypoglycemia. Metformin improves sensitivity of tissues to insulin and thus reduces blood glucose without increasing plasma insulin levels. This action is very beneficial in insulin resistance. If used when contraindications such as renal and hepatic insufficiency exist, chances of lactic acidosis increase many fold. These conditions are more likely to exist in elderly diabetics.

Thus, selection of patients for metformin therapy is very vital. Old age is not an absolute contraindication. In a relatively younger diabetic without any major complication, metformin need not be withheld on the grounds of age as with sulfonylurea therapy, periodic monitoring of blood glucose as well as hepatic, renal, cardiac status, and general condition is mandatory. Metformin is administered immediately after the food, 2-3 times a day in dosage of 250-500 mg. If required, total daily dosage can be increased up to 2 g daily. GI disturbances are common with metformin therapy. The incidence and severity of GI disturbances are reduced by administering metformin after food and by starting with a smaller dosage and gradually increasing it up to 2 g daily if required. About 5-10% of patients do not tolerate metformin even if these precautions are observed. Alternatively, slow release preparations can be used to reduce GI side effects.

*Alpha-glucosidase inhibitors (AGIs):* These reversibly inhibit intestinal α-glucosidase enzymes and slow down digestion of complex carbohydrates, and thus delay absorption of glucose into circulation. When used alone, AGIs do not cause hypoglycemia. Alpha-glucosidase inhibitors can be used alone in mild diabetics, or can be combined with insulin or oral agents if required. AGIs are administered 2-3 times a day along with major meals. Abdominal distention and diarrhea are common side effects, thus it is advisable to start with a small dose and gradually increase it.

*Pioglitazone:* It has no specific contraindications in elderly. However, impaired left ventricular function, which is a specific contraindication to the use of glitazones, is more likely to be present in this age group. Thus, patients should be thoroughly evaluated before putting them on pioglitazone. Carcinoma of urinary bladder is also more common in elderly. Thus, elderly patients with hematuria or history of hematuria should be evaluated in details to rule out carcinoma of bladder before starting pioglitazone therapy. If they develop hematuria while on pioglitazone, it should be discontinued and investigations for carcinoma of bladder should be started. Pioglitazone can be reintroduced if carcinoma of bladder is ruled out.

*Dipeptidyl peptidase-4 inhibitors ($DPP_4Is$) and glucagon-like peptide-1 receptor agonists ($GLP_1RAs$):* Both these subgroups, particularly $DPP_4Is$, are ideal for use in elderly diabetics. $DPP_4Is$ are oral agents and comparatively far less expensive than injectable or oral $GLP_1RAs$. Freedom from hypoglycemia and weight gain; and relative cardiovascular safety profile makes them very suitable for first add-on agent in elderly diabetics. $DPP_4Is$ are often used as initial agents in monotherapy in elderly.

*Insulin:* Elderly patients are likely to make substantial errors in insulin mixing and administration techniques. Hence, premixed insulin should be used as far as possible. In affording patients insulin injection devices should be used.

Once daily injections improve compliance; however, in those requiring >20 units daily, twice daily injections should be recommended to reduce incidence of night-time hypoglycemia.

Glargine, glargine 300, and degludec given once daily topped up with premeal sulfonylureas or nonsulfonylurea insulin secretagogues or $DPP_4$ Is are good alternatives. In those who can afford, glargine 300 or degludec the peak less insulin with lower incidence of hypoglycemia, particularly nocturnal hypoglycemia should be used.

When prandial insulin is required to control postprandial rise of blood glucose, rapid-acting insulin analogs should be preferred over short-acting human insulin in affording patients. The main advantages of rapid-acting insulin analogs are: (1) lesser prevalence of hypoglycemia, (2) option to inject insulin after meal instead of 30 minutes before meal, so that the dose can be reduced or withheld in case reduced quantity of meal is consumed or meal is skipped.

## CONCLUSION

Prevalence of diabetes in elderly is increasing at rapid rates. Elderly diabetics have special problems and require patient attention of diabetologist. The management needs to be individualized depending upon associated complications and handicaps.

# CHAPTER 17

# Prescribing Antidiabetic Medications in Renal Impairment

## INTRODUCTION

Diabetic patients, particularly those who have diabetes for long duration and who are having inadequate glycemic control over long periods, are likely to have varying degrees of renal impairment. In order to slow down the rate of further deterioration of their renal function, one needs to maintain their glycemic control along with blood pressure control. Many antidiabetic medications are excreted by the kidneys and thus have altered pharmacokinetics in presence of renal impairment. If an adjustment in dosage and/or frequency of medications eliminated by the kidneys is not made, depending upon the severity of renal impairment, the patient is exposed to the risk of hypoglycemia. Hypoglycemia in long-standing elderly diabetic patients carries higher morbidity and mortality due to precipitation of acute vascular events, particularly in those who have underlying macrovascular disease. Of course, one also needs to consider various other factors responsible for pulling glycemic control in opposite directions. In addition to delayed excretion of some antidiabetic medications, factors, such as poor food intake due to loss of appetite and vomiting, impaired capacity of the kidneys for gluconeogenesis, tend to shift blood glucose to lower levels while insulin resistance associated with renal impairment tends to partially neutralize the tendency for hypoglycemia due to factors mentioned above. Glycemic efficacy of sodium-glucose cotransporter-2 ($SGLT_2I$) is progressively reduced with reducing glomerular filtration rate (GFR).

In order to make dosage adjustments, one needs to estimate renal functions periodically (once a year till renal function is in normal range, once in 6 months in mild renal impairment and more frequently in moderate-to-severe renal impairment depending on individual situation).

One needs to calculate estimated GFR (eGFR) by applying a mathematical formula to serum creatinine value or by downloading eGFR calculators on desktops/laptops/smartphones. The method of estimating creatinine clearance is a bit more time-consuming and involves estimation of serum creatinine, 24 hours urine volume, and urine creatinine; and then calculating creatinine clearance.

Now, let us look at individual antidiabetic agents.

## METFORMIN

*Estimated glomerular filtration rate >60 mL/min/1.73 $m^2$*: Administer full dose and perform yearly estimation of eGFR.

*Estimated glomerular filtration rate 45-60 mL/min/1.73 $m^2$*: Full dose with 3-6 monthly estimation of eGFR.

*Estimated glomerular filtration rate 30-45 mL/min/1.73 $m^2$*: 50% reduction in dose with 3-6 monthly reviews. If eGFR is between 45 and 30 mL/min/1.73 $m^2$, do not initiate metformin.

Discontinue if eGFR is <30 mL/min/1.73 $m^2$.

## SULFONYLUREAS

*Glipizide and gliclazide:* No dose adjustment is required in any degree of renal impairment.

*Glimepiride:* Start conservatively with 1 mg/day, uptitrate conservatively.

*Glibenclamide:* It is an agent with very long duration of action, which is further prolonged in renal impairment. It has two metabolites: M1 and M2, both have hypoglycemic action.

Avoid glibenclamide if eGFR is <60 mL/min.

## NONSULFONYLUREA INSULIN SECRETAGOGUES

*Repaglinide:* Estimated glomerular filtration >30 mL/min/1.73 m² —full dose.

*Estimated glomerular filtration rate <30 mL/min/1.73 m²:* Initiate and uptitrate conservatively.

## PIOGLITAZONE

No dosage adjustment required; however, by the time patients develop significant renal impairment, pioglitazone is likely to become unsuitable from various other points of view, e.g., (1) in edematous patients and (2) associated cardiac failure.

## ALPHA-GLUCOSIDASE INHIBITORS

The literature on the use of α-glucosidase inhibitors—acarbose and voglibose in renal insufficiency is inadequate and divergent views are expressed. Thus, it is advised to follow manufacturer's recommendations of avoiding these agents in "severe renal impairment (serum creatinine >2 mg%)."

## INSULIN

Short-acting insulin and rapid-acting insulin should be preferred over longer-acting insulin, which should be used in addition to short-acting insulin in selected cases, failing to reach acceptable fasting glycemic goals with short-acting insulin regimen. In severe renal impairment, rapid-acting analogs have marginal advantage over short-acting insulin as their half-life is insignificantly affected.

## $DPP_4I$'S AND $GLP_1RA$'S

Dose adjustment of dipeptidyl peptidase-4 inhibitors ($DPP_4Is$) in renal impairment is based on pharmacokinetic profiles to maintain drug concentrations at the same level as in patients with normal renal function and not on safety or efficacy parameters, which remain unchanged in renal impairment **(Table 1)**.

**TABLE 1:** DPP$_4$Is in renal impairment.

| Agent | Dose (mg) eGFR >60 | Dose (mg) eGFR 30–60 | Dose (mg) eGFR <30 |
|---|---|---|---|
| Sitagliptin | 100 OD | 50 OD | 25 OD |
| Saxagliptin | 5 OD | 5 OD | 2.5 OD |
| Linagliptin | 5 OD | 5 OD | 5 OD |
| Vildagliptin | 50 BD | 50 OD | 50 OD |
| Teneligliptin | 20 OD | 20 OD | 20 OD |
| Alogliptin | 6.25–25 OD | 6.25–25 OD | 6.25–12.5 OD |

(DPP$_4$Is: dipeptidyl peptidase-4 inhibitors; eGFR: estimated glomerular filtration rate)

## Glucagon-like Peptide-1 Receptor Agonists

Exenatide and exenatide extended release (XR) are contraindicated in those with eGFR <30 mL/min/1.73 m². No dose adjustment is required in milder renal impairment.

No dose adjustment is required for other glucagon-like peptide-1 receptor agonists (GLP$_1$RAs) in any degree of renal impairment.

## Sodium-glucose Cotransporter-2 Inhibitors

Generally, these agents are not recommended in those with eGFR <45 mL/min/1.73 m², as glycemic efficacy goes down with the reduction of eGFR and side effects increase. However, the exact level of eGFR beyond which these agents are prescribed keeps on changing slightly from time-to-time and varies from country-to-country as per the guidelines set by respective regulatory authority. The trend is towards reducing eGFR levels. Based on DAPA CKD and empagliflozin CKD studies, these two agents are prescribed by nephrologists as pure nephroprotective drugs in diabetics as well as nondiabetics, in those with eGFR>25 and 20 mL/min/1.73 m², while canagliflozin is based on CREDENCE trial is being prescribed as nephroprotective agent in diabetic nephropathy up to eGFR of 30 mL/min/1.73 m². Some loss of glycemic efficacy should be accepted in such situations and should be managed through other antidiabetic agents.

## Bromocriptine

No adjustment in dosage required in any degree of renal impairment **(Table 2)**.

*Notes*: eGFR is estimated glomerular filtration rate in mL/min. One of the commonly used methods of calculation uses modification of diet in renal disease (MDRD) formula:

$$eGFR = 175 \times (\text{serum creatinine})^{-1.154} \times (\text{age})^{-0.203} \times (0.742 \text{ if female}) \times (1.212 \text{ if Afro-American})$$

There are few other formulas which are commonly used.

Some laboratories give eGFR values by default with every serum creatinine report.

Estimated glomerular filtration rate calculators can be downloaded on smartphones/laptops.

**TABLE 2: Classification of renal impairment based on eGFR values.**

| Renal function | eGFR in mL/min/1.73 m$^2$ |
| --- | --- |
| Normal | >90 |
| Mild impairment | 60–90 |
| Moderate impairment | 30–60 |
| Severe impairment | <30 |

(eGFR: estimated glomerular filtration rate)

# 18
## CHAPTER

# Acute Metabolic Complications of Diabetes

## INTRODUCTION

Diabetes is a lifelong metabolic disorder characterized by inability of β-cells in pancreatic islets of Langerhans to secrete adequate insulin and resistance of tissues to insulin, resulting in hyperglycemia. Diabetic patients suffer from various complications, which have high mortality and morbidity and impart a heavy economic burden on the patient, his immediate family as well as society. Diabetes is an expensive disease. It is estimated that global expenditure including direct as well as indirect costs for treatment of diabetic patients was approximately ₹80 lakh crores in 2021 ($USD 1,000 billion). About 50% of direct expenditure was on management of complications of diabetes. India has about 74 million diabetic patients and it is estimated that by the end of 2045, the population of diabetic patients in our country will grow to 134 million. Thus, it is very important to impart basic knowledge of diabetes and its complications to the patient, his immediate family and healthcare workers at all the levels.

Complications of diabetes can be divided into acute complications and gradual onset complications. Based on affected tissues or causative factors, the complications are divided into: (1) vascular, (2) metabolic, (3) infective, and (4) connective tissue complications.

## ACUTE METABOLIC COMPLICATIONS

These can occur at any point in a diabetic patient, even in early stage. In fact, in some cases the presenting symptoms of diabetes are due to the underlying complications such as diabetic ketoacidosis or nonketotic hyperosmolar state.

The main acute metabolic complications of diabetes are:
- Hypoglycemia
- Diabetic ketoacidosis and coma
- Nonketotic hyperosmolar state
- Lactic acidosis

## HYPOGLYCEMIA

Severe hypoglycemia is the most common metabolic emergency and the most common setting for hypoglycemia is that of a diabetic on oral medications, insulin, or on various combination therapies. In the period between 1993 and 2005, 5 million visits to the emergency services were recorded in the USA for hypoglycemia; 25% needed hospitalization. Forty-four percent of those who were hospitalized were above the age of 65 years. But for hypoglycemia, therapy for diabetes would have been as simple as that of Addison's disease or hypothyroidism. Hypoglycemia is one of the main barriers coming in the way of diabetic patients reaching their glycemic targets. It develops in a diabetic who is on inappropriate dosages of antidiabetic medications or due to mistakes in taking these medications, inappropriate food intake or exercise. Severe hypoglycemia is defined as a condition in which assistance of other person is required. Hypoglycemic coma, convulsions, drowsiness, need to administer glucose by intravenous (IV) route, and need for hospitalization are some of the examples of severe hypoglycemia. For the diagnosis of hypoglycemia, the random blood glucose during the symptomatic stage should be 70 mg or below. Hypoglycemia can occasionally be fatal, thus should be never taken lightly.

The symptoms of hypoglycemia depend upon the rate of fall of blood glucose and the severity of hypoglycemia. The blood glucose levels at which symptoms appear are variable and depend upon previous metabolic control. In poorly controlled patients, symptoms appear at higher plasma glucose levels as compared to those who are tightly controlled. The early symptoms are known as adrenergic symptoms because they are due to reflex secretion of extra quantities of adrenalin in the circulation as a biofeedback mechanism to control hypoglycemia. These include palpitations, tremors, anxiety, sweating. Every patient does not get all the symptoms during the hypoglycemic episode but usually the same symptoms are present, whenever hypoglycemia occurs again. These symptoms serve as a warning signal and if recognized, the patient can immediately take some carbohydrate containing food items, such as biscuits, bread, sandwich, or sugar, to correct hypoglycemia. In milder cases, the symptoms are automatically corrected due to rise in blood glucose following secretion of extra quantities of counter regulatory hormones (Table 1).

Hence, at every follow-up visit, particularly in well-controlled diabetics, the attending doctor should pointedly ask about such adrenergic symptoms, particularly before meal timings and if present, hypoglycemia should be confirmed by doing random blood glucose test at appropriate times and the dosage of anti-diabetic medications should be reduced. If blood glucose continues to fall further, brain is deprived of glucose—its only fuel and a new set of symptoms develop. These include hunger, headache, fainting, abnormal behavior, rowdiness, altered consciousness, and ultimately coma. Some may develop hemiparesis mimicking

**TABLE 1: Hormonal response during hypoglycemia.**

| Glycemic threshold (mg/dL) | Response | Role in prevention/correction of hypoglycemia |
|---|---|---|
| 80–85 | ↓Insulin | First defense against hypoglycemia |
| 65–70 | ↑Glucagon | Primary glucose counter regulatory factor |
| 65–70 | ↑Epinephrine | Critical when glucagon is deficient |
| 65–70 | ↑Cortisol, growth hormone | Not critical |
| 50–55 | Symptoms | Prompt behavioral defense (food ingestion) |
| <50 | ↓Cognition | Compromises behavioral defense |

cerebrovascular accident while others may get convulsions. These symptoms are known as neuroglycopenic symptoms because they are due to deficiency of glucose in neurons **(Table 2)**.

In many long-standing elderly diabetic patients and in those who are very tightly controlled over a long period, warning adrenergic symptoms are absent and they straightaway develop neuroglycopenic symptoms. This condition is known as "hypoglycemia unawareness" or "hypoglycemia-associated autonomic failure". Hence, every acute neuropsychiatric episode in a diabetic, on antidiabetic therapy with insulin and/or insulin secretagogue therapy (sulfonylureas and newer agents such as repaglinide) should be treated as hypoglycemia unless proved otherwise.

Whenever hypoglycemia is suspected, random blood glucose should be estimated with properly stored, valid dry strips, and periodically calibrated reliable glucometer. For confirmation of hypoglycemia in a symptomatic patient, blood glucose of 70 mg% or below should be documented and symptoms should disappear after correction of hypoglycemia. Such documentation is important, particularly in situations where symptoms are mild, recurrent, nonspecific, and if symptoms develop at times when

**TABLE 2: Symptoms of hypoglycemia.**

| Neurogenic | Neuroglycopenic |
|---|---|
| *Adrenergic:* | • Cognitive impairments |
| • Palpitations | • Behavioral changes |
| • Tremor anxiety/arousal | • Psychomotor abnormalities |
| *Cholinergic:* | • Seizure |
| • Sweating | • Coma |
| • Hunger | |
| • Paresthesia | |

*Note:* Factors affecting glycemic thresholds are poorly controlled type 1 diabetes mellitus (T1DM) and type 2 diabetes mellitus (T2DM), tight glycemic control in T1DM, and older age.

*Sources:*
1. Cryer PE. Hypoglycemia, functional brain failure, and brain death. J Clin Invest. 2007;117(4):868-70.
2. Cryer PE, Davis SN, Shamoon H. Hypoglycemia in diabetes. Diabetes Care. 2003;26(6):1902-12.
3. Meneilly GS, Cheung E, Tuokko H. Altered responses to hypoglycemia of healthy elderly people. J Clin Endocrinol Metab. 1994;78(6):1341-8.

hypoglycemia is unlikely (e.g., after meals). It is not uncommon to come across patients having many vague symptoms, which they attribute to hypoglycemia and reduce the dosage of their antidiabetic medications or even stop these medications without consulting their doctor, thus resulting in poor metabolic control.

## Rebound Hyperglycemia (Somogyi Effect)

It refers to hyperglycemia that follows severe hypoglycemia and can last for 12–24 hours. It is due to exaggerated and prolonged compensatory response triggered by counterregulatory hormones ("overshoot effect"). The hypoglycemic symptoms may be ignored or absent. It is often seen in patients on insulin in whom insulin dosages are increased very rapidly in an eagerness to swiftly achieve good metabolic control, in those patients in whom large dosage of insulin is given once a day, and in those patients in whom only short-acting insulin is used and fasting blood glucose control is attempted by increasing predinner dose of short-acting insulin, instead of adding intermediate-acting or long-acting insulin. Thus, it is important to remember, particularly in patients on a large dosage of insulin, that occasionally, hyperglycemia, particularly fasting hyperglycemia is due to inappropriate use of insulin and in such circumstances injecting less insulin but more frequently and using long-acting or intermediate-acting insulin to provide for basal insulinization of tissues, particularly liver will reestablish blood glucose control.

## Management of Hypoglycemia

*Prevention:* All diabetic patients on insulin and/or oral hypoglycemic agents (sulfonylureas and glinides) should be informed about symptoms of hypoglycemia and should be asked to carry some sweets in their pocket/purse along with their diabetes identity card. They should be trained to maintain fixed-meal timing, avoid fasting, consume extra food during extra-physical activity, and consume a carbohydrate containing snack or sweets in case warning adrenergic symptoms develop. After recovery from an episode of hypoglycemia, the patients should critically analyze the events and identify their mistakes and correct them to avoid future hypoglycemic episodes. If hypoglycemia occurs in spite of absence of any identifiable mistake, and particularly if it is recurrent, the patients should immediately contact their doctor who will reduce the dosage of their antidiabetic medications. Patients should be trained about availability of insulin in two strengths (U/40 and U/100, containing 40 and 100 units of insulin per milliliter, respectively), and about using U/40 syringe for U/40 insulin and U/100 syringe for U/100 insulin. If U/100 insulin is filled in U/40 insulin syringe, the patient will end up receiving two and half times the intended dose and will obviously have severe hypoglycemia. This blunder is actually happening in a day-to-day practice!

- U/100 insulin syringes have orange caps and black marks and figures.
- U/40 insulin syringes have red caps and red marks and figures **(Figs. 1A and B)**.

## Treatment of Severe Hypoglycemia

If the patient is conscious and alert, he should be asked to take three teaspoons of sugar or glucose. If there is no improvement in 15 minutes, he should repeat three teaspoonfuls of sugar and wait for another 15 minutes. If there is no recovery in another 15 minutes or worsening of symptoms, patients should seek medical attention. If he is unconscious, drowsy or rowdy, 50 mL of 25% glucose should be given as IV bolus. In case a patient is on long-acting sulfonylureas, such as glibenclamide, IV bolus of 25% glucose should be followed by a pint of 5% glucose, which should be continued till his blood glucose is stabilized.

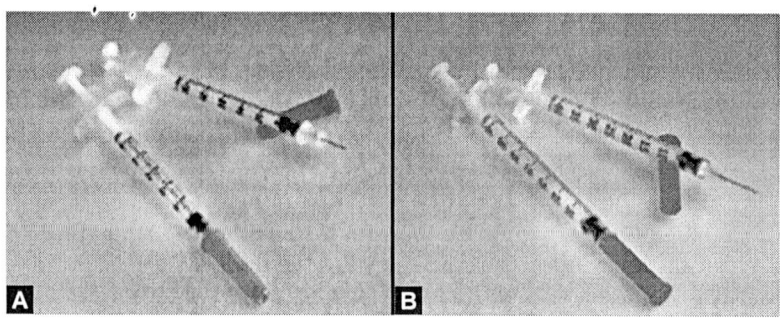

**FIGS. 1A AND B:** (A) U/100 syringe and (B) U/40 syringe. *(For color version, see Plate 5)*

These patients can have a prolonged or recurrent hypoglycemia and thus require close observation and repeated blood glucose estimations up to 48 hours. If IV access is difficult, 1 mg of glucagon should be injected subcutaneously or intramuscularly (IM). The relatives of patients prone to get severe hypoglycemia, particularly those who do not have warning hypoglycemic symptoms, should be instructed to keep a vial of glucagon handy and inject it during hypoglycemic emergency.

The management of diabetes is a balancing act between tight glycemic control and episodes of hypoglycemia. Tighter the control, lesser the complications—but at the cost of higher chances of hypoglycemia as clearly shown in the graph **(Fig. 2)**. The treating clinician should be shrewd and experienced to set individual goals depending upon variables, such as age, comorbid conditions, life expectancy, patient's attitude and support system, etc., and then achieve the goal by carefully selecting antidiabetic agents to suit individual needs and giving detailed education about lifestyle from the point of view of avoiding hypoglycemia **(Fig. 3)**.

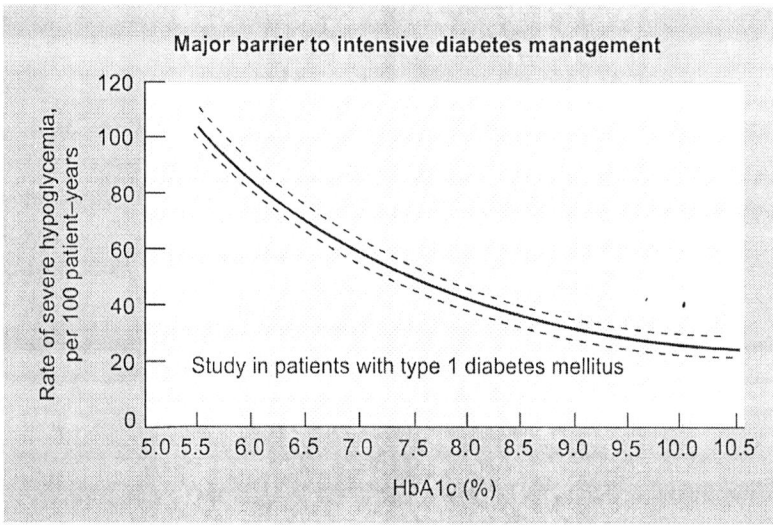

**FIG. 2:** Rate of severe hypoglycemia increases as glycated hemoglobin (HbA1c) levels decrease in patients with diabetes.

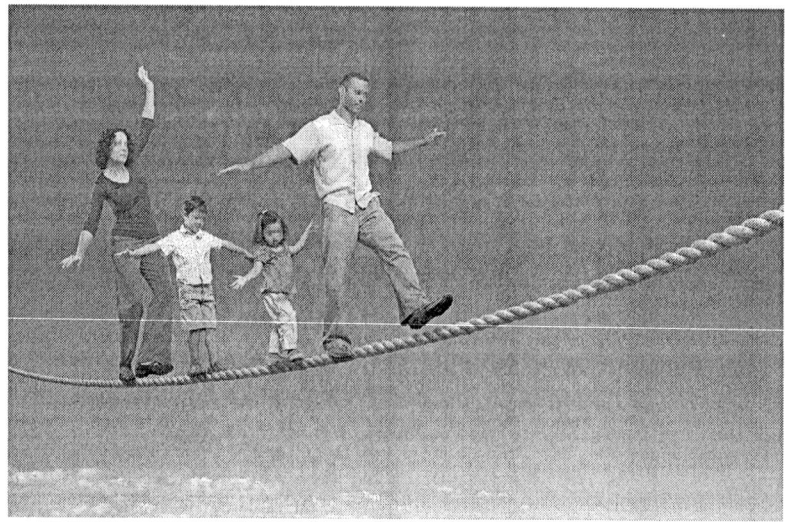

**FIG. 3:** The management of diabetes is balancing tight glycemic control and hypoglycemia.

## DIABETIC KETOACIDOSIS AND COMA

This complication is much more common in type 1 diabetes mellitus (T1DM) as compared to type 2 diabetes mellitus and occurs when insulin is withdrawn or when diagnosis is delayed. Sometimes, it develops in poorly controlled type 2 diabetic patients when severe insulin resistance develops as a result of serious complications such as myocardial infarction, septicemia, or disseminated tuberculosis, particularly during poor glycemic control. The patients present with symptoms of poor control, such as polyuria, polydipsia, extreme weakness, in addition to symptoms of associated complication. In addition, they have deep rapid breathing due to acidosis.

If the condition is not swiftly diagnosed and treatment is delayed, dehydration and hypotension set in leading to poor tissue perfusion, electrolyte disturbances, multiorgan failure, and ultimately coma. Patients in diabetic ketoacidosis and coma require immediate hospitalization in a well-equipped hospital and expert management. The four cornerstones of management are: (1) correction of fluid deficit, (2) administration of insulin in IV infusion, (3) correction of electrolyte imbalance, and

(4) identification and management of associated underlying factor. Hourly monitoring of blood glucose, blood pressure, central venous pressure, urine output, level of consciousness and frequent monitoring of electrolytes, creatinine, and blood gases is required. As this book is aimed at family physicians and general duty medical officers working in outpatient setup, details of indoor management of diabetic ketoacidosis are beyond its scope. We will tackle diagnosis and immediate management while awaiting hospitalization.

## Diagnosis of Diabetic Ketoacidosis

In a dehydrated, hypotensive, ill-looking diabetic patient, random blood glucose, urine for glucose, and ketones should be done on the spot. Dry strips and reliable glucometer for blood glucose estimation and dry strips for urine glucose and ketone estimation should form part of essential equipment in every outpatient clinic outside hospital setup and should be carried in emergency bag when on visit. Under the above-mentioned setting, severe hyperglycemia, glycosuria, and ketonuria indicate diabetic ketosis. Even if urine is not available for examination, severe hyperglycemia under such a setting is an indication for immediate hospitalization for confirmation of diagnosis and further management. Since occasionally, ketoacidosis can be a first manifestation of T1DM, one should estimate random blood glucose in every seriously ill patient soon after he is brought in the clinic.

## Treatment while Awaiting Hospitalization

- After confirming severe hyperglycemia and glycosuria, six units of short-acting insulin should be given IM or IV while awaiting hospitalization (subcutaneous insulin is absorbed very slowly in a hypotensive patient).
- Intravenous access should be established and normal saline should be started at a rapid rate. In severely dehydrated and shocked patient, first pint should be given over 1 hour. In elderly and in those with cardiac decompensation, the infusion rate should be slower. The second pint should run over 2 hours. The rate of administration of IV normal saline should be guided by blood pressure, urine output, and tolerance to IV fluids. Ideally, the patient should reach hospital within <1 hour.

**TABLE 3:** Differential diagnosis of diabetic and hypoglycemic coma.

| Characteristics | Hypoglycemia | Diabetic coma |
|---|---|---|
| Onset | Sudden | Slow |
| Skin | Moist | Dry |
| Signs and symptoms | Tremors, sweating, hunger, confusion, weakness | Nausea, vomiting, rapid breathing, dehydration |
| Blood glucose | <50 mg% | High |
| Urine glucose | Usually absent | ++++ |
| Urine ketones | Absent | Present |

- In febrile patient and in those having obvious infective focus, a full dose of appropriate antibiotic should be administered IV.
- Administration of sodium bicarbonate is contraindicated unless the patient is severely hypotensive and/or has severe acidosis (pH <7.1) **(Table 3)**.

*Note:* In case of doubt and nonavailability of blood glucose monitoring equipment, do not hesitate, shoot 50 mL 25% glucose. Swift recovery would confirm hypoglycemic coma while lack of any significant improvement would rule it out and indirectly support the diagnosis of diabetic coma without significantly worsening it.

## NONKETOTIC HYPEROSMOLAR HYPERGLYCEMIC STATE

This complication is less common than diabetic ketoacidosis and always develops in type 2 diabetic patients and can occasionally be its first manifestation. It is not as rare as many clinicians believe. Many cases are missed due to lack of awareness about the condition as well as laboratory tests required to diagnose it. Myocardial infarction, stroke, septicemia, and drugs, such as diuretics and mannitol, are some of the precipitating causes. The characteristic features of nonketotic hyperosmolar hyperglycemia (NKHH) are:
- *Severe hyperglycemia:* Blood glucose is usually above 600 mg%, values above 1,000 mg% are not uncommon.
- Ketoacidosis is conspicuous by absence. Urinary ketone is either absent or present in insignificant quantity. Thus,

acidotic breathing is absent. In these patients, there is severe insulin resistance which, in association with β-cell defect, is responsible for severe hyperglycemia. However, the small amount of insulin secreted by β-cells, even though not sufficient to control blood glucose, is sufficient to prevent excessive fat breakdown because fat cells are not severely insulin resistant in these cases, thus ketoacidosis does not develop. This also explains why NKHH develops only in type 2 diabetic patients and not in type 1 diabetic patients because in the latter, there is no endogenous insulin to prevent fat breakdown.

- *Profound dehydration:* NKHH is associated with breakdown of thirst mechanism, thus dehydration is profound and associated with hypotension and inadequate tissue perfusion. Many patients present with acute neurological manifestations that include confusion, irritability, abnormal behavior, hemiplegia, convulsions, and ultimately coma.
- *High plasma osmolarity:* In NKHH, plasma osmolarity is >340 mOsm/L. In case, facilities to estimate osmolarity are not available, it can be derived from following formula.

Plasma osmolarity = 2 (Na + K) in mEq/L + blood glucose in mg%/18 + blood urea nitrogen in mg%/2.8

## Clinical Features

One should suspect NKHH in elderly diabetic patients with severe dehydration, hypotension, and acute neurological manifestations associated with severe hyperglycemia and absence of severe ketonuria. One should also keep in mind that occasionally, it could be the first manifestation of diabetes. If one does random blood glucose on the spot in all medical emergencies, irrespective of whether there is a history of diabetes or not, one can pick up cases of NKHH, which carry much higher mortality as compared to diabetic ketoacidosis and coma.

## Management of Nonketotic Hyperosmolar Hyperglycemia

Immediate hospitalization in well-equipped setup is mandatory. Once hospitalized, dehydration should be rapidly corrected by administering 0.45% saline. However, in those with significant hypotension, normal saline should be infused initially. First 1 L should be infused over 1 hour and next liter over 2-3 hours. Subsequent infusion rate should be adjusted as per central venous pressure, urine output, and blood pressure. Average fluid loss is around 9 L. Insulin should be given in IV infusion form. Usually, 5-6 units/h are required in the initial period. IV insulin infusion should be preceded by administering 8 units of insulin bolus intravenously.

General principles of management and monitoring of NKHH are same as diabetic ketoacidosis.

## LACTIC ACIDOSIS

Acidosis due to excessive accumulation of lactic acid in blood is known as lactic acidosis. For diagnosis of lactic acidosis, blood pH should be 7.2 or less, blood lactate concentration persistently above 5 mm and symptoms of acidosis should be present. Mere transient rise in blood lactate level is not sufficient for the diagnosis of lactic acidosis. There are many conditions which lead to lactic acidosis. Severe tissue hypoxia following shock (e.g., cardiogenic shock and septicemic shock) and biguanide administration are some important causative factors in the field of diabetology. Lactic acidosis is extremely rare but life-threatening complication of biguanide therapy. Among the biguanides, it is six times more common with phenformin as compared to metformin. Thus, phenformin was either banned or voluntarily withdrawn from most of the countries including India. Italy is the only advanced country where it is still available. If 33,000 patients are treated with metformin for 1 year, one patient is likely to develop metformin-induced lactic acidosis. In the western countries, mortality of biguanide-induced lactic acidosis is 50-60%, even after quick diagnosis and immediate treatment. In our country, it is believed that due to lack of awareness about the condition, some cases are being missed.

Lactic acidosis is more common in those on phenformin than metformin. In most cases, biguanide-induced lactic acidosis has developed following use of these agents, in spite of contraindication to their use or their use in supratherapeutic dosages. Hepatic and renal failure, heavy consumption of alcohol while on biguanides, significantly compromised left ventricular function, and severe bronchial asthma and chronic obstructive pulmonary disease (COPD) (acute exacerbation in patients with these disorders produces tissue hypoxia, which acts as predisposing factor for lactic acidosis in patients on biguanides) are contraindications to the use of biguanides. A noteworthy feature about phenformin-induced lactic acidosis is that, in an occasional case, it has occurred even in those patients in whom phenformin was correctly prescribed. As far as metformin is concerned, in all the cases of documented lactic acidosis, metformin was used either when clear contraindications to its use existed or it was used in high dosages and thus lactic acidosis was avoidable. While phenformin is lipophilic and is metabolized in liver before its excretion from the kidneys, metformin is less lipophilic and is directly excreted by the kidneys. These pharmacological differences between the two biguanides explain the relative safety of metformin over phenformin as regards lactic acidosis. Thus, phenformin was banned or voluntarily withdrawn from the market in most of the advanced countries between 1978 and 1980.

## Clinical Features and Laboratory Investigations

Symptoms of biguanide-induced lactic acidosis are nonspecific. Restlessness, upper abdominal discomfort, vomiting, deep rapid acidotic breathing, and drowsiness are common. Unless the clinician is aware of the condition, he is unlikely to arrive at the diagnosis. Thus, whenever a diabetic on biguanides presents with abovementioned symptoms or presents with unexplained deterioration in general condition, biguanide-induced lactic acidosis must be considered in differential diagnosis.

Plasma lactate and pyruvate should be estimated in suspected cases. They are elevated in lactic acidosis. If facilities to measure lactate and pyruvate are not available, acidosis should be confirmed by estimating blood pH and diabetic ketoacidosis and uremia should be ruled out by estimating blood glucose, urine or blood ketones, and serum creatinine. If these conditions are ruled out and if there is no history suggestive of aspirin poisoning, diagnosis of lactic acidosis can be confidently made. Even at a district level hospital, one can make a diagnosis of lactic acidosis with reasonable certainty. This is how one should proceed: Estimate sodium, chlorides, and bicarbonates in blood and calculate "anion gap".

$$\text{Anion gap} = [(Na) - (Cl + HCO_3)] \text{ in mEq/L}$$

The normal value is <16. Values >22 are suggestive of metabolic acidosis. In a diabetic patient on biguanides and having anion gap of >22, if diabetic ketoacidosis and uremia are ruled out, one can confidently make a diagnosis of lactic acidosis.

## Prevention of Biguanide-induced Lactic Acidosis

Since the mortality of this condition is 50–60%, in spite of prompt diagnosis and immediate treatment in well-equipped setup, the emphasis should be on its prevention.
Following precautions should be taken to prevent biguanide-induced lactic acidosis.

- Do not use biguanides in hepatic and renal insufficiency and in those consuming large amount of alcohol.
- Monitor serum creatinine and estimated glomerular filtration rate (eGFR) yearly and discontinue biguanides when GFR falls below 30 mL/min.
- Use minimal effective dose of biguanides and try to reduce it in well-controlled patients.
- Avoid use of biguanides in those with severe proliferative diabetic retinopathy because usually these patients have diabetic nephropathy and serum creatinine is not a sensitive test to detect early nephropathy.

## Treatment of Suspected Cases of Biguanide-induced Lactic Acidosis in Clinic Setup

Promptly withdraw biguanides and send the patient to well-equipped hospital. While awaiting hospitalization, diabetic ketoacidosis, and hypoglycemia should be ruled out and cardiovascular system should be assessed clinically and electrocardiogram should be taken. If diagnosis of acidosis is confidently made on clinical grounds and ketoacidosis ruled out, 50 mL of 7.5% sodium bicarbonate should be given intravenously.

After hospitalization patient should be assessed in details and sodium bicarbonate should be repeated as required. In some centers, IV glucose-insulin infusion is given, while in other centers, tris-hydroxymethyl aminomethane (THAM) and methylene blue are used as buffers. If required, patients should be put on urgent hemodialysis.

# CHAPTER 19

# Chronic Complications of Diabetes

## INTRODUCTION

These are usually seen in long-standing and poorly controlled diabetics. They are classified as follows: (1) microvascular complications, (2) macrovascular complications, (3) Nonalcoholic fatty liver disease (NAFLD), (4) associated infections, and (5) musculoskeletal complications.

A brief information on various chronic complications of diabetes follows. Please note that while discussing the management of these complications, the emphasis in on preventive management which has to be continuously carried out in primary care physician's clinic. The discussion on specific therapeutic management of complications is beyond the scope of this book and thus not discussed here [e.g., details about vitrectomy, dialysis, cardiac interventions, etc.]. Primary care physician is an important member of team and has a role to play in the form of coordination between a system specialist and the patient.

## MICROVASCULAR COMPLICATIONS

Microvascular disease in a diabetic is a specific complication affecting the small blood vessels predominantly in the retina (diabetic retinopathy), kidneys (diabetic nephropathy), and nerves (diabetic neuropathy including autonomic neuropathy). From a histopathological point of view, the lesions are specific and not reproduced in any other disorder. Essentially, they consist of thickening of capillary basement membrane. The microvascular complications of diabetes have high morbidity and mortality.

Microvascular complications develop about 5 years after the onset of diabetes, particularly if metabolic control is inadequate. Thus, first screening for microvascular complications should be done 5 years after the onset in type 1 diabetic patients. Since type 2 diabetes mellitus (T2DM) is slowly progressive disease, it can remain undetected for a few years after the onset. Thus, in these patients, screening for microvascular disease should be done immediately after the diagnosis. About 30% of type 2 diabetic patients show some evidence of microvascular disease at the time of diagnosis.

It has now been proved beyond any doubt that these microvascular complications can be prevented or postponed by continuous meticulous control of blood glucose [Diabetes Control and Complications Trial (DCCT) and United Kingdom Prospective Diabetes Study (UKPDS)]. This information should be given to all diabetic patients from time-to-time, in order to motivate them for regular follow-up **(Fig. 1)**.

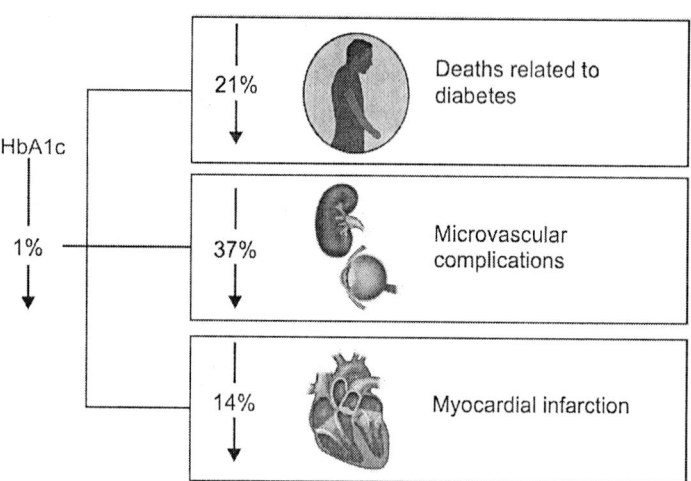

**FIG. 1:** Result from United Kingdom Prospective Diabetes Study (UKPDS): lowering glycated hemoglobin (HbA1c) reduces the risk of complications.

*Source:* Stratton IM, Adler AI, Neil HA, Matthews DR, Manley SE, Cull CA, et al. Association of glycemia with macro vascular and micro vascular complications of type 2 diabetes (UKPDS 35): prospective observational study. BMJ. 2000;321(7258):405-12.

## Management of Diabetic Retinopathy

### Prevention

- Maintain continuous metabolic control by appropriate treatment with diet, exercise, and medication [fasting and premeal blood glucose <110 mg%, postmeal blood glucose <180 mg%, and glycated hemoglobin (HbA1c) <7%]
- Meticulous control of hypertension [blood pressure (BP) should be <130/80 mm Hg)]
- All diabetic patients should undergo yearly ophthalmic evaluation so that early retinopathy is detected. At the appropriate time, patients having significant retinopathy should undergo laser photocoagulation to prevent further deterioration in visual acuity.
- Antiplatelet agent—aspirin, angiotensin-converting enzyme (ACE) inhibitors, such as ramipril and statins have some role in prevention of diabetic retinopathy.
- Primary care physician should coordinate between the patient and his retinologist for further treatment [intravitreal injection of vascular growth factor inhibitors such as ranibizumab (Lucentis) and bevacizumab (Aventis) and for surgical procedures such as vitrectomy].

## Management of Diabetic Nephropathy

- Continuous meticulous control of blood glucose
- Control of blood pressure
- Yearly serum creatinine and glomerular filtration rate (GFR), and urinary albumin/creatinine ratio
- In those who have borderline or high serum creatinine, avoid all nephrotoxic drugs, i.e., aminoglycosides (gentamicin, amikacin, etc.), and nonsteroidal anti-inflammatory drugs.
- Prompt control of urinary tract infections
- In those in whom nephropathy has developed, low protein, and potassium diet should be given (reduce milk, meat, *dal*, citrus fruits, and coconut water). Avoid potassium-sparing diuretics (e.g., spironolactone), if in a given patient, one is not able to keep serum potassium at desired level.

- All patients with diabetic nephropathy should be jointly managed in consultation with a diabetologist and a nephrologist. Review all the antidiabetic medicines and discontinue those contraindicated in renal insufficiency. In patients with advancing renal insufficiency, antidiabetic medications including insulin undergo slow metabolism and hence the dosage needs to be reduced. These patients are likely to develop repeated hypoglycemia if regular blood glucose estimation and adjustment of insulin and SU dosage are not done. In those with end-stage renal failure, kidney transplantation or repeated hemodialysis (usually 2–3 times a week) is required. Continuous ambulatory peritoneal dialysis is an alternative to hemodialysis.

- Those with raised urinary albumin/creatinine ratio should be put on small dose of ACE inhibitors or angiotensin receptor blockers (ARBs), even if blood pressure is within normal limits. This will help to prevent or slow down progression to macroalbuminuria and frank diabetic nephropathy. In those already in early nephropathy stage, use of these agents will delay the onset of end-stage renal failure. ACE inhibitors have stronger evidence in type 1 diabetes mellitus (T1DM), while ARBs have stronger evidence in T2DM.

Sodium-glucose cotransporter-2 inhibitors ($SGLT_2Is$) have excellent renoprotective properties and they should be added to slow down the deterioration of diabetic nephropathy. If the blood glucose control is good, one can reduce the dose of other antidiabetic medications to create a space for $SGLT_2I$. It should be noted that these agents loose part of their glycemic efficacy in patients with renal impairment.

*Finerenone*: This is the latest mineralocorticoid receptor antagonist (MRA) with a structure which is nonsteroidal, thus side effects such as gynecomastia are lower than spironolactone. Its excellent renoprotective properties have been recently proved in a major trial: Finerenone in prevention of progression or diabetic kidney disease and cardiovascular events, in T2DM patients with DKD. It was given in the dosage of 10–20 mg once a day. One needs to closely monitor serum potassium levels and finerenone has to be discontinued if hyperkalemia develops, it also significantly reduced composite of cardiovascular death, nonfatal myocardial infarction, nonfatal stroke and hospitalization for heart failure. We will hear a lot on this promising agent in future. It is being used along with $SGLT_2I$ and renin-angiotensin-aldosterone system (RAAS) blockers for renoprotection and cardiovascular protection, particularly for heart failure protection in T2DM patients with DKD. Recently, finerenone was introduced in India, soon after its international launch.

## Management of Diabetic Neuropathy

- Meticulous blood glucose control
- For control of paresthesia, antidepressants, and antiepileptics such as carbamazepine are often useful. Duloxetine and pregabalin are effective in controlling painful symptom.
- *Control of postural hypotension*:
  - Train the patient to stand up gradually in three steps:
    1. Move the lower limb up and down in lying down position 5-6 times
    2. Sit up and move the legs forward and backward
    3. Gradually stand up
  - Use of elastic crepe bandages from ankle to the knee during the daytime
  - While sleeping, the head should be propped up so that when getting up in the morning, the degree of postural drop in BP is reduced.
  - Use antihypertensive agents which do not aggravate the postural drop (e.g., ACE inhibitors).
  - Use of 5-fludrocortisone orally
  - Meticulous foot care (refer to appendix)

## MACROVASCULAR COMPLICATIONS OF DIABETES

Prevalence of coronary artery disease, peripheral vascular disease as well as cerebrovascular disease is much higher in diabetic patients as compared to nondiabetic patients. The basic underlying factor for all these complications is atherosclerosis, which is accelerated in diabetic patients, thus leading to increased prevalence of macrovascular disease.

In addition, hypertension is also much more common in diabetic patients than in nondiabetic patients and it further accelerates macrovascular disease. Uncontrolled diabetes is associated with an atherogenic dyslipidemia consisting of low high-density lipoprotein (HDL) cholesterol, high triglycerides, and high small dense low-density lipoprotein (LDL) particles, thus further aggravating the problem. Many T2DM patients have insulin resistance at tissue level, which leads to hyperinsulinemia, which further aggravates atherosclerosis.

## General Principles of Management of Macrovascular Disease in Diabetics

- Meticulous control of blood glucose and plasma lipids by prudent diet, exercise, weight reduction, and appropriate antidiabetic and lipid-reducing medications.

Since we know that hyperinsulinemia could accelerate atherosclerosis and many type 2 diabetic patients have inbuilt hyperinsulinemia, we should take care to prevent further aggravation of this problem by producing therapeutic hyperinsulinemia. Hence, the selection of the medication is important. In insulin-requiring diabetics, we should judiciously use insulin and should have patience while increasing the dosage of insulin, in order to avoid hyperinsulinemia. Moreover, since obesity is associated with insulin resistance, it is very important to prescribe appropriate diet and exercise so as to control weight and insulin resistance. As far as oral antidiabetic drugs (OADs) are concerned, metformin, and dipeptidyl peptidase-4 inhibitors ($DPP_4Is$) are weight neutral, while glucagon-like peptide-1 receptor agonists ($GLP_1RAs$) and $SGLT_2I$ significantly reduce weight. Sulfonylureas (SUs), pioglitazone, and insulin are associated with weight gain.

- Meticulous control of hypertension (if present). Selection of antihypertensive medication is very important (please refer to Chapter 21).
- Avoidance of tobacco in any form.

In addition to general measures which are applicable to all patients having macrovascular diseases, specific treatment should be carried out, depending upon the organ and site involved.

## NONALCOHOLIC FATTY LIVER DISEASE

Nonalcoholic fatty liver disease (NAFLD) is a condition in which excess fat is accumulated in the liver. This build-up of fat is not caused by heavy alcohol use. When heavy alcohol use causes fat to build-up in the liver, this condition is called alcohol-associated liver disease (heavy alcohol use is defined as >21 standard drinks/week in men and >14 standard drinks/week in women in the USA, and >30 g of alcohol/week in men and >20 g of alcohol/week in women in Europe).

Nonalcoholic fatty liver disease has struck the globe in the form of pandemic and unlike COVID pandemic; it is not going to abate in near future. It is a chronic progressive lifestyle metabolic diseases and is closely associated with other lifestyle and metabolic disorders such as obesity, T2DM, metabolic syndrome, etc. In many countries, NAFLD has already become the most common chronic liver disease. It is estimated that the global prevalence of NAFLD is 32.4% in general population and 55.5% in T2DM patients. Since obesity and insulin resistance are the main drivers of NAFLD, it is not at all surprising that it is strongly associated with T2DM. We do not have national level data on prevalence of NAFLD in our country.

The main underlying pathophysiological feature is insulin resistance. Excessive lipolysis, increased synthesis of triglycerides, and increased uptake in liver leads to fatty infiltration of liver. Many share features of metabolic syndrome. In T2DM patients with similar HbA1c, it is more common in those who have higher insulin resistance.

If adequate precautions are not taken to improve the faulty lifestyle, NAFLD progresses through following steps:
- *Fatty infiltration of liver*: In this stage, there is excessive fat accumulation in the liver but inflammation is absent. Patients are usually asymptomatic and hepatomegaly is picked up on routine physical examination and on abdominal ultrasound examination. Liver function tests are normal or liver enzymes, particularly serum glutamic pyruvic transaminase (SGPT) is mildly elevated.

- *Nonalcoholic steatohepatitis (NASH)*: In this stage, there are inflammatory changes in the liver and enzymes are usually raised mildly. Many patients are still asymptomatic at this stage; some may have mild pain in right hypochondrium and indigestion.
- *Hepatic fibrosis*: In this stage, some of the liver parenchymal cells are destroyed and replaced by fibrous cells, which do not have any capacity to carry out liver functions. Consistency of liver is changed from soft to firm and the size starts shrinking. The functional capacity of liver gradually deteriorates, serum albumin level goes down, and prothrombin time may be elevated. Increased levels of liver fibrosis can be picked up by ultrasound examination and more precisely by liver fibroscan.
- *Cirrhosis of liver*: Liver fibrosis is an irreversible process but it can be halted by adequate measures including weight reduction through aggressive diet and exercise and simultaneous management of glycemic derangement. If these parameters are unsuccessfully managed, fibrosis progresses and cirrhosis of liver results. Further worsening leads to gradually increasing portal hypertension, which is manifested through splenomegaly, anemia due to blood loss from esophageal varices, and thrombocytopenia resulting from hypersplenism. Cirrhosis of liver is a predisposing factor for subsequent development of hepatocellular carcinoma.

At all stages, patients with NAFLD are more prone to develop atherosclerotic cardiovascular disorders.

## Diagnosis of NAFLD

Clinically NAFLD is picked up in patients with soft hepatomegaly after ruling out other possibilities by history and appropriate investigations. Elevation of liver enzymes including SGPT is not very sensitive or specific test for diagnosis of NAFLD. Ultrasound examination of abdomen done for some other reason or done as a routine screening tests in health checkup picks up many patients. Many fibrosis scoring systems based on clinical and laboratory parameters are used. Elastography is an enhanced form of ultrasonography which is semiquantitative measure of liver elasticity which is proportionately affected depending upon degree of fibrosis. MRI elastography is more sensitive. Liver biopsy is a gold standard but being invasive procedure, is rarely performed in real world situations.

## Management of NAFLD

Aggressive lifestyle changes through diet and exercise to reduce weight are important preventive steps.

For those with established disease, there are no approved or recommended drugs and several agents including almost all antidiabetic agents have been studied with varying degree of success. Among non-antidiabetic agents, vitamin E, vitamin A, omega-3 fatty acids, obeticholic acid, and ursodeoxycholic acid have some promise. Vitamin E however, has failed to show any benefits in those with diabetes. Among antidiabetic agents, metformin, $DPP_4I$, $SGLT_2I$, and $GLP_1RAs$ have all shown some beneficial effects based on soft assessment methods such as biochemical, ultrasound, or fibrosis scoring parameters. Pioglitazone has been assessed with liver biopsy and has shown more promise, but it was tried only in relatively advanced biopsy proved cases and thus, this findings cannot be extrapolated in mild cases of NAFLD.

## Conclusion

NAFLD is very strongly associated with T2DM as both share insulin resistance as underlying pathophysiological factor. If not treated with measures to reduce weight through lifestyle changes such as diet and exercise, it progresses to cirrhosis of liver and occasionally to hepatocellular carcinoma. It is associated with acceleration of atherosclerotic cardiovascular disorders. Thus, making primary care physician aware of NAFLD and make early diagnosis and implement aggressive preventive measures is the need of the day.

## INFECTIONS IN DIABETES

Both acute and chronic infections are more common in diabetes. Hyperglycemia, defective immunity due to impaired function of polymorphonuclear leukocytes, and vascular lesions in the infected organs are some of the underlying factors for increased prevalence of infections in diabetes.

## Bacterial Infections

Some of the common infections in diabetes are as follows:
- Acute and chronic cholecystitis, including a fulminant variety called emphysematous cholecystitis **(Fig. 2)**
- Urinary tract infections, including lower urinary tract infections such as cystitis and upper urinary tract infections such as pyelonephritis, including a fulminant variety called emphysematous pyelonephritis
- Tuberculosis, including pulmonary tuberculosis. Peculiarities of pulmonary tuberculosis in a diabetic patient:
  ○ Lower lobe involvement is more common than nondiabetic patients.
  ○ As compared to the magnitude of symptoms of pulmonary tuberculosis, the size of radiological appearance on chest X-ray is larger and is suggestive of consolidation.
  ○ Drug resistance more common than nondiabetic patients.
- Skin and soft tissue infections such as cellulitis, necrotizing fasciitis, furuncles, abscess, Fournier's gangrene of the skin of scrotum, carbuncles, etc. **(Figs. 3 to 5)**.
- Diabetic foot infections **(Fig. 6)**

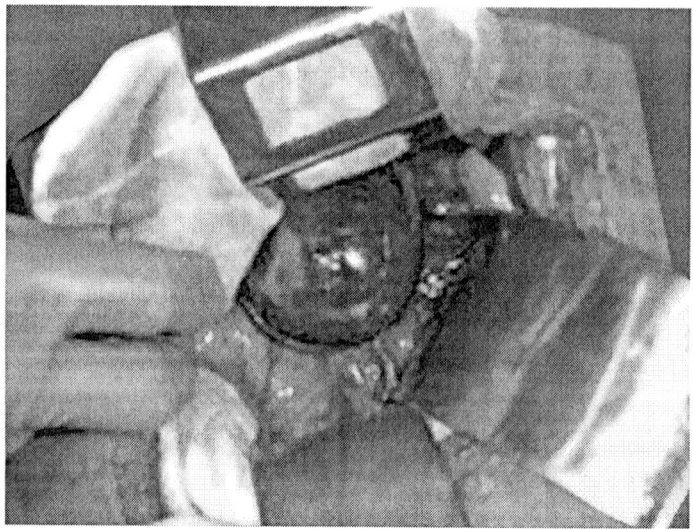

**FIG. 2:** Fulminant, gangrenous cholecystitis. *(For color version, see Plate 6)*

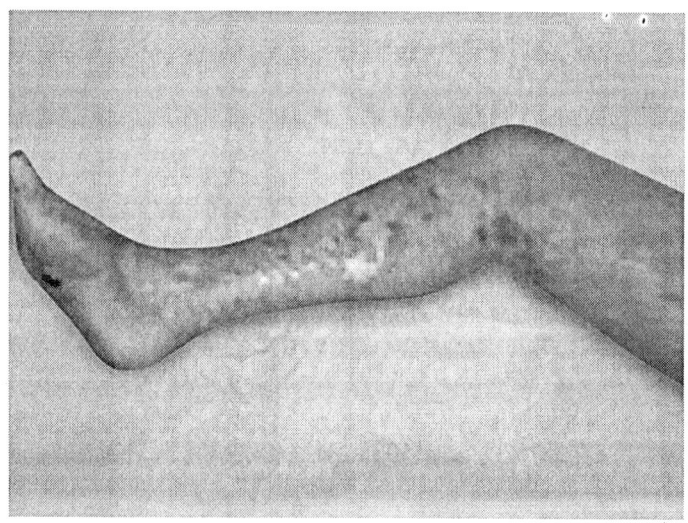

**FIG. 3:** Necrotizing fasciitis of right leg. *(For color version, see Plate 6)*

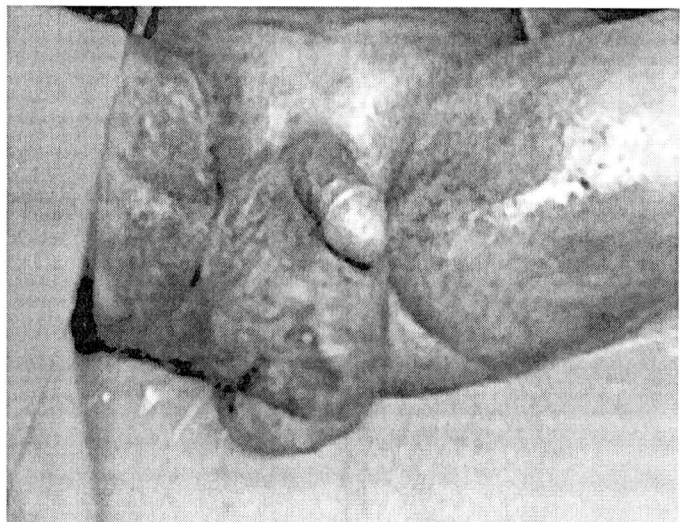

**FIG. 4:** Fournier's gangrene of scrotum. *(For color version, see Plate 7)*

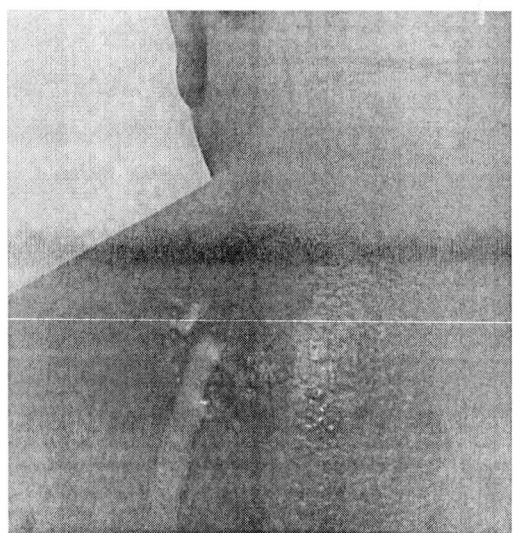

FIG. 5: A large carbuncle on the back. *(For color version, see Plate 7)*

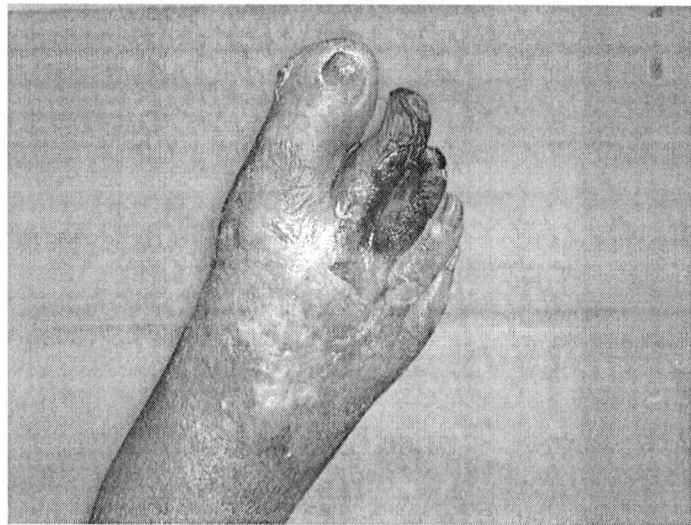

FIG. 6: Right foot abscess with gangrene of second and third toes. *(For color version, see Plate 8)*

## Fungal Infections

- Interdigital web space infections in feet and infections at skin-folds such as inguinal area and axilla
- Rhinocerebral mucormycosis
- Balanitis and balanoposthitis

## General Principles of Management of Infections in Diabetes

Infections worsen glycemic control due to resultant insulin resistance and poor glycemic control interferes with recovery from infections. To quickly pull the patient out of this vicious cycle, quick establishment of tight metabolic control is of paramount importance. Early initiation of insulin therapy in those not yet on insulin and intensification of insulin in those on insulin is needed. The general principles of management are same as in nondiabetic patients. These include appropriate empirical antibiotic administration (parenteral antibiotics should be preferred unless infection is mild and localized), adequate and early drainage whenever pus is present, dispatch of biological material for culture and change of antibiotics if required after receiving culture report, along with rest and elevation whenever appropriate as in lower limb infections.

## MUSCULOSKELETAL AND RHEUMATOLOGIC COMPLICATIONS OF DIABETES

Several musculoskeletal and connective tissue disorders are associated with diabetes. Usually, long-standing, poorly controlled diabetics are affected. Glycosylation of various proteins, including collagen, micro- and macrovascular involvement of affected organs are some of the underlying pathophysiological factors.

Some of the common musculoskeletal and connective tissue disorders associated with diabetes:
- Diabetic stiff hand syndrome, also known as diabetic cheiroarthropathy or limited joint mobility syndrome. The skin of hand and fingers is stiff, waxy, and shiny and mobility

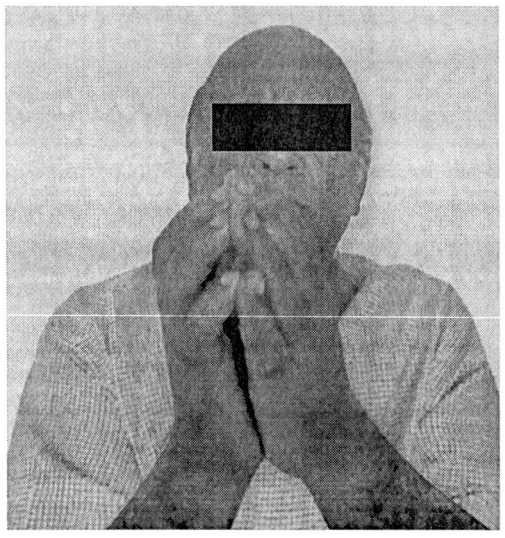

**FIG. 7:** *Namaste* sign: Cheiroarthropathy and limited joint mobility in a long-standing diabetic, leading to inability to fully extend the fingers at interphalangeal joints. This is best demonstrated as in picture above, by asking the patients to place the palms of both hands together. *(For color version, see Plate 8)*

*Note:* Inability to attain classical *Namaste* posture.

of small joints of hands is limited. When the patient tries to hold both hands in *"Namaste"* position, a gap remains between the fingers of both hands due to limited joint mobility (positive *Namaste* sign) **(Fig. 7)**
- Flexor tenosynovitis of fingers in hand
- Dupuytren's contracture of fingers of hand results from shortening and fibrosis of palmar fascia
- Frozen shoulder or adhesive capsulitis of shoulder joint. This is one of the most common musculoskeletal involvements in a diabetic patient, affecting about 20% of the patients. It is due to reversible contracture of capsule of glenohumeral joint.
- Charcot foot (diabetic osteoarthropathy, also known as neuropathic arthropathy) is a condition involving destructive and lytic joint changes. It is a severe form of degenerative arthritis, resulting from loss of sensation due to underlying diabetic neuropathy in the involved joints. Pedel bones are most

commonly affected. Loss of sensation leads to inadvertent and unnoticed repeated microtrauma to the joints, which leads to degenerative changes.

## CONCLUSION

Diabetes commonly affects the musculoskeletal system, resulting in significant morbidity. These manifestations may go unrecognized or simply be overlooked in daily clinical practice. However, many of these rheumatological complications are treatable (to varying degrees), with resultant improvements in quality of life and more independence in activities of daily living. Thus, clinicians should be aware of the possible musculoskeletal complications of diabetes, in order to intervene and provide the best care for affected patients.

# CHAPTER 20

# The Diabetic Foot

## INTRODUCTION

The diabetic foot is one of the common complications of diabetes, often requiring prolonged hospitalization. Due to several factors including ignorance, apathy, poverty, etc., our patients having diabetic foot lesions reach appropriate specialized healthcare professionals with expertise, experience, and availability of infrastructural facilities required to treat complex diabetic foot, in more advanced stage of the disease as compared to those in developed world. Nearly 20% of the admissions for diabetic patients are for diabetic foot. Approximately 5–10% of all diabetic patients develop foot ulcers at least once in their lifetime and >50% of nontraumatic amputations of lower limbs are for foot complications in diabetic patients. Amputation of a part of lower limb is 15 times more common in diabetic patients as compared to general population. The morbidity and cost of treating foot complications are extremely high. In a developing and poor country like India, where very few people are covered by health insurance, such an expensive treatment is out of reach of most of the people. Thus, there is an urgent need to focus attention on prevention and early appropriate treatment of diabetic foot. So also is the need to do research on diabetes healthcare economics, and basic as well as clinical research.

## ETIOPATHOGENESIS

Since the etiology of lower limb complications in diabetic patient is multifactorial, the term "diabetic foot" has been coined to encompass a multitude of leg and foot presentations, where the underlying disease is diabetes mellitus. The major factors involved in the causation are poor metabolic control, ischemia, neuropathy, infection, and delayed wound healing. Most of the patients with diabetic foot have chronic, poorly controlled metabolic status. The atherosclerotic process in diabetics is accelerated, multisegmental with predilection for vessels below popliteal artery. The process is often bilateral. Dyslipidemia and tobacco consumption, if present, further worsen the problem. Diabetic peripheral neuropathy leads to impaired sensations in the lower limb. This makes the foot vulnerable to trauma due to mechanical, chemical, and thermal factors, leading to ulceration. Loss of proprioception and muscle atrophy due to motor neuropathy leads to foot deformities. The change in foot configuration with new pressure points leads to callous formation and subsequent ulceration. Autonomic neuropathy leads to dry fissured skin, offering portals of entry for microorganisms. These are important contributory factors for foot infections. The foot infections **(Fig. 1)** are the major cause of limb loss. One of the major consequences of nonhealing foot ulcer is osteomyelitis of tarsal and metatarsal bones. Mixed infections are common and often staphylococci are associated with aerobic or anaerobic streptococci, or with one of the Enterobacteriaceae, viz., *Escherichia coli, Klebsiella, Proteus, Enterobacter,* etc. **(Fig. 2)**.

## PREVENTION

Since diabetic foot considerably increases affected patient's economic burden, as regards direct as well as indirect costs, prevention and prompt treatment of minor diabetic foot lesions by taking appropriate foot care are vital. Persistent tight metabolic control is important to prevent or slow down progression of

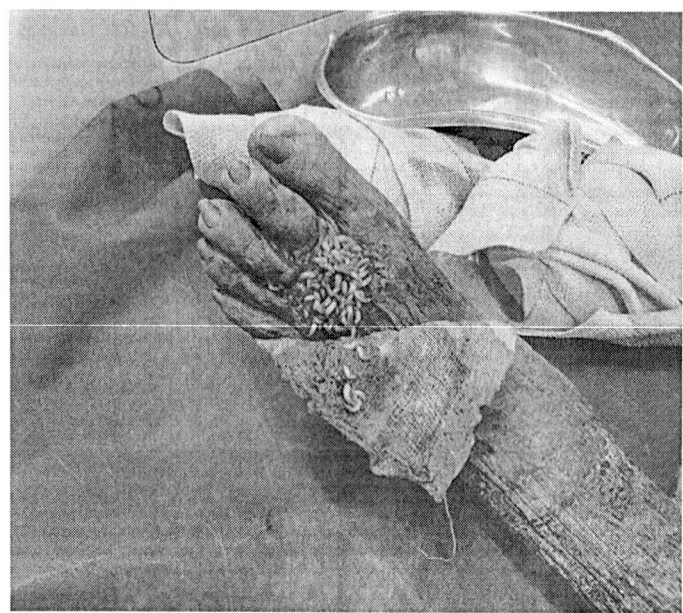

**FIG. 1:** Diabetic foot infested with maggots. *(For color version, see Plate 9)*

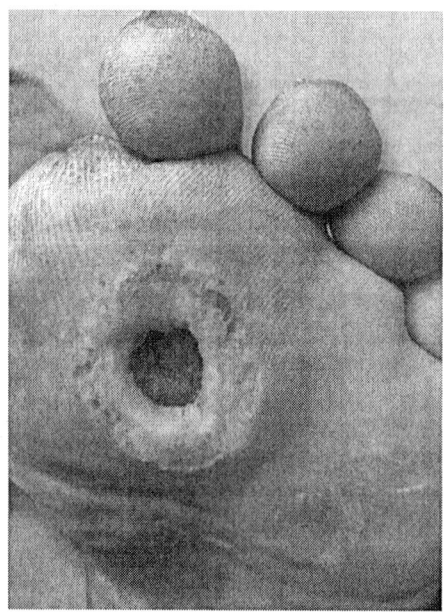

**FIG. 2:** A classical neuropathic foot ulcer on left sole. *(For color version, see Plate 9)*

diabetic neuropathy. Normalization of blood pressure in those who are hypertensive, correction of dyslipidemia, if present, and abstinence from tobacco will go a long way in controlling atherosclerotic process. Thus, the role of structured, therapeutic, and in-depth patient education program need not be stressed.

## MANAGEMENT

Management of diabetic foot requires multidisciplinary approach and needs to be individualized depending upon the case. Those who are nontoxic and afebrile at presentation and in those who do not have deep-seated infection, osteomyelitis, or gangrene, can be treated on outpatient basis with oral antibiotics, rest, elevation of affected part, and appropriate wound care. However, since clinical picture is often deceptive in diabetic foot infections, a close watch is often mandatory. Deterioration of metabolic status, persistence of leukocytosis, and lack of improvement in clinical status are indications for indoor treatment. Some patients with apparently minor lesions with mild visible signs of inflammation, absent evidence of bone involvement on X-ray but persistent leukocytosis, nonhealing of overlying ulcer, if present, need further investigations such as magnetic resonance imaging (MRI) of the affected area, lower limb arterial Doppler, and lower limb arterial angiography. Hospitalization and parenteral antibiotics are required in patients who are toxic and acutely ill and have complicated infections with osteomyelitis and in those who have failed to respond to oral antibiotics. The choice of antibiotics will depend on clinical judgment regarding the severity, duration, rate of progression, and the probable pathogenic flora. Since, the mixed infections are common, it is prudent to administer a combination of antibiotics. Besides immobilization and elevation of the affected limb, early surgical incision and adequate drainage are very important. It provides material for bacterial culture and antibiotic sensitivity, and releases pressure, thus improving local circulation. The surgical procedure should be performed early, preferably within 24–48 hours after hospitalization. The intervening period should be utilized to establish reasonable blood glucose control and correction of ketosis, if present, with insulin administration, and to assess the status of various organs, and to stabilize cardiovascular system. It is not necessary to wait for ideal blood glucose control, which in any case is difficult, unless infection is controlled with adequate drainage and appropriate antibiotics. Many of the severely infected diabetic foot cases have multiple complications at the time of admission. These include renal impairment, cardiac failure, septicemia, anemia, and acute respiratory distress syndrome (ARDS). Multidisciplinary team in intensive care units should manage these patients. After quick assessment and treatment with insulin and appropriate antibiotic combinations, the surgical procedures should be preferably carried out under local/regional anesthesia. Waiting too long in order to get ideal preoperative status and inadequate drainage are the major pitfalls. During the healing process, prevention of weight bearing is vital. Even when the foot lesion has healed, the job is not complete. The underlying conditions, such as foot deformities, calluses, and increased pressure, are still present. Thus, detailed training regarding foot care and prescription of appropriate footwear, considering the case-specific problems, is essential. The use of reconstructive surgery has evolved as a response to help lower the incidence of amputations of the lower limb in diabetic patients. Reconstructive surgery is indicated in following circumstances: (1) infection has been adequately drained and treated but the ulcer has not healed, (2) the arterial flow has been adequate initially or has been restored by bypass or angioplasty but the ulcer failed to heal, (3) pressure relieving techniques have not been successful, (4) in those who present very late with nonviable tissue, quick decisions regarding timing, and level of amputations are vital. When tissues are nonviable, early amputation at appropriate level saves life, and duration and cost of hospitalization. A joint assessment for operative fitness should be carried out and the informed consent should be taken. An anesthetist, experienced in diabetic foot cases, should be involved. Hyperbaric oxygen therapy (HBOT), rendered in specially designed chambers, is an adjunct to medical and surgical treatments in difficult and problematic cases with delayed wound healing. "vacuum-assisted closure (VAC)" suction therapy is a new modality increasingly used nowadays to expedite wound healing. In this method, surgically treated and debrided wound is sealed with foam dressing and is attached through suction tube to vacuum suction machine especially designed for the purpose. Continuous low pressure suction quickens separation of slough and leads to faster wound healing.

## CONCLUSION

Diabetic foot lesions are common in developing country like India. They reduce quality of life and drastically increase economic burden of the diabetic patient, and his family. A massive patient and primary physician education program for prevention and treatment at primary care level is the need of the day. Similarly, development of multidisciplinary teams at tertiary care centers and national collaborative clinical research programs on various aspects of diabetic foot are urgently required.

# CHAPTER 21

# Hypertension in Diabetes

## DEFINITION

Hypertension is defined as sustained systolic blood pressure of 130 mm Hg or greater and/or diastolic blood pressure of 80 mm Hg or greater. Hypertension is frequently associated with diabetes mellitus (DM). The prevalence of hypertension in diabetic population is twice that in nondiabetic population. Hypertension is recognized as a major risk factor for cardiovascular disease, so is diabetes. When both coexist, the risk is not merely added up, but compounded.

The pathogenesis of hypertension in type 1 diabetes mellitus (T1DM) differs from that in type 2 diabetes mellitus (T2DM). While in the former it is correlated to the onset of diabetic nephropathy, in the latter it is often present before the diagnosis of diabetes. It is often associated with insulin resistance and compensatory hyperinsulinemia, which leads to hypertension through a variety of mechanisms. Hypertension in diabetes is associated with increased mortality and morbidity from macrovascular as well as microvascular complications of diabetes.

Although lowering elevated blood pressure (BP) has beneficial effects in reducing hemorrhagic stroke and congestive heart failure, it may not extend equal beneficial effects as regards controlling progression of atherosclerosis. Ideal antihypertensive therapy should be effective to reduce BP to target of 130/80 mm Hg or below. It should be well tolerated and inexpensive. It should not worsen glycemic control and lipid levels and it should not adversely affect concomitant disorders, like peripheral vascular disease, gout, or bronchospastic disorders, such as bronchial asthma and chronic obstructive lung disease [chronic obstructive pulmonary disease (COPD)].

## BLOOD PRESSURE MEASUREMENT

Blood pressure should be measured in sitting position after 5 minutes rest. Patient's feet should be on ground and arm supported. Appropriate-sized cuff should be used. At initial visit, BP should also be recorded 2 minutes after standing for verification of postural hypotension. Subsequently, frequency of standing BP measurement should be individualized. BP should be recorded at each visit. Home BP monitoring should be strongly recommended to verify presence of "white coat hypertension" (high readings in medical settings, but BP readings in normal range at home), which is often overdiagnosed by the patient partly on imaginary basis without actually measuring the BP repeatedly at home; and also "masked hypertension" (BP in normal range at medical setting but in high range outside). In selected cases ambulatory BP monitoring should be advised.

## NOTE ON 8TH JOINT NATIONAL COMMITTEE GUIDELINES

In Joint National Committee (JNC) 8 guidelines, the focus has shifted from classification of hypertension to management of hypertension **(Table 1)**. These guidelines have diluted primacy given to thiazide diuretics as first-line treatment for hypertension and have listed thiazides, angiotensin-converting enzyme (ACE) inhibitors, angiotensin receptor blockers (ARBs), and calcium channel blockers (CCBs) as equal agents and advocated that any one of these four groups can be used as first-line agents, depending upon underlying situation. These guidelines recommend that BP should be brought down to <150/90 mm Hg in those above 60 years of age and <140/90 mm Hg in those who are younger than 60 years. There is no separate recommendation for diabetic patients. American Diabetes Association (ADA) recommends BP goal of <130/80 mm Hg in all diabetic patients irrespective of age.

**TABLE 1: Classification of blood pressure for adults as per Joint National Committee (JNC) 7 guidelines.**

| JNC 7 BP category | SBP (mm Hg) | DBP (mm Hg) | Treatment |
|---|---|---|---|
| Normal | <120 | and <80 | |
| Prehypertension | 120–139 | and 80–89 | Lifestyle change |
| Hypertension: Stage 1 | 140–159 | and/or 90–99 | Single drug |
| Hypertension: Stage 2 | ≥160 | and/or ≥100 | Two drugs |

*Note*: Utility of this table: Start with one-drug therapy for stage 1 hypertension and two-drug therapy for stage 2 hypertension.
(BP: blood pressure; DBP: diastolic blood pressure; SBP: systolic blood pressure)

## EPIDEMIOLOGY

Diabetes mellitus and hypertension are common disorders and prevalence of both rises with increase in age. They are frequently seen together in the same individual, suggesting a common pathogenic mechanism. Hypertension is twice as common in individuals with DM as compared to normal persons. In SL Raheja Hospital, Mumbai, hypertension was noted in 40% of all type 2 diabetic patients attending the outpatient department. In a survey done by the All India Institute of Medical Sciences at New Delhi and at Bengaluru in age-group 34–65 years, 25% men and 23% women had hypertension. Twenty percent of hypertensives and 7–8% normal people had diabetes. In Helsinki study, prevalence of hypertension was 30% in type 2 diabetic patients and 14% in normal population. Below the age of 50 years, prevalence of hypertension is higher in diabetic men than in women but after the age of 50 years, prevalence is higher in women than in men.

## TYPES OF HYPERTENSION IN DIABETES MELLITUS

Hypertension in patients with diabetes is divided in following subgroups:
- *Surgically curable hypertension ("adrenal hypertension") as in Cushing's disease, primary hyperaldosteronism, and pheochromocytoma*: In these conditions, both hypertension and diabetes

result from hyperfunction of endocrine organ and surgical treatment, leading to correction of hyperfunction which leads to normalization of both BP and blood glucose. This is rarest type of hypertension.

Hypertension due to renal artery stenosis can also be treated surgically or by nonsurgical intervention (renal artery angioplasty). In diabetes, atherosclerosis is accelerated and renovascular hypertension is more common than in general population.

- *Hypertension without diabetic nephropathy*:
  - *Isolated systolic hypertension:* Systolic BP of 160 mm Hg or more with diastolic BP below 90 mm Hg is defined as isolated systolic hypertension (ISH). ISH is more common in diabetic patients because of associated advanced atherosclerosis and resultant loss of arterial elasticity.

    In past, ISH was taken lightly by the medical profession due to prevailing belief that it is not as important as elevated diastolic blood pressure in pathogenesis of vascular complications. As per the current recommendations, ISH should be as aggressively treated as diastolic hypertension.
  - *Essential hypertension:* This is the most common type of hypertension in type 2 diabetic patients. The diagnosis of hypertension may precede, follow, or coincide with that of diabetes. Its pathogenesis is similar to that of essential hypertension in nondiabetics; however, additional factors may operate. In recent years, the role of insulin resistance in genesis of hypertension has evoked considerable interest.

    Insulin resistance results in hyperinsulinemia which predisposes to hypertension through a variety of mechanisms such as: (1) increased sympathetic activity, (2) increased sodium and water retention, (3) vascular smooth muscle proliferation, (4) altering sensitivity of vasculature to vasoactive substances, etc.
- *Hypertension in those with diabetic nephropathy:* Renal damage in diabetic nephropathy is responsible for hypertension. It is seen in pure form in type 1 diabetic patients with diabetic nephropathy. In middle-aged and older type 2 diabetic patients

with nephropathy, the etiology of hypertension is often mixed. The earliest manifestation of diabetic nephropathy is microalbuminuria. At this stage, the systemic BP is usually in prehypertension range but intraglomerular pressure is elevated. Administration of ACE inhibitors and ARBs leads to reduction in intraglomerular pressure and reversal of microalbuminuria.

- *Orthostatic hypotension with supine hypertension:* When hypertensive diabetic develops severe autonomic neuropathy, he develops postural hypotension but he remains hypertensive during the time he is resting in supine position.

## MANAGEMENT OF HYPERTENSION IN DIABETICS

Nonpharmacological measures should be introduced in prehypertension stage and continued along with pharmacological agents, if by themselves, they are not sufficient to bring BP down to the target of 130/80 mm Hg or below. Weight reduction in overweight patients by prudent diet control and appropriate dynamic exercise (30–40 minutes walk daily at brisk pace) is very effective and proven nonpharmacological measure. It also helps in achieving goals for metabolic control. Hypertensive patients should restrict salt intake to 5 g/day and refrain from smoking.

### Pharmacological Agents

If nonpharmacological measures do not bring down BP to target, antihypertensive agents should be added. Even though, the general principles of antihypertensive therapy are same in diabetic patients and nondiabetic patients, there are certain special, considerations while selecting an agent in diabetic hypertensive individual. The agent should not worsen metabolic control, it should have beneficial effects on vascular complications of diabetes and it should improve the quality of life, and should not cause orthostatic hypotension. One has to study the needs of an individual patient depending upon presence or absence of various vascular complications of diabetes and other conditions which could be associated [e.g., COPD/bronchial asthma and congestive cardiac failure (CCF)], and select appropriate agent. It is to be noted that in many diabetic patients a combination of two or three antihypertensive agents representing different classes is required to reach the target BP.

## Thiazide Diuretics

These are one of the agents of choice in stage 1 diabetic hypertensive without microalbuminuria. Hydrochlorothiazide in dosage of 12.5 mg daily is safe, effective and inexpensive. Its role in preventing vascular complications such as stroke is proved beyond doubt. In the dosage mentioned above, it does not significantly increase blood glucose, cholesterol, and uric acid levels. Of late, chlorthalidone is preferred over hydrochlorothiazide in view of stronger evidence supporting its cardiovascular protective properties. Sustained release indapamide, a thiazide-like diuretic is also commonly used and is considered more suitable because of lesser metabolic interference on blood levels of glucose, potassium, and cholesterol. If patient has stage 2 hypertension or if monotherapy with thiazide is not sufficient to reach target BP, second agent (ACE inhibitor/ARB/CCB) is added.

One should keep a watch on electrolyte disturbances and glucose and cholesterol levels.

## Angiotensin-converting Enzyme Inhibitors

These agents are particularly suited for use in diabetic hypertensive patients because when given to those who have microalbuminuria, urinary albumin excretion can be reverted to normoalbuminuria. These agents can be administered even in prehypertensive diabetic patients with microalbuminuria. At this stage, intraglomerular pressure is high and its reduction leads to reduction in albumin excretion rate. Among various ACEIs, ramipril has undergone extensive research as regards its protective effect on endothelium in patients with macrovascular diseases with or without diabetes [Heart Outcomes Prevention Evaluation (HOPE) study]. Through vasculoprotection, ACEIs offer action beyond BP control in diabetic hypertensive as well as prehypertensive with microalbuminuria. Thus, ADA used to recommend ACEIs along with ARBs as the drugs of first choice to initiate treatment of hypertension in diabetic patients, while JNC 8 recommends any one of the following four groups as the first-line antihypertensive in diabetic patients as well as nondiabetic patients. They do not have separate recommendations for diabetic patients. The four groups are: (1) ACEIs, (2) ARBs, (3) CCBs, and (4) thiazide diuretics. Recently, ADA has made slight change in guidelines, ACEIs/ARBs are indicated as drugs of first choice in those hypertensives with micro-/macroalbuminuria, in others any one of the four groups can be selected for first-line therapy. ACEIs/ARBs can be combined with thiazide diuretics or CCBs, if required in sequential manner or as primary combination in those with stage 2 hypertension. Combinations of various ARBs/ACEIs with 12.5 mg of hydrochlorothiazide/chlorthalidone and CCBs are available in single pill in two-/three-drug combinations.

Captopril, enalapril, lisinopril, and ramipril are the members of ACEI available in our country. Severe hyperkalemia, bilateral renal artery stenosis, pregnancy, and lactation are contraindications for use of ACEIs. About 10–15% patients have to discontinue ACEIs due to intractable cough.

### *Angiotensin Receptor Blockers*

These agents act on renin angiotensin system at a step beyond the site of action of ACEIs. They also provide renoprotective action. Like ACEIs, they also have the ability to convert those having microalbuminuria to normoalbuminuria. If started in diabetic patients who already have diabetic nephropathy, they slow down the rate of advancement of nephropathy. The time taken to reach end-stage renal failure as well as to double serum creatinine value, as compared to baseline value at the beginning of ARB therapy, is doubled as compared to those who do not take ARBs. Losartan was the prototype introduced in our country more about two decades back. In a major trial in hypertensive patients, losartan was found to provide vasculoprotective action. Candesartan, irbesartan, azilsartan, olmesartan, valsartan, and telmisartan are other ARBs available in our country. Their indications and contraindications are same as those of ACEIs. Their use does not lead to cough hence they can replace ACEIs in those who develop troublesome cough. Valsartan has been found to have beneficial effects in patients suffering from CCF. Even though, ARBs have action at a site separate from that of ACEIs on renin–angiotensin–aldosterone system (RAAS); and even though, both actions are complementary to each other, a large trial on combination of telmisartan and ramipril was unable to demonstrate any additional beneficial effects in those on combination therapy, however, side effects were higher in those on combination therapy [Ongoing Telmisartan Alone and in Combination with Ramipril Global Endpoint Trial ("ONTARGET") study]. Thus, ACEIs should not be combined with ARBs. Telmisartan and olmesartan are two of the most commonly prescribed ARBs in our country. The contraindications for use of ARBs are same as those of ACEIs.

## Calcium Channel Blockers

This antihypertensive drug class is made up of a few chemically different subclasses, all sharing antihypertensive properties but differing in other actions on cardiovascular system (e.g., diltiazem and verapamil reduce heart rate while nifedipine tends to increase it). Dihydropyridine subclass of CCBs is most commonly used as antihypertensive agents. The following agents from this class are available in our country: amlodipine, cilnidipine, nifedipine, benidipine, azelnidipine, and efonidipine. These agents neither have adverse metabolic effects, nor are they contraindicated in bronchospastic disorders and peripheral vascular disease, but at the same time, unlike ACEIs and ARBs, they do not offer any specific advantage for the treatment of diabetic hypertensive. However, in some trials, antiatherosclerosis effect and endothelial protection have been attributed to amlodipine. Some degree of renal protection is also provided by many CCBs. The mechanism of action involves blocking the entry of calcium from the extra-cellular space to inside the smooth muscle cells on the arterial wall through calcium channels and thus producing vasodilation. Edema over feet is the most common side effect. CCBs can be added to any other antihypertensive agent. Even though, usually, they are not the agents of first choice to start the treatment, CCBs are commonly employed in combination with other agents in diabetic patients. Cilnidipine has become a popular CCB of late because of its dual calcium channel blocking properties. It blocks N-type as well as L-type channels. It is less likely to cause pedal edema.

### Beta-blockers

Beta-blockers are not preferred as antihypertensive agents in plain hypertension without any cardiovascular comorbidity. They are strongly indicated in postmyocardial infarction, angina pectoris, and heart failure (carvedilol is the beta blocker of choice in heart failure). In patients with diabetes and abovementioned cardiovascular conditions, β-blockers need not be proscribed and if these patients also have hypertension, dosage of other antihypertensive agents can be adjusted as required. Till two decades back, atenolol was very commonly used antihypertensive agent and is still used at some centers particularly in small town India. Absence of any cardioprotective evidence in spite of its efficacy as an antihypertensive agent and presence of such evidence with selective β-blockers such as metoprolol and nebivolol led to shift from atenolol to these selective β-blockers. Nonselective β-blockers such as propranolol mask the symptoms of hypoglycemia and thus delay diagnosis and treatment. Thus, selective β-blockers such as metoprolol, nebivolol, or bisoprolol should be preferred. Large doses of β-blockers can increase serum cholesterol levels. Thus, if a moderate dose (e.g., 50–100 mg of metoprolol) is insufficient to bring down BP to target, an agent from other antihypertensive group should be added instead of stepping up the dose of β-blockers. Beta-blockers are not suitable in patients with associated bronchospastic disorders, bradyarrhythmias and severe peripheral vascular disease.

Many of our diabetic hypertensive patients, particularly young ones, have significant sympathetic overdrive and have hypertension associated with tachycardia, in such situations β-blockers can be used upfront in the management of hypertensive diabetic patients. Furthermore, BP-reducing efficacy of β-blockers was never in doubt. In clinical practice, a situation often arises where one of the preferred antihypertensive agent is unsuitable or contraindicated and others together are not able to bring down BP to the goal, in such situation, unless clear-cut contraindications exist, such as advanced degree of heart block, β-blockers can be always used as antihypertensive agents in diabetic patients. Also keep in mind that ACEIs and ARBs cannot be combined together thus, from point of view of availability for prescription, there are only three preferred antihypertensive agent groups and not four. These are some of the reasons explaining very common use of β-blockers in diabetic patients in a day-to-day practice in India. Metoprolol, nebivolol, bisoprolol, and carvedilol are some of the commonly used β-blockers in our country.

## *Alpha-blockers*

These agents are metabolically neutral, improve insulin resistance, improve symptoms of prostatism, and are not contraindicated in patients having bronchospastic disorders and peripheral vascular disease. These are their plus points while choosing antihypertensive agent in diabetic hypertensive. However, postural hypotension is a common side effect, which could be very troublesome in elderly long-standing diabetic having autonomic neuropathy, which itself causes postural hypotension. In ALLHAT study on cardiovascular outcomes in patients having hypertension and diabetes, incidence of combined cardiovascular disease, and heart failure was more with those put on doxazosin (an α-blocker), as compared to those on chlorthalidone. Thus, α-blockers are no more used as preferred agents but one has to use them in moderate dosages if other antihypertensive drugs are not able to bring down BP to target. Prazosin is a commonly used α-blocker agent in our country.

## *Aldosterone Antagonists (Mineralocorticoid Receptor Antagonists)*

Spironolactone and eplerenone are commonly used agents. They block the effect of aldosterone on renal distal tubule and increase the secretion of sodium and water and reduce the excretion of potassium. These agents are useful in the management of resistant hypertension, which is defined as uncontrolled hypertension in spite of use of maximal doses of three antihypertensive agents belonging to different classes, one of them being a diuretic. Adverse events include hyperkalemia, gynecomastia, and erectile dysfunction. Eplerenone is a bit safer. Baseline and periodic potassium and creatinine monitoring should be advised. One should be more careful when prescribing these agents to those on ACEIs/ARBs as these agents are also liable to cause hyperkalemia.

### Centrally Acting Agents

Alpha-methyldopa and clonidine belong to this class of agents. These agents are rarely used nowadays due to availability of a wide range of agents which are better tolerated and equally efficacious. Drowsiness, postural hypotension, and weakness are some of the common side effects of these agents. Alpha-methyldopa is still extensively used in the management of hypertension in pregnancy as its safety in this situation is proved beyond doubt. Sometimes, these agents are used in combination with other antihypertensive agents in diabetics with severe hypertension with associated problems, making some of the commonly used agents unsuitable.

## STEPWISE MANAGEMENT OF HYPERTENSION IN DIABETICS

*Stage 1*: Start with nonpharmacological measures, if target BP is not reached, add thiazides/ACEIs/ARBs (if microalbuminuria is present, ACEIs/ARBs should be preferred). If target BP is reached, continue, otherwise, add thiazides to ACEIs/ARBs or vice versa (for gradation of hypertension, refer **Table 2**).

*Stage 2:* Start with any two of the following groups: thiazides/ACEIs/ARBs/CCBs. Usually, thiazides should be one of the agents chosen. ACEIs and ARBs should not be used together. In those with microalbuminuria, ACEIs/ARBs should be preferred while those with angina pectoris or tachycardia should be put on β-blockers. If contraindications for use of any of the agents are present, other agents should be used (e.g., if a patient has severe peripheral vascular disease and bilateral renal artery stenosis, CCBs should be used along with thiazides). If target BP is not reached with a combination of two different agents, third agent from different group should be added. If three agents are not sufficient, fourth agent from different group should be added. Patients with stubborn hypertension are likely to have

**TABLE 2: Maximum recommended doses of commonly used antihypertensive agents.**

| Diuretics: | | ACE inhibitors: | |
|---|---|---|---|
| Hydrochlorothiazide | 25 mg | Enalapril | 40 mg |
| Indapamide | 25 mg | Captopril | 50 mg |
| Chlorthalidone | 25 mg | Lisinopril | 40 mg |
| | | Ramipril | 20 mg |
| ARBs: | | CCBs: | |
| Losartan | 100 mg | Amlodipine | 20 mg |
| Valsartan | 160 mg | Felodipine | 20 mg |
| Candesartan | 300 mg | Nifedipine | 80 mg |
| Irbesartan | 300 mg | Diltiazem | 480 mg |
| Olmesartan | 120 mg | Verapamil | 480 mg |
| Telmisartan | 160 mg | Cilnidipine | 40 mg |
| Beta-blockers: | | Alpha-blockers: | |
| Atenolol | 100 mg | Prazosin | 10 mg |
| Metoprolol | 450 mg | Doxazosin | 10 mg |
| MRAs: | | | |
| Spironolactone | 100 mg | | |
| Eplerenone | 50 mg | | |

(ACE: angiotensin-converting enzyme; ARBs: angiotensin receptor blockers; CCBs: calcium channel blockers; MRAs: mineralocorticoid receptor antagonists)

complications and other associated conditions, leading to inability to employ some of the mainline antihypertensive agents. In such circumstances, one may resort to use of α-blockers and occasionally, even centrally acting agents such as α-methyldopa. One should start with a moderate dose of an antihypertensive agent and gradually uptitrate the dose if required. Before adding an agent from different antihypertensive group, adequate trial should be given. In stage 1 hypertension, uptitration can be done at 2 monthly intervals while in stage 2 hypertension, it can be done at monthly interval unless there are compelling reasons for rapid reduction of BP **(Table 2)**. **Flowchart 1** summarizes the stepwise management of hypertension is diabetes.

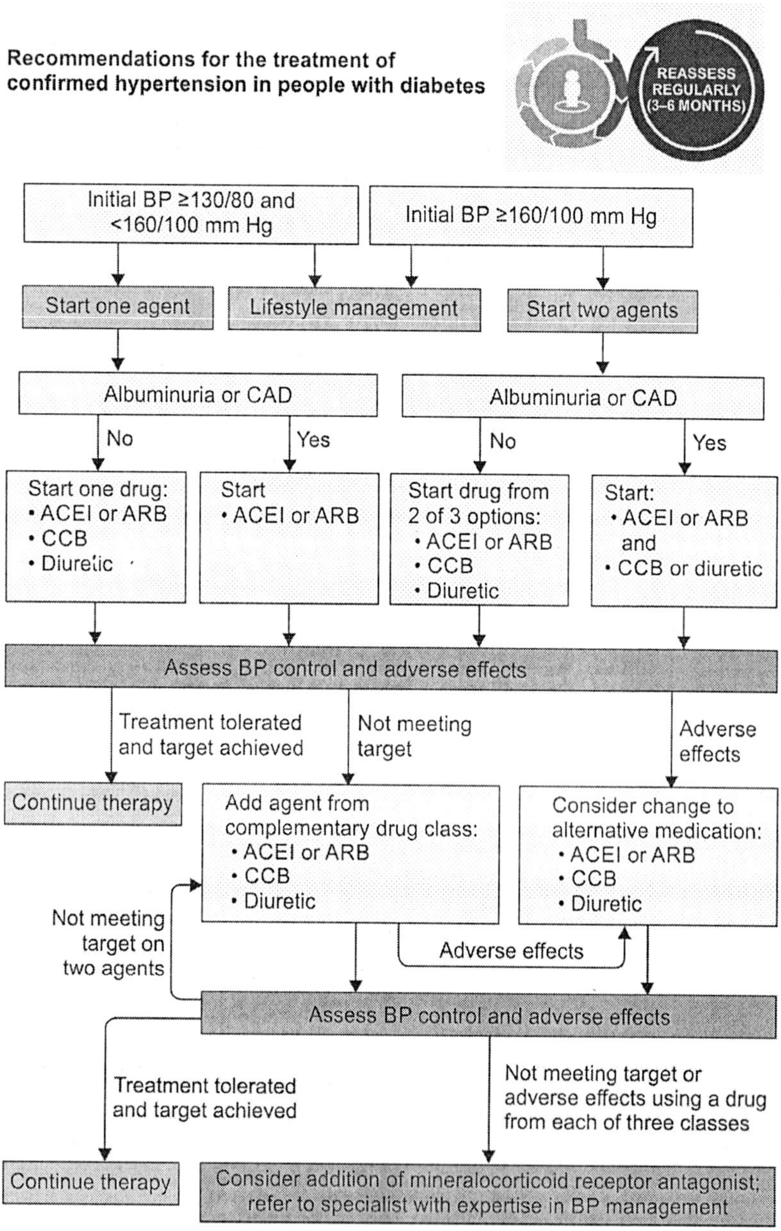

# Hypertension in Diabetes

**Recommendations for the treatment of confirmed hypertension in people with diabetes**

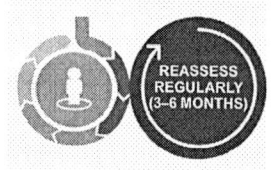

**FLOWCHART 1:** ADA guidelines for stepwise management of hypertension in diabetes.

(ACEI: angiotensin-converting enzyme inhibitor; ADA: American Diabetes Association; ARB: angiotensin receptor blocker; BP: blood pressure; CAD: coronary artery disease; CCB: calcium channel blocker)

*Source*: Diabetes care 2023;46(Suppl 1):S158–S190.

## SUMMARY

Hypertension is common in diabetic patients. Antihypertensive therapy has proved to be beneficial beyond any doubts in reducing morbidity and mortality associated with cardiovascular disease. Antihypertensive therapy in the presence of diabetic nephropathy slows down the decline in renal functions. It also reduces progression of diabetic retinopathy.

However, benefits are obtained only in those patients who reach the target BP. Hypertension in diabetic patients is stubborn and many patients require two or three different antihypertensive agents to reach the target. Many diabetic patients refuse to accept that they have real high BP and attribute higher readings in clinics to "white-coat hypertension" without actually taking BP readings at home in structured manner. Thus, noncompliance with antihypertensive pill prescription is high. It is the duty of treating clinician to record BP at every visit and to aggressively treat hypertension till the set goal is reached. (Refer to Rule of 33% below). The management includes meaningful dialog with the patient to remove misconceptions from his mind and ascertain drug compliance.

---

*Rule of 33%*
- 33% of hypertensives are diagnosed, 67% are undiagnosed.
- 33% of diagnosed hypertensives are on drug treatment.
- 33% of those on drug treatment are at their BP goal.

# CHAPTER 22

# Management of Dyslipidemia and Cardiovascular Risk in Diabetes Mellitus

## INTRODUCTION

The type of dyslipidemia in diabetes depends upon the subtype of diabetes. Type 2 diabetes mellitus (T2DM) is often typically associated with high triglyceride levels and low high-density lipoprotein (HDL) cholesterol levels. Their low-density lipoprotein cholesterol (LDL-C) values are same as in local community, and are often in normal range. However, small dense LDL particles, which are more atherogenic, are in higher concentration. This peculiar combination of lipid abnormalities is known as "diabetic dyslipidemia" or atherogenic dyslipidemia. The pathophysiological features leading to T2DM and diabetic dyslipidemia are interwoven. Type 2 diabetic patients have two- to fourfold higher chances of developing coronary artery disease and cerebrovascular disease as compared to nondiabetics. The higher prevalence is seen even in those patients who achieve persistent tight blood glucose control. It is believed that coexisting dyslipidemia significantly contributes to higher prevalence of macrovascular disease and thus needs to be aggressively managed along with hyperglycemia and hypertension, if present.

The lipid levels in type 1 diabetic patients are same as those in local community and in fact, in those patients with well-controlled blood glucose, HDL cholesterol values are higher than nondiabetics. Large scale observational or interventional studies on dyslipidemia in type 1 diabetes mellitus (T1DM) are lacking.

If dyslipidemia persists after controlling blood glucose, it should be treated as in type 2 diabetics. We will thus concentrate on management of dyslipidemia as well as primary and secondary prevention of atherosclerotic cardiovascular disease (ASCVD) in type 2 diabetic patients. Dyslipidemia is very common in type 2 diabetic patients and its aggressive management along with blood glucose control and management of other risk factors is rewarding. While isolated tight blood glucose control helps to prevent or reduce microvascular complications at all stages, same approach does not give equivalent protection against macrovascular disease, unless aggressive management of dyslipidemia along with other associated risk factors, such as hypertension and obesity is carried out simultaneously as conclusively proved in Steno-2 study. In type 2 diabetics, the desirable level of LDL-C, the most crucial of all the components of lipid profile, is lower than general population, particularly in those with associated ASCVD **(Table 1)**. Furthermore, several international studies have proved that lower the level of LDL-C, stronger is the protection from ASCVD even in those who have already reached the lipid goals. Thirty mg reduction in LDL-C is associated with 30% reduction in risk of coronary heart disease (CHD) **(Fig. 1)**. Thus, the scope of this chapter is wider than mere reduction of lipid number to get at the lipid goal, but its end goal is reduction of cardiovascular risk through primary and secondary prevention.

**Figure 2** clearly shows results of primary and secondary CHD prevention trials with various statins. Please note that irrespective of statin used and baseline LDL-C levels, statins reduced the risk for CHD, both in primary and secondary prevention studies.

**TABLE 1: Desirable level of LDL cholesterol in T2DM.**

| Clinical status | Desirable LDL cholesterol (mg%) |
|---|---|
| No ASCVD/risk factors | <100 |
| ASCVD/risk factors + | <70 |
| Advanced ASCVD | <55 |

(ASCVD: atherosclerotic cardiovascular disease; LDL: low-density lipoprotein; T2DM: type 2 diabetes mellitus)

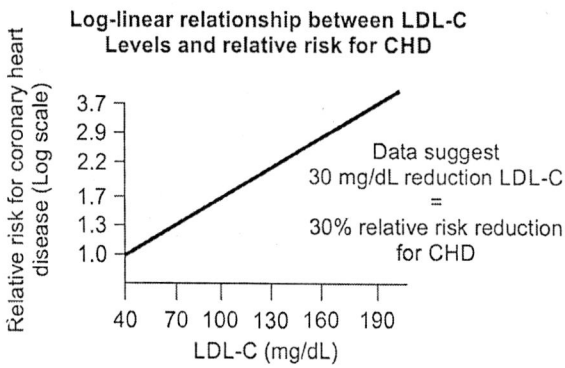

**FIG. 1:** Linear relationship between LDL-C and relative risk of CHD.

(CHD: coronary heart disease; LDL-C: low-density lipoprotein cholesterol)

*Source*: Grundy SM, Cleeman JI, Merz CN, Brewer HB Jr, Clark LT, Hunninghake DB, et al. Implications of recent clinical trials for the National Cholesterol Education Program Adult Treatment Panel III guidelines. Circulation. 2004;110(2):227-39.

Now you will understand why all the guidelines are recommending statins in all T2DM patients >40 years including those who are already at their LDL-C goal.

The desirable HDL cholesterol values should be >40 mg% in men and >50 mg% in women and triglycerides level <150 mg%. If this goal is reached along with the goals for glycemic control and blood pressure, prevalence of macrovascular complications can be significantly reduced as shown in multiple risk factor reduction in type 2 diabetic patient's trial (Steno-2 study). However, to get maximum benefit, one must attain and reach the LDL goals early in life and then maintain it throughout. Reaching and then maintaining LDL goals in 30s can lead to around 55% relative risk reduction from ASCVD, while achieving the goal in 70s reduces ASCVD risk by only 20% (legacy effect).

Even though, high triglyceride and low HDL cholesterol levels are very strongly associated with coronary artery disease, we do not have a strong evidence in the form of interventional trial proving association between increase of HDL cholesterol and reduction in incidence of coronary artery disease. As regards triglycerides, till recently such evidence was lacking. Recent

# Management of Dyslipidemia and Cardiovascular Risk in Diabetes Mellitus

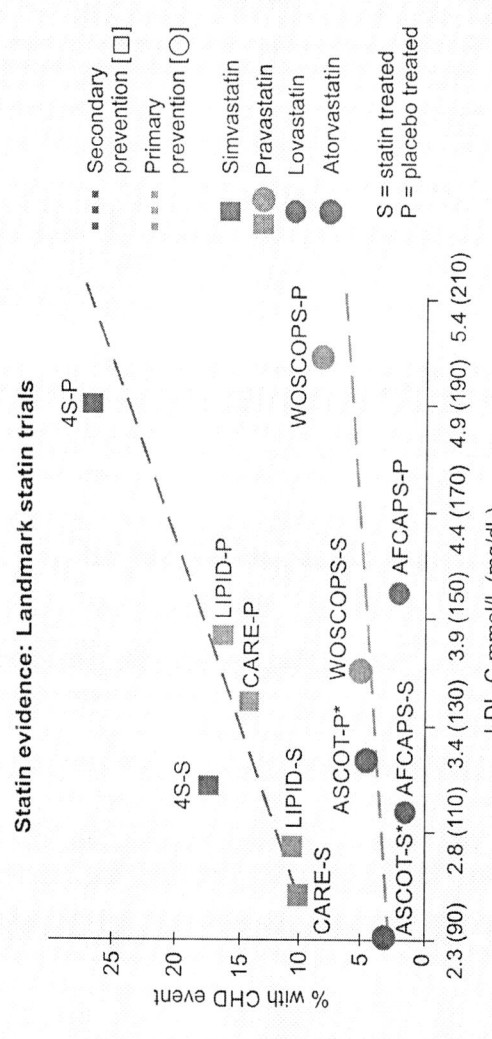

*Extrapolated for 5 years.

**FIG. 2:** Landmark statin trials for primary and secondary prevention of CHD. *(For color version, see Plate 10)* (CHD: coronary heart disease; LDL-C: low-density lipoprotein cholesterol)

*Source:* Adapted from Kastelein JJ. The future of best practice. Atherosclerosis. 1999;143 (Suppl 1):S17-21.

clinical study, "REDUCE-IT", proved the cardiovascular protective properties of icosapent ethyl, a purified chemical derived from marine fish oil in patients with ASCVD or high risk for it and already on a statin and having normal level of LDL-C and raised triglycerides. Till the publication of this report, several trials with varying levels of purification of fish oil in varying dosages, had failed to show any beneficial effect. Icosapent ethyl is not available in India. Thus, in management of dyslipidemia in diabetes, primary goal is to reduce LDL-C to <100 mg% (<70 mg% in those having established macrovascular disease), and secondary goal is to reduce triglycerides to <150 mg% and to increase HDL cholesterol to >40 mg% and >50 mg% in men and women, respectively. Hypertriglyceridemia is often associated with reduced HDL cholesterol levels and increased small dense LDL particle levels. Total LDL-C levels may not be elevated.

## INVESTIGATIONS

Diabetic dyslipidemia does not commonly present with typical signs such as xanthelasmatas, tendon xanthomas, and corneal arcus (refer to **Fig. 3** for classical butter fly xanthelasma in middle-aged T2DM patient with dyslipidemia). Thus, lipid profile following 12 hours fast should be done at yearly interval as long as the goals are met. In those with abnormal values, it should be repeated at 3–6 monthly intervals depending upon individual situation. The first estimation of lipid profile should be done a few weeks after the diagnosis of diabetes and initiation of treatment (usually at the time of first or second follow-up).

## MANAGEMENT OF DYSLIPIDEMIA AND CV RISK

### Nonpharmacological Treatment

Diet control, regular physical activity, and weight reduction in overweight persons should be aggressively perused. Total caloric intake should be decided after giving consideration to the type of work and current weight. Fat should provide 25% of the calories and saturated fat should provide 7% of the calories (refer to the Chapter 12). Dynamic exercise such as 30 minutes of brisk walk daily should be encouraged (refer to Chapter 11).

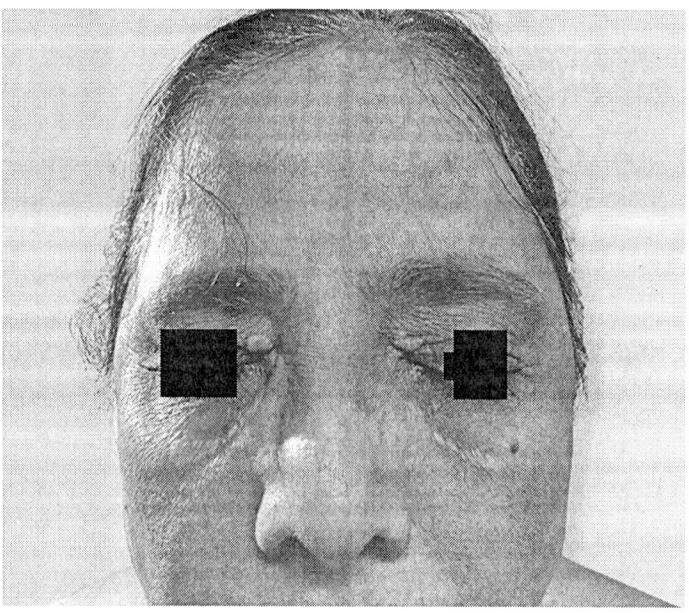

**FIG. 3:** Typical "butterfly rash" around eyes in middle-aged type 2 diabetic patient with dyslipidemia *(For color version, see Plate 11).*

*Cessation of smoking:* Smoking and tobacco in any form should be totally avoided. This will help to increase in HDL cholesterol in those who are tobacco consumers.

## Pharmacological Treatment

Large number of interventional studies on the role of statins in primary and secondary prevention of ASCVD in diabetic patients including the patients at the goals (**Fig. 2**), and lack of such data with other lipid-lowering agents has led to establishment of statins as the mainstay of management of dyslipidemia and in primary and secondary prevention of ASCVD in diabetes. Depending upon the potency to reduce LDL-C, the statins are classified in two subgroups, high-intensity statins (ability to reduce LDL-C by 50% or more) and moderate-intensity statins (ability to reduce LDL-C by 30–50%) (**Table 2**).

All type 2 diabetic patients with overt ASCVD or high risk for it should receive high-intensity statin therapy.

| TABLE 2: High-intensity and moderate-intensity statin therapy.* ||
|---|---|
| **High-intensity statins** | **Moderate-intensity statins** |
| • Atorvastatin 40–80 mg<br>• Rosuvastatin 20–40 mg | • Atorvastatin 10–20 mg<br>• Rosuvastatin 5–10 mg<br>• Simvastatin 20–40 mg<br>• Pitavastatin 1–4 mg |

*Only statins available in India are mentioned.

Those above 40 years without ASCVD or high risk for it should be started on moderate-intensity statins irrespective of baseline LDL-C level.

In those with lesser cardiovascular risk (absence of ASCVD/high risk for it and age <40 years), the first goal is to reduce LDL-C to <100 mg%. If LDL-C levels are >130 mg%, pharmacological treatment should be started simultaneously with lifestyle measures. If LDL-C is between 100 mg% and 130 mg%, nonpharmacological treatment should be started and lipids should be repeated after 3 months. If goals are not reached at that time, pharmacological treatment should be added. For isolated rise in LDL-C, monotherapy with statins should be preferred.

### *Indications for Statins in Combination with Other Lipid-lowering Agents*

*Ezetimibe*: It acts by reducing absorption of cholesterol from the gut and is usually well tolerated. Its dose is 10 mg once a day orally. It reduces LDL-C level by 15–20%. In "IMPROVE-IT" study on T2DM, patients having an episode of acute coronary insufficiency within last 10 days, addition of ezetimibe to ongoing simvastatin therapy led to significant cardiovascular risk reduction as compared to placebo plus simvastatin.

### Indications of Statin–Ezetimide Combination

- In those on statin with intolerance to the prescribed dose, ezetimibe can be added and statin dose reduced. If a statin is not tolerated at all, ezetimibe can replace statin.
- In those not reaching LDL goals in spite of using statin in recommended dose, ezetimibe can be added and statin continued in full dose.

## PCSK9 Inhibitors

The PCSK9 inhibitors are injectable agents and require dosing at 2-4 weekly intervals. Both evolocumab and alirocumab have proved their efficacy as regards ability to significantly reduce LDL-C and offer cardiovascular protection in patients with T2DM (Fourier study, Odyssey outcome study). Though available in India, their use is very limited due to exorbitant cost. The indications are same as those for ezetimibe.

## Bempedoic Acid

Bempedoic acid is the latest lipid-lowering agent, introduced in India in 2022. Its efficacy to reduce LDL-C is similar to that of ezetimibe. It blocks the LDL-C synthesis in liver one step prior to the site of action of statin. It has significantly lesser side effects on muscular system. Rise in serum uric acid level is seen and occasionally it can lead to gout. Patients on bempedoic acid require periodic uric acid monitoring. Rupture of tendons such as tendo-Achilles is seen occasionally. It is available as 180 mg tablet to be administered once a day. In recently concluded CLEAR outcome Clinical Trial published on 4th March, 2023 in New England Journal of Medicine, it was concluded that among statin intolerant patients requiring pharmacotherapy for primary or secondary prevention of ASCVD, 180 mg of bempedoic acid daily resulted in significant 13% risk reduction in primary endpoint event (death from cardiovascular diseases, nonfatal myocardial infraction, nonfetal stroke or coronary revascularization) as compared to placebo after a median of 40.6 months of follow-up. It can be used as an alternative to ezetimibe as an adjuvant to statin or along with ezetimibe in those who are totally intolerant to statin and monotherapy with ezetimibe is not sufficient to reach LDL-C goals.

## Bile Acid Sequestrants

In patients having contraindications to use of statins or intolerance to statins, bile acid sequestrants can also be used. Gastrointestinal disturbances and tendency to raise triglyceride levels are some of the limitations of these agents. They are not freely available in India.

## Monitoring of Statin Therapy

Higher doses and use of high potency statins are associated with increased chances of side effects such as hepatotoxicity, myopathy, and occasionally, rhabdomyolysis. Female sex, renal failure, hypothyroidism, and concomitant use of other agents such as fibrates, particularly gemfibrozil are other risk factors. However, on the whole, the serious side effects are extremely rare. In a meta-analysis including 180,000 patients from 21 studies of at least 3 years duration, incidence of myalgia was 1.5–3.0%, myopathy 5/100,000 cases, and rhabdomyolysis 1.6/100,000 cases. Statins are life-protecting and lifesaving agents. Many patients are deprived of their advantages due to reluctance of a clinician to prescribe them on account of misconceptions about high prevalence of their side effects; furthermore, often they are summarily withdrawn when a patient gets vague aches and pains. All these aches and pains in a patient on statin are not necessarily statin induced. All the patients should undergo liver function test (LFT) before starting statin therapy. These investigations should be repeated as per the need based on individual case. There are many causes for a slight rise in serum glutamic-oxaloacetic transaminase (SGOT) and serum glutamic-pyruvic transaminase (SGPT) levels, many drugs can cause a transient and mild rise of levels of these enzymes in blood. Thus a rise up to twice the higher limit of normal is not an indication for withholding or immediate discontinuation of the medication. A small rise in SGPT and SGOT is common in nonalcoholic fatty liver disease (NAFLD), which is present in a majority of T2DM patients. Presence of NAFLD, with or without slight rise in hepatic enzymes, is not a contraindication for statin therapy. Those with significant derangement of LFTs should be investigated further and appropriate decisions about withholding or withdrawing statins should be taken as per individual case. Creatine kinase (CK) levels need not be measured as a routine before starting statin therapy. In selected cases, when complications such as myositis or rhabdomyolysis are suspected (severe muscle pains, significant rise of hepatic enzymes, passing of "coca cola" colored urine, etc.), CK levels should be measured and statins should be promptly withheld if CK is more than 10 times upper limit of normal. Statin therapy is continued over a very long-term period (usually lifelong). In patients who are intolerant to a statin but with CK levels <10 times upper limit of normal one can reduce the dose of a statin or try an alternate statin after a gap of few days.

Associated mild to moderate hypertriglyceridemia is tackled by statin monotherapy. Rosuvastatin is preferred over atorvastatin and simvastatin in mixed dyslipidemia.

### Secondary Goals

After tackling LDL-C attention should to be focused on attaining goals for HDL cholesterol and triglycerides.

*HDL cholesterol*: The goal is HDL cholesterol >40 mg% and 50 mg% in men and women, respectively. Nonpharmacological measures such as cessation of smoking and physical exercise should be aggressively pursued. Consumption of moderate quantities red wine, almonds, wallnuts, and grapes may help. Pharmacological agents have safety and efficacy issues. None of the dedicated HDL-specific agents such as nicotinic acid or its derivatives have stood the test of time. Statins and fibrates increase HDL cholesterol to some extent.

## HYPERTRIGLYCERIDEMIA

Till recently, there was no solid proof based on a large interventional study for use of pharmacotherapy in diabetics with mild isolated hypertriglyceridemia (triglycerides 151–399 mg%). In such situations, the standard therapy is lifestyle management along with measures to improve blood glucose control. Change of statin to rosuvastatin and using it in higher doses is one of the commonly employed strategies. Abstinence from alcohol, or if it cannot be avoided, consumption in limited quantity (not more than a peg a day), is required. Search should be made to find out possible underlying cause (hypothyroidism, renal failure, drugs, etc.) and tackle it. Tight blood glucose control itself helps to significantly reduce serum triglyceride levels but LDL-C levels are not significantly reduced merely by controlling blood glucose.

Pharmacotherapy should be promptly started if serum triglyceride is 400 mg% or above, to protect the patient from acute pancreatitis. Among the commonly available time tested agents, fibrates are the drugs of choice, and should be prescribed in combination with statins. It should be remembered that combination therapy with statins and fibrates carries higher risk of drug-induced side effects. Thus, these patients should be under close clinical and biochemical monitoring for muscle pain, weakness, exhaustion, and periodic LFT and CK estimation. Among the fibrates, based on its ability to reduce serum triglyceride level, fenofibrate in the dosage of 160 mg once daily is preferred. Gemfibrozil and bezafibrate are also available in our country. While the former has a slightly better action on LDL-C levels, the latter also has a mild hypoglycemic action. Gemfibrozil should not be used in combination with statins as side effects associated with this combination are significantly higher than those with fenofibrate-statin combination. Addition of fibrates to statin does not lead to additional cardiovascular risk reduction, over and above that produced by statin monotherapy, as observed in major trials such as FIELD and ACCORD. However, in subgroups with high baseline triglyceride levels associated with low HDL cholesterol levels (triglyceride >200 mg% and HDL cholesterol <34 mg%), some beneficial effects were observed.

Recent clinical study, "REDUCE-IT", proved the cardiovascular protective properties of icosapent ethyl, a purified chemical derived from marine fish oil in patients with ASCVD or high risk for it and already on a statin and having normal level of LDL-C and raised triglycerides level. Till the publication of this report, several trials with varying levels of purification of fish oil in varying dosages, had failed to show any beneficial effect. Icosapent ethyl is not available in India. Once available, this agent will be used in those with triglycerides level >400 mg% to reduce acute pancreatitis risk as well as in those with moderate hypertriglyceridemia associated with low HDL cholesterol levels not responding to nonpharmacological measures and statin therapy.

Recently, a new agent, saroglitazar was introduced in India. Saroglitazar belongs to a new class of agents which have combined peroxisome proliferator-activated receptor (PPAR) α- and γ-agonist activity. It is a first agent of this class and India is the first country to have it in a day-to-day clinical practice. Through its PPAR α-agonist activity, it reduces triglyceride levels and works like fibrates, while PPAR γ-agonist activity leads to some improvement in glycemic control. It is more potent than fenofibrate in its ability to reduce triglycerides. Long-term longitudinal trials to study its effects on hard cardiovascular end points are not available. It can be considered as an alternative to fenofibrate, as an adjuvant to statin in those with severe hypertriglyceridemia, not responding to statin monotherapy.

## CONCLUSION

Dyslipidemia is a strong cardiovascular risk factor and is commonly associated with T2DM. Both lead to accelerated atherosclerosis and early onset of diffuse macrovascular disease. When both are present together, risk is not merely added up, but compounded. Aggressive management of high LDL-C is associated with reduced new incidence of macrovascular disease as well as reduced morbidity and mortality in those who already have macrovascular disease. However, the scenario in actual day-to-day practice is depressing. A large number of diabetic patients are not subjected to periodic lipid profile estimation. In those with abnormal lipid profile, often no or inadequate lifestyle and pharmacological measures are implemented, thus lipid goals are not reached. Even in those who are taking lipid-reducing agents, there are failures as regards reaching target lipid levels. Clinicians, in charge of management of diabetic patients, should be more aggressive as regards monitoring and management of lipid abnormalities in their patients. It should be remembered that management of diabetes goes far beyond a mere blood glucose management. It involves efficient screening and management of other risk factors such as dyslipidemia.

> *"Aggressive cardiovascular prevention must be a priority in subjects with diabetes mellitus, as most will die of cardiovascular disease. In diabetes mellitus some of many risk factors associated with vascular disease have multiplicative rather than additive effect and this reinforces the importance of correcting even minor abnormalities of factors such as dyslipidemia.*
> 
> *Moreover, much of atherogenic potential of diabetic dyslipidemia is due to relatively subtle abnormalities that may appear unimpressive or simply missed by routine biochemical screening of fasting samples."*

Source: Pickup's Textbook of Diabetes.

# CHAPTER 23

# Surgery in a Diabetic Patient

## INTRODUCTION

Patients with diabetes undergoing surgical treatment are a common situation in a day-to-day practice. Several factors are responsible for high rate of various surgeries in diabetic patients.

- Rapidly increasing prevalence of diabetes
- Gradually increasing longevity of patients with diabetes
- Diabetes-related complications requiring surgical treatment
- Emergence of surgical procedures, such as coronary artery bypass graft (CABG) and renal transplant, as alternatives to medical management of coronary artery disease and end-stage renal failure, respectively.
- Rapidly emerging prevalence of morbid obesity and acceptance of bariatric surgery as an effective treatment option.

It is estimated that in the USA, around 50% patients with diabetes undergo at least one surgical procedure in their lifetime.

Apart from CABG and renal transplants, other common surgeries in patients with diabetes are different types of foot surgeries (minor abscess drainage to bypass graft surgeries and amputations), eye surgeries (cataract extraction, vitreoretinal surgeries), cholecystectomy, etc.

When patients with diabetes undergo surgery, the complication rate is higher than nondiabetics in same age-group. Besides metabolic abnormalities of diabetes, associated macrovascular and microvascular complications, both known and silent, and thus undiagnosed are responsible for increased morbidity and mortality associated with surgery in a diabetic patient. Coronary artery disease, cardiac autonomic neuropathy, and reduced capacity to fight micro-organisms are some of the underlying factors.

However, with meticulous preoperative workup, with attainment of good and steady metabolic control, and with coordinated intraoperative and postoperative management, the mortality and morbidity associated with surgery in a diabetic patient can be reduced nearly to levels seen in nondiabetic patients.

## METABOLIC EFFECTS OF SURGERY AND ANESTHESIA

Stress associated with surgery and anesthesia causes a lot of metabolic alterations, the degree of which depends on the amount of surgical trauma and duration of surgery.

Increased secretion of counter regulatory hormones, which opposes the action of insulin, decreased secretion of insulin, and increased insulin resistance are the main metabolic changes. This leads to severe hyperglycemia unless patient is adequately insulinized. Uncorrected hyperglycemia leads to osmotic diuresis and dehydration, which results in hypotension and inadequate tissue perfusion, leading to organ ischemia. Also associated with hyperglycemia are protein breakdown and lipolysis. Along with these changes, there is a loss of body mass with negative nitrogen balance and impaired wound healing with decreased resistance to infections. The magnitude of these catabolic changes will depend upon duration of surgery, amount of surgical trauma, severity of underlying disorder and degree of metabolic control achieved during perioperative period.

## ANESTHETIC AGENTS AND ANESTHESIA

Following points should be noted:
- Ether, a commonly used agent of past, had many side effects (hyperglycemia, hyperketonuria, and acidosis). Modern anesthetic agents such as halothane and enflurane are safer.
- Patients in whom spinal anesthesia is given are more prone for hypotension and hyperglycemia due to "chemical sympathectomy".
- High doses of epidural anesthesia can lead to hypoglycemia.

- Diabetic patients having significant autonomic neuropathy are prone to develop cardiac arrest during the surgery.
- Diabetic patients are more sensitive to narcotics than non-diabetic patients.
- Endotracheal intubation may be occasionally difficult due to limited mobility of atlanto-occipital joint.
- Light balanced anesthesia has minimal side effects.

## PREOPERATIVE EVALUATION

This is absolutely necessary to avoid complications. The main aims are to establish good metabolic control and to anticipate complications and to take preventive measures.

Preoperative evaluation starts with the proper identification of type of diabetes. The previous metabolic control should be assessed by estimating blood glucose levels as well as glycated hemoglobin (HbA1c) levels. Presence of complications such as diabetic nephropathy and autonomic neuropathy should be identified by carrying out appropriate investigations and clinical examinations [serum creatinine, blood urea nitrogen (BUN) for assessment of kidney functions, and BP response to postural changes and study of RR intervals during inspiration and expiration on electrocardiogram]. Cardiovascular evaluation for ischemic heart disease (IHD), hypertension, and congestive cardiac failure should be made.

The investigations for preoperative evaluation are given in **Table 1**.

## INSULIN THERAPY

Patients undergoing major surgery should be admitted 48–72 hours before surgery for final assessment and fine-tuning of antidiabetic therapy. In all patients who were on insulin, it should be continued.

In those type 2 diabetic patients with inadequate control [fasting blood sugar (FBS) >150 mg%], insulin should be started. Sometimes, it is advisable to start insulin in preoperative period even in well-controlled type 2 diabetic patients as insulin treatment is very flexible.

Three dosages of premeal short-acting insulin with supplementation of long-acting or intermediate-acting insulin at bedtime

**TABLE 1: Preoperative investigations in patients undergoing major surgery.**

| For all patients | • FBS, PPBS<br>• HbA1c<br>• X-ray chest<br>• Electrocardiogram<br>• Serum creatinine, BUN<br>• Serum electrolytes<br>• Complete hemogram<br>• Routine urine examination |
|---|---|
| Additional investigations for selected patients | • Treadmill stress test<br>• 2D echocardiogram with color Doppler<br>• Coronary angiography<br>• Coagulation profile |

(BUN: blood urea nitrogen; FBS: fasting blood sugar; HbA1c: glycated hemoglobin; PPBS: postprandial blood sugar)

for basal insulin requirement provide good round the clock metabolic control.

If patients are on metformin, it should be discontinued 2 days prior to surgery to avoid metformin-induced lactic acidosis in perioperative period. Intraoperative or postoperative hypotension and resultant tissue hypoxia increase the chances of metformin-induced lactic acidosis. Long-acting sulfonylureas such as glibenclamide should be discontinued 2–3 days prior and short-acting sulfonylureas such as gliclazide and glimepiride and other agents such as repaglinide should be discontinued on a day prior to surgery to avoid hypoglycemia.

## ON THE DAY OF SURGERY

Fasting for at least 12 hours is required to guard against undiagnosed diabetic gastroparesis. Surgery should be scheduled in the morning session as far as possible. Frequent blood glucose monitoring with reliable glucometer should be done (initially on hourly interval and subsequently on 2-hourly interval).

Glucose or glucose-insulin drip should be started in the ward before shifting the patient to the theater. 5% or 10% dextrose should be infused at the rate of 100 mL/h. In elderly or in those with left

**TABLE 2: Insulin infusion rates.**

| Plasma glucose (mg%) | Insulin infusion (units/h) or glucose bolus amount |
|---|---|
| <70 | 20 mL 25% glucose bolus |
| 71–100 | 1.0 |
| 101–150 | 1.5 |
| 151–200 | 2.0 |
| 201–250 | 3.0 |
| 251–300 | 4.0 |
| >300 | 6.0 |

ventricular dysfunction, infusion rate should be reduced to 60–75 mL/h. Use of central line would be ideal in such situations. Daily serum electrolytes should be monitored and potassium replacement should be given accordingly till patient is stabilized and oral feeds are resumed.

Insulin infusion should be given through separate microdrip, which can be "piggybacked" on dextrose drip. Fifty-five units of short-acting human insulin should be added to a pint of normal saline. At this concentration, 10 microdrops/min will deliver 1 unit/h. The rate of microdrip is to be adjusted as per insulin requirement. If infusion pump is available, 100 units of short-acting human insulin should be added to 100 mL of normal saline and rate of infusion adjusted as per requirement (1 mL/h will deliver 1 unit of insulin per hour). Infusion pumps deliver accurate quantity of fluid and also reduce fluid overload. This is important particularly in those who require large doses of insulin and in those who have left ventricular dysfunction. Insulin requirement will depend on several factors including degree of insulin resistance, type of surgery, state of β-cell function, etc. Insulin requirement is higher during surgeries such as CABG and renal transplantation.

Table 2 gives details about insulin infusion rates.

## ALTERNATIVE INSULIN REGIMENS

*Standard cocktail (glucose-insulin-potassium infusion)*: In standard cocktail, 10% glucose plus 15 units of short-acting insulin plus 20 mEq of potassium chloride is infused at 100 mL/h till patient

**TABLE 3: Guidelines for selection of infusion fluid.**

| Blood glucose in mg% | Infusion to be administered |
|---|---|
| <100 | Plain 10% glucose + KCL |
| 101–150 | 10% glucose + KCL + 10 units of insulin |
| 151–250 | 10% glucose + KCL + 15 units of insulin |
| 251–300 | 10% glucose + KCL + 20 units of insulin |
| >300 | Change to variable insulin infusion regimen |

resumes oral feeds. This regimen is less flexible as compared to variable rate insulin infusion described above. However, it is easier to administer. The flexibility can be increased by making four infusion sets, containing 0, 10, 15, and 20 units of insulin while keeping glucose and potassium chloride concentration fixed. Each infusion container should be labeled depending upon units of insulin mixed in it. The infusion should be selected as per blood glucose value, which should be monitored hourly during intraoperative stage and initial postoperative period, and subsequently at 2-hourly intervals. **Table 3** gives guidelines for selection of infusion fluid.

## Subcutaneous Insulin

Even though not an ideal regimen, it may be employed if intravenous (IV) insulin infusion regimens cannot be employed due to lack of experienced paramedical staff and resident doctors on the wards. Patient's daily insulin requirement during immediate preoperative period is calculated. One-third of total insulin dose is given as short-acting preoperative dose subcutaneously and 5% glucose infusion is started at the rate of 100 mL/h. Blood glucose is monitored hourly and small doses (4–6 units) of short-acting insulin are given subcutaneously every 3–4 hourly if blood glucose is above 200 mg%.

## MINOR SURGICAL PROCEDURES

In insulin-treated patients, subcutaneous short-acting insulin in the dose of one-third of total daily dose of insulin is given preoperatively and 5% glucose infusion is started at 100 mL/h. Glucose infusion is discontinued when patient starts oral feeds and original subcutaneous insulin regimen is reintroduced prior to first postoperative oral feed.

In patients on oral antidiabetic agents, morning pills should not be given and 5% glucose infusion should be started preoperatively and infused at 100 mL/h. Infusion should be discontinued when patient resumes oral feeds and regular oral antidiabetic drug therapy should be reintroduced simultaneously. Even in patients undergoing minor surgical procedures, fasting and preoperative, postoperative, and pre first postoperative feed blood glucose should be estimated and abovementioned plan should be modified if required. In stable diabetics undergoing very short procedures who are likely to resume oral feeds soon after the procedures, preoperative insulin, and intra- and immediate postoperative glucose infusion may not be required (e.g., cataract extraction, minor incision, drainage procedures, and other procedures carried out under local anesthesia).

## POSTOPERATIVE CARE

Careful monitoring of blood glucose and appropriate adjustments in insulin infusions, monitoring of vital functions, intake and urine output, and ensuring adequate hydration and at the same time avoiding over hydration, particularly in elderly and in those with impaired left ventricular function are important during postoperative period. Appropriate antibiotic therapy for infective conditions and prophylactic antibiotic for prevention of secondary infection in noninfective conditions are recommended. Careful and detailed attention to above mentioned points would go a long way in prevention of postoperative complications. The common postoperative complications are listed here:

- Metabolic (diabetic ketoacidosis, hyperosmolar nonketotic state, hypoglycemia, and electrolyte disturbances)
- Cardiovascular (myocardial infarction, left ventricular failure, cardiac arrhythmias, hypotension, and stroke particularly after CABG)
- Renal (acute renal failure and fluid overload)
- Infections

## SPECIAL SITUATIONS

- *Emergency surgeries in poorly controlled patients*: Ask for 4–6 hours for critical assessment, preoperative investigations, correction of dehydration, and metabolic derangement. Start the patient on IV insulin infusion and normal saline infusion through separate lines to correct hyperglycemia and fluid deficit; add potassium chloride to the pint of normal saline if there is hypokalemia. Sometimes diabetic ketoacidosis presents with symptoms mimicking acute surgical abdomen. Prompt correction of hyperglycemia and fluid and electrolyte imbalance leads to rapid disappearance of symptoms. Keep this in mind when you come across abovementioned clinical situation, insist for adequate time for correction of metabolic derangement and reassessment.
- *Coronary artery bypass graft*: Insulin requirement during intraoperative period is usually very high, 10 units/h is not uncommon. Hypothermia, liberal use of inotropic drugs and dextrose solution are some of the underlying conditions leading to high insulin requirement.
- *Renal transplantation*: Insulin requirement is high due to infusion of large volume of fluids including dextrose, dexamethasone and β-agonist agents. Similarly, during cesarean section the requirements of insulin go up due to β-adrenergic agonists and use of dexamethasone.

## CONCLUSION

Careful preoperative assessment, well planned and coordinated intraoperative, and postoperative monitoring and management of diabetes, anticipation and preventive measures for complications go a long way in decreasing perioperative mortality and morbidity in a diabetic patient undergoing surgical treatment.

# CHAPTER 24

# COVID-19 and Diabetes

## INTRODUCTION

Three years have passed since the tsunami of the severe acute respiratory syndrome coronavirus 2 (SARS-CoV-2) [coronavirus disease 2019 (COVID-19)] virus has struck the globe. After originating in the city of Wuhan in China toward the end of 2019, the virus was first isolated in Chinese laboratories in December, 2019 and spread rapidly across the globe prompting World Health Organization (WHO) to declare it as a pandemic in March, 2020. Initial epidemiological data suggested that rich countries were affected more than poorer countries, though part of the disparity could be due to paucity of diagnostic facilities and relatively infrequent traveling in poorer countries. It spread from China to the USA via Europe and soon the pandemic spread globally and India was not spared. First case of COVID-19 in India was reported from Kerala on January 27, 2020 and till December 19, 2022, 44,676,087 (roughly 4.46 crore) cases have been diagnosed in our country. Till the same date, 534,674 deaths due to COVID-19 have been reported. Thus, our COVID-19 mortality rate is 1.2%. Many believe that both the incidence as well as mortality figures have been grossly under reported and there are multiple obvious reasons leading to under reporting.

When COVID-19 affects people with diabetes, chances of developing severe pneumonia, acute respiratory distress syndrome (ARDS), need for intensive care unit admission, invasive ventilatory support, arterial thrombosis (coronary, cerebral, and pulmonary), acute kidney injury, prolonged hospitalization, etc., are higher than in nondiabetic patients. The overall morbidity and mortality are higher in people with diabetes. Tough it was initially thought that the chances of developing COVID-19 were not higher in those with diabetes, subsequent epidemiological data suggested that incidence of COVID-19 was higher in countries with high prevalence of diabetes even after accounting for income disparities between the countries. Massive amount of published work on various aspects of COVID-19 is available and systematic review of these publications has revealed that among the patients affected by COVID-19, those with diabetes are 3.6 times more likely to require hospitalization and 2.3 times more at risk of death. The reasons are obvious. Syndromic nature of the disease, associated comorbidities such as hypertension, obesity, renal failure, atherosclerotic cardiovascular disease, proinflammatory and procoagulant nature of the disease, older age of patients with diabetes, etc., are partly responsible for higher hospitalization rate and increased mortality. However, even after adjusting for age, sex, comorbidities mentioned above, relative risk for mortality is higher in those with diabetes. Though, initial studies on effect of diabetes on hospitalization, mortality and morbidity were exclusively done in patients with T2DM, subsequent studies done in type 1 diabetes mellitus (T1DM) showed similar trends in these patients.

In order to avoid getting infected with COVID-19 or to get complications needing hospitalization and intensive treatment, if infection is not avoidable, a person with diabetes should optimize lifestyle changes and use appropriate antidiabetic medications in appropriate doses as per his individual needs and under advice of treating physician. The role of frequent self-monitoring and periodic laboratory tests is obvious. The aim is to persistently maintain tight glycemic control and remain one step ahead of SARS-CoV-2 virus.

There has been considerable work done on role of glycemic status in relation to need for hospitalization, ventilatory support, development of complications, mortality, etc. Poorer the glycemic control, worse is the outcome as regards the parameters discussed above. Glycemic status at the onset of disease is equally important. Higher glycated hemoglobin (HbA1c) at hospitalization is associated with higher morbidity and mortality.

Thus, those with diabetes, as well as their caregivers should work extra hard to maintain persistent good glycemic control. Remaining complacent till getting infected with COVID-19 and then working harder to establish tight glycemic control is detrimental.

## ANTIDIABETIC MEDICATIONS AND COVID-19

No antidiabetic medication is totally contraindicated [beyond usual contraindications, e.g., metformin in grade 5 chronic kidney disease (CKD)], in patients with COVID-19 and diabetes, similarly no antidiabetic medication is the drug of choice in patients with COVID-19 and diabetes, the emphasis is on individualization, as in those without COVID-19.

Following discussion on individual antidiabetic agents or groups will help the clinician to choose *"horses for courses."*

### Metformin

Ambulatory patients with adequate oral intake and stable hemodynamic status can continue to take metformin. Hospitalized patients, particularly if having respiratory complications or if hemodynamically unstable, should not be prescribed metformin as any condition leading to hypoxia increases the likelihood of lactic acidosis, which otherwise is extremely rare but life-threatening complication of metformin therapy. Metformin is contraindicated if glomerular filtration rate (GFR) is <30 mL/min/1.73 m². Some studies have shown beneficial effect on mortality in COVID-19 through suppression of inflammation and cytokine storm.

### Dipeptidyl Peptidase-4 Inhibitors

Dipeptidyl peptidase-4 ($DPP_4$) is present on epithelial cells of respiratory tract in ample quantity and it helps to facilitate entry and multiplication of SARS-COV-2 virus in the respiratory tract. Thus, according to a hypothesis, not conclusively proved, blocking of $DPP_4$-by-$DPP_4$Is can potentially help prevent the spread of this virus. These agents have excellent gastrointestinal (GI) tolerance, require minimum preinitiation assessment including monitoring of renal parameters. Thus, they can be continued in those with good metabolic control and started in appropriate drug naive patient or added to existing antidiabetic medications as per the need. The abovementioned features have increased the popularity of these agents among the clinicians particularly for prescribing during teleconsultation.

## Sulfonylureas

In stable, ambulatory, uncomplicated, well-controlled patients with normal renal function and reliable oral intake, these agents can be continued or started in appropriate drug naive patients or added to other agents as per the need as in those without COVID-19 infection.

Sulfonylureas (SUs) are insulin secretagogues and unlike $DPP_4Is$ and glucagon-like peptide-1 ($GLP_1$) agonists, their action is not glucose dependent, thus incidence of hypoglycemia, which can be severe, serious or prolonged in elderly patients is significantly higher as compared to those on antihyperglycemic agents. In elderly, unstable patients, particularly with renal impairment and in those whose oral intake is unpredictable, SUs, particularly glibenclamide, should be avoided.

## Sodium-glucose Cotransporter-2 Inhibitors

Use of sodium-glucose cotransporter-2 inhibitors ($SGLT_2Is$) leads to a minor increase in lactic acid production resulting in slight reduction of intracellular pH, which is postulated to help host defense against COVID-19. However, these agents should be avoided in hospitalized patients with COVID, particularly in elderly, debilitated, hypovolemic, hypotensive patients, and in those patients with vomiting or inadequate and unpredictable oral intake. In such situations, there is increased likelihood of patients developing normoglycemic ketoacidosis, a rare but potentially lethal complication of $SGLT_2I$ therapy.

## Pioglitazone

Pioglitazone has no specific advantages or disadvantages as regards management of diabetes with associated COVID-19.

## Glucagon-like Peptide 1 Agonists

Gastrointestinal side effects, particularly in initial phase of treatment, and the need for frequent monitoring and dosage adjustment, make this group, a bit unsuitable for fresh prescription. However, those ambulatory, stable patients with mild COVID can continue with these agents.

## Insulin

Those with diabetes have insulin deficiency, absolute or relative, thus insulin therapy has no contraindications. In hospitalized patients with COVID-19 and diabetes, particularly those in ICU set up, those on steroids, insulin has no alternative. Patients already on insulin will naturally require continuation of insulin, while many others, who did not require insulin before they were infected with SARS-CoV-2 virus would require insulin, at least temporarily. The selection of type, dose, and frequency of insulin will depend upon individual situation as in those without SARS-CoV-2 infection.

In short, the general principles of management of diabetes in those with COVID-19 are not different from management of diabetes in general. In critically ill, ICU patients, noninsulin antidiabetic medications have hardly any role to play in the management of hyperglycemia. As the patient becomes noncritical and hemodynamically stable, gradually other agents can be added, starting with $DPP_4Is$ followed by metformin and subsequently other agents, simultaneously, particularly in those who did not require insulin before COVID-19 infection, insulin dosages and frequencies can be gradually reduced and then discontinued as per the individual situation. The *mantra* for attainment of success is thorough individualization using common sense.

## EFFECT OF COVID-19 ON GLYCEMIC CONTROL

Effect of COVID-19 on glycemic control is not as thoroughly studied as effect of diabetes on COVID-19. Severe SARS-CoV-2 infection is associated with stress hyperglycemia, new onset diabetes as well as worsening of glycemic control in a known diabetic. SARS-CoV-2 virus can damage β-cells directly or indirectly through cytokine storm and toxemia which can lead to new onset diabetes. Higher incidence of new onset T1DM has also been reported. Stress of severe infection and steroid administration can lead to worsening of diabetes or temporary stress hyperglycemia. Development of full-blown diabetic ketoacidosis has been reported in patients with COVID-19 infection.

## COVID-19 VACCINATION FOR PATIENTS WITH DIABETES

Diabetes is not at all a contraindication for full immunization with COVID-19 vaccine. In fact, they are more vulnerable to be affected by COVID-19 and develop complications. Thus, patients with diabetes should be preferentially immunized. All patients with diabetes, unless they are acutely ill or have specific allergy issues with COVID-19 vaccines should be vaccinated. Presence of mild to moderate elevation of blood glucose or blood pressure should not be treated as an excuse for postponement or contraindication for vaccination.

In conditions such as severe thrombocytopenia or coagulation disorders, and in those with history of severe allergy in past, domain experts such as hematologists and allergy specialists should be consulted and vaccination can be carried out under their guidance in an institution with well-equipped emergency department as stand by.

Though whether to get vaccinated or not is not an issue at all, there are some unresolved issues such as choice of vaccine, gap between recovery from active COVID-19 infection and vaccination.

A precautionary note regarding the underlying circumstances during which some of the studies on various aspect of COVID-19 were done and published will not be out of place here. The period was extremely stressful. Medical infrastructure was extremely overstretched and was bursting at the seams. During initial phase of pandemic, scientific documentation on COVID-19 was conspicuous by absence. Though many excellent top quality research works were published on COVID-19, as regards, some of the published work on diabetes and COVID-19, the design, planning, execution, and writing was obviously not done under ideal or optimal condition, many studies were descriptional and were published in extra quick time as everybody was thirsty for guidance from scientific data on COVID-19. While interpreting the data, this aspect should be considered. For the medical research workers across all the disciplines, the COVID-19 experience would be handy in future.

# CHAPTER 25

# Travel and Diabetes

## INTRODUCTION

The ever-increasing trend toward travel, both short term and over a longer period, domestic as well as international travel, for various purposes such as leisure travel, adventure travel, religious travel, or travel for study or work has further accelerated due to more and more people participating in "revenge travel." As the end of prolonged corona virus disease of 2019 (COVID-19) pandemic is in sight, everybody, including people with diabetes are expressing their freedom through traveling. The possibilities for travel today are endless, and multiple modes of transport are available to the traveler.

During travel, people with medical conditions such as diabetes have to face many challenges **(Fig. 1)** such as carrying medications and other diabetes supplies, access to healthy and appropriate food on time, storage of insulin and supplies such as glucometer strips and overall management of blood glucose levels, access to healthcare facilities if needed; and last but not the least, possibilities of medical emergencies.

Due to challenges in managing blood glucose levels and higher possibilities of developing medical conditions and emergencies while traveling, particularly if one has a long-standing diabetes or in elderly people with diabetes, they tend to avoid or skip the travel plan. But diabetes should not be a barrier to travel. The good news is that people with diabetes, who have reasonably stable blood glucose control and stable heart and kidney status, can travel

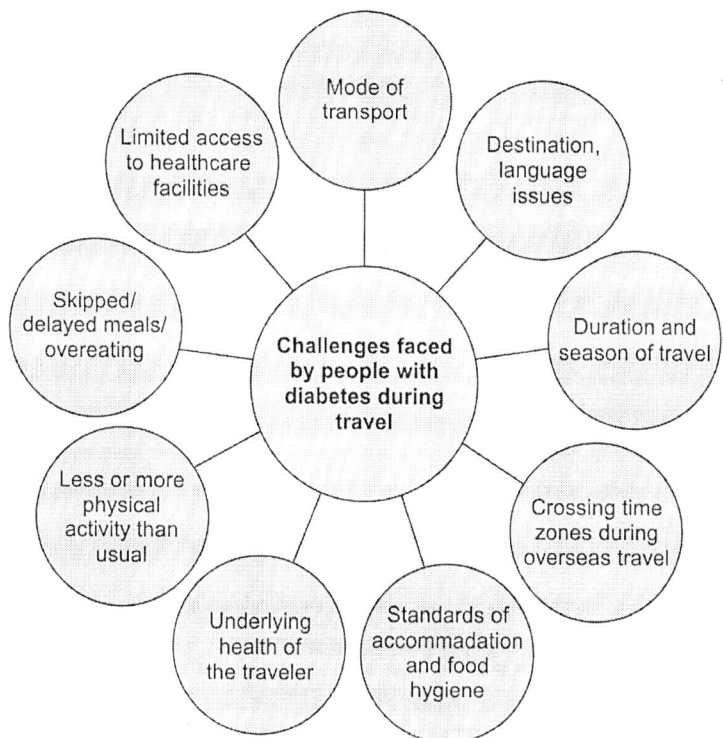

**FIG. 1:** Challenges faced by people with diabetes during travel.

without any fear or stress if they meticulously plan their trip with respect to the diabetes supplies, proper storage of insulin/blood glucose estimating strips, and access to healthy meals.

Below are a few handy tips for people with diabetes embarking on travel.

The tips are particularly useful for those planning long-term international travel and those with long-term diabetes and associated with comorbidities.

## BEFORE GOING

1. A visit to the treating physician is a must at least 1–2 weeks prior to the trip to ensure that the person with diabetes is fit to travel. The individual should also be counseled on the following point.

- How the planned activities could affect glucose levels and how to manage during those times.
2. *If traveling to places in a different time zone, use following guidelines for insulin dosage and time adjustments*:
    - **Flying East (days are shorter):** Adjustment of basal or long-acting insulin (Lantus, Tresiba, Toujeo, etc.), when difference between time at departure and arrival cities is 3 hours or more.
        - On the day before departure, give the usual dose at the usual time of day, e.g., if you are injecting 10 units of Lantus at 10 PM, take same dose at the same time on the day prior to travel.
        - When you begin travel, keep your watch set to your departure country time (do not change time on your watch at the start of the journey) and give half of the normal dose at the usual time, i.e., 5 units at 10 PM while in travel.
        - After giving this half dose, change your watch to the destination time (you can find this out from the flight attendant or from the world clock on your smartphone, Googling airline ticket (difference between time of departure and the time of arrival minus actual flying time, this information is always on your ticket, though boarding pass does not mention actual flying time). If you are wearing a smart watch such as Apple watch, it will automatically get adjusted to arrival city time immediately after arrival.
        - According to your destination time, give the remaining half of the long-acting (basal) insulin at the same hour you are accustomed to giving insulin (in your case, 5 units of Lantus at 10 PM, take your Lantus at 10 PM local time at the city of arrival).
        - The next day keep to the destination time and give the usual full dosage at the usual time, in your case 10 units of Lantus at 10 PM local time. Give short- or rapid-acting insulin before meals as usual.
    - **Flying West (days are longer):** Adjustment of basal or long-acting insulin (Lantus, Tresiba, Toujeo, etc.), when difference between time at departure and arrival cities is 3 hours or more.

The day before departure, give the usual dose at the usual time of day, in your case, 10 units of Lantus at 10 PM.
- When you begin travel, keep your watch set to time of departure city and give 80–90% of regular dose at the usual time, 8 or 9 units of Lantus at 10 PM in your case [10% reduction if time difference is relatively short (3–4 hours), and/or current glycemic control is not very tight].
- After giving this reduced dose, change your watch to the destination city time.
- According to your destination time, give the usual full dose of insulin at the hour you are accustomed to (in your case 10 units of Lantus at 10 PM).
- Give short- or rapid-acting insulin before meals as usual. These insulin do not require any adjustment for time zone changes, but they will require usual adjustments for food timing and amount. Since the days are longer, you will consume at more times during your flight and this will need an additional cover by injecting short- or rapid-acting insulin, preferably later.

- **Using twice-daily premixed insulin (Mixtard, Novomix, Ryzodeg, etc.):** If you use twice-daily premixed insulin, then take your usual insulin before departure at the normal time., If you are taking 10 units of Novomix before breakfast and dinner, take the last predeparture dose as usual, e.g., 10 units of Novomix before breakfast. On the flight carry a pen of rapid-acting insulin, e.g., Novorapid, Apidra, etc. This type of insulin lasts in circulation for 3–4 hours. Check your blood glucose every 4 hours on flight. If it rises above 250 mg, give yourself 4 units rapid-acting insulin every 4 hours (preferably with a meal), e.g., 4 units of Novorapid, until it is time for your usual second injection of premixed insulin as per destination city time after arrival, in your case 10 units of Novomix before breakfast/dinner as per the time of arrival and subsequently continue Novomix 10 units twice a day before breakfast and dinner.
  - Please note these are simplified guidelines and will need some modifications in an individual case. The key is to check your blood glucose levels frequently.
  - To carry a brief resume of medical status including age, duration of diabetes, and associated medical conditions,

and also a detailed prescription which should include all the medications, their dosages and chemical names of all the proprietary drugs; and supplies such as glucometers, test strips, lancets, injection devices, etc., preferably typed on the doctor's letterhead. Such information will be of immense help for local doctor in case of traveler developing medical emergency.
    - Certificate of vaccination against relevant infectious conditions (COVID-19 for current situation, yellow fever if traveling to African continent) should be carried and kept with other travel documents such as passport.
3. Have a ready list of pharmacies and medical facilities close to the hotel.
4. Wear medical Diabetes ID bracelet.
5. Buy an adequate and appropriate travel insurance plan to cover a medical emergency during the trip.
6. For the flight, order a special diabetes-friendly meal in advance or carry meals from home.
7. *Packing*:
    - Carry all diabetes supplies in a carry-on bag (cabin baggage) as insulin may get too cold in check-in-luggage. Divide medicines and supplies in two separate sets in separate bags. Keep one set always with you wherever you go, (e.g., in a small pouch in computer bag or purse in case of women travelers. These two bags are allowed as an additional piece of luggage besides main carry-on bag by all airlines). The second pouch of supplies can be carried in main carry-on bag. So, carry additional small bag even if you are not carrying laptop computer. Often, when flight is fully booked, main carry-on bags of passengers boarding toward the end are taken away from them right at the boarding gate or aircraft door and sent to luggage compartment of aircraft and they are asked to collect them from the luggage belt after arrival. Passengers are likely to forget to remove medicines and supplies for in-flight consumption before handling over the luggage at the last possible moment.
    - Pack twice the quantity of medicines and supplies.
    - Ensure to pack adequate quantities of healthy snacks and nuts. Be prepared for a delay in in-flight food service due to

turbulent air condition or nonavailability of specific food you had ordered before boarding the flight.
8. *Airport security*:
    - In many countries, people with diabetes are exempted from the 100 mL liquid rule for medicines, fast-acting carbs such as juice and gel packs to keep insulin cool.
    - Ask for hand inspection in case of a continuous glucose monitor or insulin pump as medical devices can be damaged while going through the X-ray machine. Those wearing these instruments are advised to carry the pertinent literature to clear the doubts, if any of security personnel is there—asks for it.

## WHILE TRAVELING

1. In case of a road trip, carry a cooler with healthy food and plenty of water to drink.
2. Store insulin in the insulin coolant pouch. Avoid keeping it at a hot place or directly on ice.
3. Avoid leaving blood glucose monitor, test strips, insulin pump, and other diabetes equipment close to heat (hot car, car's dashboard, storage area near gearbox, locked car after you disembark, sunlight, and beach), as it can get damaged.
4. Opt for healthy food options at the airport or a roadside restaurant such as:
    - Salads, greens, fruit (limited quantity), nuts, plain unsweetened yogurt
    - *Chana chaat*, roasted *chana*, unsalted *kurmura*
    - Boiled eggs and brown bread
5. Every hour or two, stop and get out of the car or walk up and down the aisle of the plane or train to keep blood glucose level under control and avoid blood clotting in veins of legs due to stagnation. While traveling in plane during long distance travel, ensure to keep yourself well-hydrated. Remember dehydration during long distance air travel due to excessive insensible perspiration is common and is one of the common causes of developing blood clots in leg veins.
6. Set an alarm on the phone for medication reminders, especially if traveling across time zones.
7. Remember to carry all hygiene and COVID protocol items such as mask and sanitizer.

## AT THE DESTINATION

1. Blood glucose levels may be out of the target range at first, but then the body adjusts in a few days and glucose levels normalize. Check blood glucose levels more frequently and then treat highs or lows as advised by the treating physician.
2. Choose healthy meals as per the recommended meal plan or if eating out of plan, it is important to exercise portion control.
3. Remain physically active.
4. If physical activity is more than usual, check the blood glucose levels before and after activity and adjust food, activity, and insulin/antidiabetes pills as needed.
5. Avoid excessive physical activity if the weather is very hot, to avoid dehydration.
6. Avoid walking barefoot especially on the road/beach/grass or temple premises.
7. In places with extreme temperatures (very hot or cold), the individual may need to check blood glucose levels more often as extreme temperature can change how the body uses insulin.
8. Learn some useful phrases such as "I have diabetes" and "where is the nearest pharmacy?" in the local language, as it may help especially during an international trip or in areas where locals do not understand your language.
9. Carry disposable wipes to clean hands before checking blood glucose levels as it will be handy when outdoors for long.

Traveling is one of the most pleasant, enjoyable, relaxing, and rejuvenating activities of life. It "recharges your batteries" and makes one more knowledgeable and experienced. Like anybody else, a person with diabetes should also participate in traveling to get immense benefits from it. If appropriately planned taking into considerations individual health-based needs and limitations, diabetes need not be a hurdle to travel and the reason for staying at home. Meticulous planning and taking all the precautions before going on a trip will help have a relaxing and more enjoyable trip without derailing the blood glucose control and general health.

Bon Voyage!

# CHAPTER 26

# Some of the Advances in the Management of Diabetes

## INTRODUCTION

Researchers across the world are working to understand different aspects of diabetes including causes, prevention, and management. Every now and then, they make important breakthroughs. It is a continuously evolving process. With the considerable advances made in diabetology over the last decade, prospects for diabetics are getting ever brighter. Let us take a look at some of the advances made in diabetes management over the last few decades.

## CONTINUOUS GLUCOSE MONITORING SYSTEMS

The monitoring systems capable of continuously monitoring interstitial fluid glucose are in clinical use for a day-to-day practice for over a decade. The disposable sensors are tucked in subcutaneous fat. They continuously monitor the tissue fluid glucose and store a mean glucose value every 5 minutes. The real-time versions have a display while those instruments which do not have real-time display facility store the data, which is retrieved as required by placing palm-sized handheld reader in close proximity of sensor or at the end of monitoring period for retrospective study. A daily graph based on 144 glucose readings is generated and 3 days data or 14 days data, depending on durability of the system is superimposed. The data is also available in the form of pie charts. One also gets to know the minimum and maximum values for a given period of 24 hours and time spent as % of 24 hours in desired range of 70–180 mg% (TIR) green color in bar, time spent above the range, above 180 mg% (TAR) yellow and orange colors in bar for range of 180–250 mg% and >250 mg% respectively, and time spent below the range, below 70 mg% (TBR) red color in bar. For an average middle-aged patient without any significant complications and comorbidity, the desired values are: around 70% in TIR, <25% in TAR, and <5% in TBR. Depending upon individualized needs of glycemic control, different times in range standards are set **(Fig. 1)**.

The system also provides an opportunity to study the relationship among variables such as food intake, exercise and antidiabetic drug administration, and their inter-relationship with interstitial fluid glucose. Hypoglycemia and hyperglycemia threshold beeps as well as trend arrows are displayed on the screens of these monitors. The systems are being upgraded by continuous research and development. The quality and durability of recently introduced sensors have improved tremendously. In fact, continuous glucose monitoring system (CGMS) is a 'Diabetologist's Holter monitor' **(Figs. 2 and 3)**. **Figure 3** shows superimposed graphs of three days. By comparing these, one can study day to day glycemic variability.

Some of the limitations include lack of accuracy, though it is continuously improving, time lag between blood glucose and interstitial fluid glucose, usually 10–15 minutes, and the cost.

Three types of CGMS are available at present:
1. *Professional CGMS*: These systems are placed on patients' body in doctor's clinics and they are active for fixed number of days, (14 days in case of Abbott's Libre system). Usually, reader is not given to the patient and at the end of 14 days, the system is removed and the doctor transfers the stored glycemic data from the sensor to software in computer via reader and gets it analyzed. Thus, it is retrospective way of studying glycemic data, deriving conclusions and then changing the management strategies as per the individualized needs of the patients. A new sensor can be applied periodically as per the need of individual patients. This system is suitable for cost-conscious developing country like India. It is also an alternative for those patients who become totally preoccupied and anxious with continuous availability of real-time data.

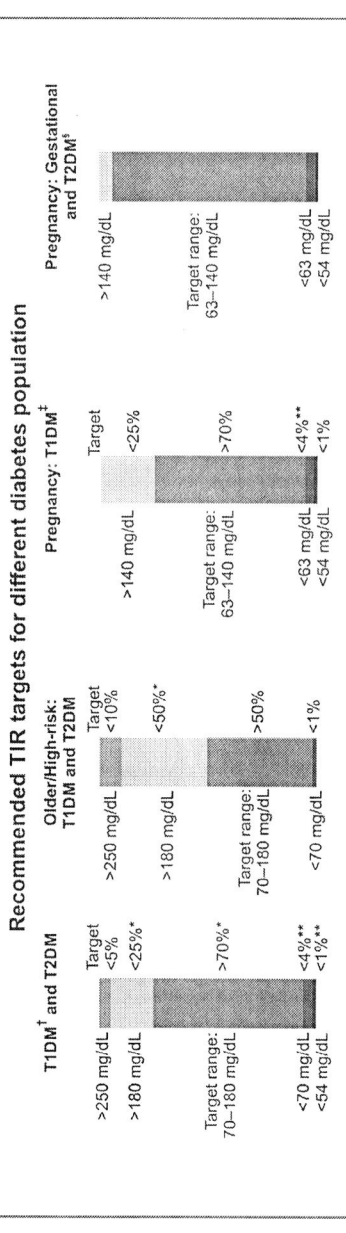

**FIG. 1:** Recommended time in range. *(For color version, see Plate 12)*

(TIR: Time in range; T1DM: type 1 diabetes mellitus; T2DM: type 2 diabetes mellitus)

†For age <25 years, if the A1C goal is 7.5%, then set TIR target to approximately 60% (See clinical applications of time in ranges section in the text for additional information regarding target goal setting in pediatric management).

‡Percentages of time in ranges are based on limited evidence. More research is needed.

§Percentages of time in ranges have not been included because there is very limited evidence in this area. More research is needed. Please see pregnancy section in text for more considerations on targets for these groups.

*Includes percentage of values >250 mg/dL (13.9 mmol/L).

**Includes percentage of values <54 mg/dL (3.0 mmol/L).

*Source:* Battelino T, Danne T, Bergenstal R, et al. Clinical Targets for Continuous Glucose Monitoring Data Interpretation: Recommendations From the International Consensus on Time in Range. Diabetes Care 2019;42:1593-1603.

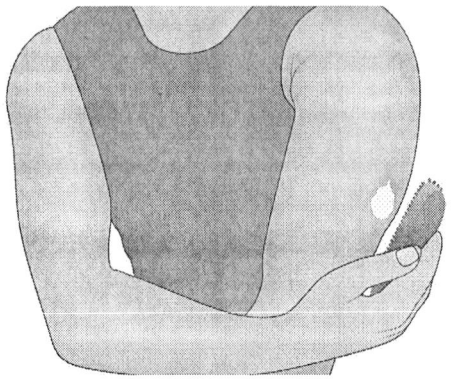

**FIG. 2:** Continuous glucose monitoring (CGM) sensor on patient's shoulder and handheld reader in right palm.

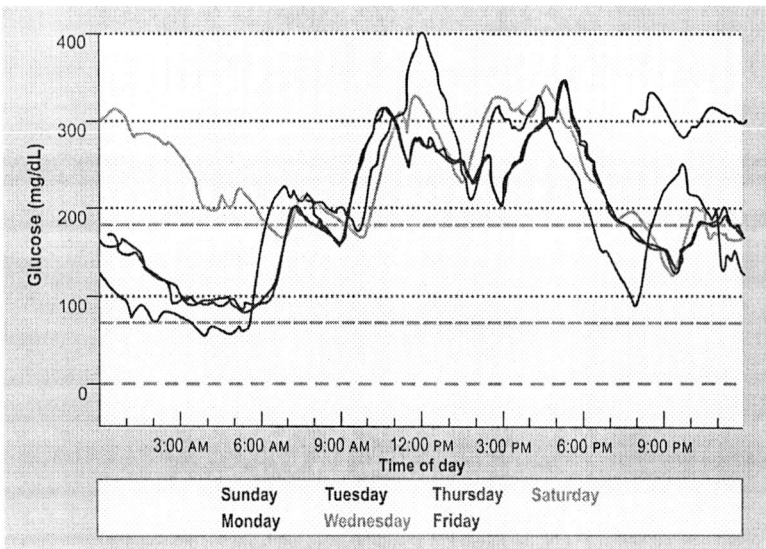

**FIG. 3:** Three days superimposed glucose graphs in continuous glucose monitoring (CGM).

2. *Intermittently scanned CGMS*: In these systems the glucose levels are continuously measured but the patient needs to periodically scan the sensor with handheld reader, usually three times daily for storage of glucose values. The reader remains with the patient and he can scan the sensor for real-time digital glucose

> **BOX 1** **Continuous glucose monitoring system report.**
>
> Mrs SP, a long-standing diabetic on thrice-a-day premixed insulin, was having poor and brittle blood glucose control with documented intraday fluctuations from <60 to >450 mg%.
> She was hooked on CGMS and glucose pattern was studied. She had a high post-breakfast peak, a slightly smaller post-lunch peak, normal post-dinner peak and a tendency for hypoglycemia in early morning. The same pattern was seen over all 3 days. She did not accept basal-bolus regimen. She was shifted to 50:50 premixed insulin before breakfast, to provide her additional rapid-acting insulin to blunt post-breakfast peak. Quicker absorption of prandial component in premixed analog also would provide additional benefit.

value flash on the screen anytime in a day and as many times he wishes.

3. *Real-time CGMS*: In these systems, the interstitial fluid glucose is continuously measured and stored.

A brief report interpreting the above displayed graphs **(Box 1)**.

## Some of the Applications of CGMS

- Type 1 diabetes mellitus (T1DM) and T2DM patients on insulin pumps or multidose insulin therapy.
- For studying glucose pattern in brittle diabetics and those prone for severe hypoglycemia.
- Whenever tight glycemic control is desired, e.g., pregnancy.
- For studying pharmacokinetics of antidiabetic medications
- For studying glycemic variability.

## INSULIN DELIVERY

Even though, rapid strides have been made in the quality of insulin, major drawbacks still remain as regards delivery of insulin. Physiologically, insulin is released round the clock in a pulsed manner directly into the portal circulation, whereas subcutaneous (SC) insulin administration leads to peripheral hyperinsulinemia and low concentration of insulin in the liver—the major site of insulin action. All the currently available delivery systems including pumps and artificial pancreas are using subcutaneous routes. Though this major obstacle has not yet been overcome, the methods of delivery of insulin through SC route have been gradually improved.

## Open-loop Delivery System

The insulin delivery systems which do not have integrated algorithm to analyze collected glycemic data and thus cannot decide about insulin dosing and automatically deliver the dose, are known as open loop systems. Insulin syringes and pens are the simplest of these systems while conventional insulin pumps as well as next generation pumps including sensor augmented pumps are also part of the open loop system.

While research in high tech open and closed-loop delivery systems is progressing, there have been some improvements in conventional subcutaneous insulin delivery systems. Insulin is commercially available, both in vials and in sealed cartridges. The latter form is available for use in pen injection devices. These devices can be carried in shirt pockets as ordinary pens. They free diabetics from the need to carry all the equipment normally required for conventional insulin injections. Several brands of patient-friendly disposable as well as reusable pens are now available in our country.

### *Insulin Pumps*

These consist of various models of portable insulin pumps, which can be attached to waist belt or kept in trouser pocket. A needle that is inserted in the SC tissue on the anterior abdominal wall is attached to the pump via polyethylene tubing. The pump case contains a syringe, the piston of which is driven by the pump. The rate of continuous insulin delivery is adjustable. In addition, there is a provision to give a premeal booster dose of insulin. By using the pump, it is possible to deliver insulin in continuous subcutaneous infusion at a rate mimicking the physiological rate of insulin delivered from the pancreas. For more than three decades a large number of patients, mostly T1DM patients, have been using these pumps and it has been shown that their use leads to better control of blood glucose level, thus postponing specific complications of diabetes as compared to conventional insulin administration. However, open-loop delivery systems have their own limitations. They administer insulin into the systemic circulation and not into the portal circulation. Another drawback of the open-loop system is the absence of a sensor to monitor blood/tissue glucose concentrations, and a computer to determine the dosage. Moreover, open-loop pump systems have their own complications such as equipment failure leading to too much or too little insulin administration with obvious consequences, cutaneous complications such as painful lumps and abscesses at the site of needle insertion, which are not very rare.

Furthermore, the cost of pumps (minimum ₹100,000) is out of reach of average Indians. However, number of Indian diabetic patients using pumps has gone up significantly over last decade.

Recently, an upgraded version of conventional insulin pump has been developed. The system contains a sensor to continuously monitor glucose levels. The glucose data is fed into pump's memory and it automatically stops delivery of insulin for a specified period of time at preset glucose level, thus preventing hypoglycemia. This is a big step forward over standalone sensors that are in use for more than a decade and pumps with sensors in a system that are not smart to suspend insulin delivery during impending hypoglycemia.

### *Smartphones*

Researchers have developed a smartphone with blood glucose estimation capability. The phone has an inbuilt glucometer with a slot to insert blood glucose estimation strip. It has a memory to store all the blood glucose estimation results and transmits the data to phone or computer of third party such as treating doctors and parents in case of minor patients.

## Closed-loop Delivery System

Insulin delivery systems which include computerized algorithms interfaced between sensors and delivery systems. The decisions about insulin dosage and delivery are partly automated in a closed loop system. These systems are also known as artificial pancreas.

### *Biostator (Artificial Pancreas)*

Biostator was the first version of artificial pancreas. It was a large-sized instrument, comparable in size to the main frame computers of early years and was used for limited time in hospitalized patients and mainly for research. It had following parts:
- Glucose analyzer for continuous monitoring of blood glucose
- A pump to deliver insulin and glucose

- A computer to determine infusion rate of insulin
- Printer to automatically record all the biochemical data.

**Current Status**

From the days of Biostator till today, there has been slow but ongoing improvement on all the fronts of artificial pancreas. The sensors, which continuously analyze interstitial fluid glucose are becoming increasingly reliable and durable. The reliability of pumps has improved while the size has dramatically reduced. The current pumps are about palm sized. The modern pumps have safety features such as automatic suspension of insulin delivery at adjustable glucose levels. The software containing algorithm which used to be housed in desktops and then laptops is now housed in a small handheld instrument and it wirelessly receives data from sensor, analyzes it, decides about insulin dosages, and wirelessly signals the pump to adjust insulin delivery rates. Many sensors are round in shape and have a diameter roughly of the size of 5 rupees coin. They are attached to skin on anterior abdominal wall or shoulder. A small filament-like projection from inner surface is placed in SC tissue where it measures interstitial fluid glucose. The palm-sized pump is attached a waist belt or a trouser pocket or kept in trouser pocket. A small tube emerging from pump delivers insulin through needle which is fixed to nearby subcutaneous tissue. The software containing device can be kept in shirt pocket. Artificial pancreas is no longer an experimental tool. In 2017 and 2018, USA and European authorities gave permission for use of specific models of artificial pancreas to commercial companies respectively and these pumps are being used by type 1 diabetic patients in those countries. Since then, lot of clinical studies have been performed comparing artificial pancreas with sensor augmented pumps and superiority of former is proved.

*Limitations of artificial pancreas*: The current version of commercially available artificial pancreas has some limitations such as:

- The system is not fully automated, but is hybrid, because manual inputs are required to adjust prandial bolus of insulin since absorption of insulin delivered to subcutaneous tissue is a slow process. (Physiologically glucose sensors sense postprandial rise insulin in seconds and extra insulin is delivered in portal circulation, not in subcutaneous tissue, in double quick time.)

- The system is not yet adequately validated in rapidly changing situations such as sudden intense physical activity.
- The durability of sensors and pump battery and insulin storage capacity of pump need improvement.
- The cost of artificial pancreas and the bureaucratic hurdles are irksome.
- Hypoglycemic episodes with artificial pancreas need to be reduced.

## FUTURE OF ARTIFICIAL PANCREAS

The ongoing research is working on all these fronts. Dual hormone systems using simultaneous delivery of glucagon or pramlintide along with insulin are being developed to reduce hypoglycemic episodes. Fed up with commercial organizations on one side and bureaucrats on the other, "Do It Yourselves" groups of T1DM patients, their parents and technocrats working on nonprofit basis have been formed. These groups are developing their own systems. They design their own algorithms and connect them with commercially available pumps and sensors. Implantable artificial pancreas offers some of the solutions such as delivery of insulin directly to the portal circulation, but has its own limitations such as need of surgery for implantation and logistics issues such as difficulties faced while changing the batteries, local reactions, etc. Modern technologies such as cloud computing and artificial intelligence are also used in design and execution of algorithm directed actions. Some progress has also been made in development of bionic artificial pancreas, which is more automated as compared to currently available systems which depend upon manual dosage adjustment during prandial period to check postprandial rise in blood glucose. The bionic artificial pancreas makes its calculations for prandial insulin requirements based on patient's body weight and artificial intelligence. It is another step nearer the ultimate aim of having totally automated pancreas.

### Pancreatic Transplantation

The application of pancreatic transplantation for the management of diabetes has been gradually increasing, following the first pancreas transplant done successfully in 1966 by Kelly and Lillehei in Minnesota, USA. This is the most physiological approach to maintain euglycemia in diabetics. However, immunological and technical problems are plenty and hence surgery can be done only at a few highly specialized centers. These problems are being gradually overcome and the success rate of pancreatic transplantation, even though at present much lower than kidney transplantation, is gradually improving. In patients with diabetic nephropathy and end-stage renal failure, pancreatic transplantation is being done simultaneously with kidney transplantation. The use of modern immunosuppressants has considerably reduced the graft rejection rates and there has been continuous improvement in surgical techniques. More than 50 institutions in the West are doing pancreas transplantation surgery and the mean 1-year survival rates of grafts are gradually improving. In most of the cases, pancreas from cadaver donors is used. Considering the cost and side effects of lifelong immunosuppression, standalone pancreatic transplantation is not recommended.

## Islet Cells Transplantation

Islet cells transplantation has been successful to some extent in humans and further research work is going on currently to improve the success rate further. There are two potential advantages of islet cell transplantation:
1. It is much simpler procedure for recipients, and
2. In vitro manipulations can be performed on islet cells before transplantation in order to reduce immunogenicity.

However, the need for lifelong immunosuppression has not yet been eliminated. Its limitations include paucity of islets cells for transplantation.

A variety of techniques to protect the transplanted islet cells from the immune system are being developed. The approach involves encapsulation of islet cells in materials that enable vascularization and oxygenation while avoiding immune cells and antibodies.

## Alternative Insulin Producing Cell Resources

Scientists are simultaneously working on several alternative strategies to overcome limitations encountered with islet cell transplantation.

## EMBRYONIC STEM CELL RESEARCH

Cells from freshly fertilized embryo from "in vitro fertilization (IVF)" can be grown in laboratory and selective growth and differentiation of pancreatic beta cells can be promoted in laboratory. Research on various aspects of this highly potential area is being carried out. If and when successful, it will offer an exciting alternative to pancreatic and islet cell transplantation. However, at present, work is in preliminary stage.

Simultaneously, work is also going on adult human pluripotent stem cell to dedifferentiate it and then transdifferentiate into functional beta cell.

## GENE THERAPY

This exciting subject has opened up the possibility of "cure for diabetes". It has been demonstrated that a gene responsible for insulin synthesis can be introduced into cells that previously did not synthesize insulin, and that these cells can be introduced in animals in which they can function in a predictable and physiological manner, which means insulin secretion as per the demand and shutting down insulin synthesis when blood glucose approaches basal normal range.

Another approach is to use the gene that determines tissue sensitivity to insulin. Mutation of the *SHIP2* gene is associated with severe reduction in tissue sensitivity to insulin, leading to diabetes. If this is tackled, insulin sensitivity can be increased and blood glucose can be normalized. Yet another approach is to use the gene that will prevent overgrowth of blood vessels in the retina which causes diabetic retinopathy, leading to blindness. Though, there are several challenges to be overcome before gene therapy in diabetes becomes a reality but it is encouraging that the possibility exists.

## NEWER INSULIN

*Insulin analogs*: Recombinant DNA technology is being used to produce several insulin analogs by the process of biological engineering. These analogs have the same biological activity as human insulin but have different pharmacokinetic profiles which are beneficial. Certain analogs are absorbed faster as compared to human insulin. They can be used with advantage in those whose postprandial blood glucose is difficult to control. Other analogs have a longer biological half-life as compared to intermediate-acting human insulin and hence are more suitable for patients having difficulty in controlling fasting hyperglycemia.

In insulin analogs, certain amino acids of insulin polypeptide chains which are not involved in the stability and biological activity of insulin are deleted or substituted to create analogs which have more desirable pharmacokinetic profiles.

In addition, in long-acting analogs, fatty acid side chains are attached to specific amino acids. These side chains help insulin crystals hold together in subcutaneous tissue for longer time and prolong the duration of action. Rapid-acting analogs (Lispro, Apidra and aspart) and long-acting analogs such as glargine, detemir and degludec insulin are already available. Fiasp is a modified version of aspart. Nicotinamide and amino acid, arginine are added to aspart in this formulation. Nicotinamide increases the speed of absorption, to make fiasp the fastest acting among all the currently available rapid-acting insulin analogs. Different groups are currently working on more rapid and long-acting analogs as well as ultralong-acting analogs aiming to develop a molecule with unique features to serve the needs of insulin requiring patients in a more efficient manner.

***Once weekly long-acting insulin [Icodec]:*** Icodec is long-acting insulin for once a week administration. It is in advanced stage of development and has already completed phase 3 studies. In 26 weeks comparative study in 526 type 2 diabetic patients, the glycemic efficacy as judged by reduction in HbA1c and time spent in range during CGM was equal to the patients in comparative group on once or twice a day long-acting insulin analogs [glargine, glargine 300; degludec]. The incidence of hypoglycemia was negligible and equal in both the groups.

In a similar comparative study done on type 1 diabetic patients, glycemic efficacy was similar but incidence of hypoglycemia was higher in icodec group, probably because of greater day to day variability of insulin requirement in type 1 diabetic patients.

Availability of once week long-acting insulin is expected to significantly improve acceptance and ease of insulin initiation and long-term compliance.

## Novel Insulin Molecules in Pipeline

*Glucose-sensitive insulin:* This novel concept is in the early stage of development. Glucose-sensitive insulin has two separate sites for host receptors, one each for insulin and mannose. Depending upon the prevailing blood glucose concentration, insulin is shunted from one to another receptor site for attachment. When blood glucose falls beyond a threshold, more insulin gets attached to mannose receptors, thus less is available for insulin receptors. In this way, hypoglycemia is avoided.

*Insulin analog 327-liver specific insulin:* This insulin analog is also in early developmental stage. It has an albumin-binding side chain, which considerably reduces its binding to insulin receptors while passing through systemic circulation and helps it to selectively concentrate in liver. Thus, it restores hepatosystemic insulin gradient and reduces episodes of hypoglycemia.

## ROUTES OF ADMINISTRATION OF INSULIN

The limitations and unphysiological nature of subcutaneous insulin administration are well known; hence continuous peritoneal infusion of insulin has been explored. This route mimics, to some extent, the normal portal to systemic circulation insulin gradient. Implantable intraperitoneal devices are used to administer insulin via this route. Obstruction of implantable catheter is a major complication.

## Inhalation Route

Ability to avoid injections and quicker onset of action than currently available rapid-acting insulin are the main attractions of inhaled insulin. The limitations are poor bioavailability, dependence on a device to inhale it and safety of suspending agents.

Strips containing dry powdered insulin are being developed. These strips are introduced in a device that releases insulin and helps the patient to inhale released insulin into the lungs. Absorption takes place in pulmonary circulation. Exubera, the first inhaled insulin for absorption through pulmonary route, was introduced in the Western markets a few years back, but was voluntarily withdrawn from the market by the manufacturer soon after its introduction. Lack of commercial success and possibility of carcinogenicity of aerosol suspending agent were the probable reasons for hasty withdrawal. Subsequently another product under the trade name Afrezza® was launched. It is user-friendly and has a better pharmacokinetic profile.

## Buccal Route

Insulin which is available in aerosol form is sprayed in buccal mucosa through which it is absorbed in circulation. The only country where this product is available for some time is Ecuador in South America. A few years back, buccal insulin made a brief appearance in India, before its withdrawal from the market as per the direction of the authorities.

## Nasal Route

Intranasal administration of insulin has been used experimentally for several years. A major problem is the adjuvants that are used to facilitate transnasal absorption of insulin, produce nasal irritation. Moreover, there are no large-scale trials to study variability of insulin absorption in diseases of the nasal mucosa. Because of abovementioned obstacles, nasal insulin research has become somewhat stagnant.

## Oral Insulin

Insulin molecule being a protein is split up into its constituent amino acids by the enzymes in upper gastrointestinal (GI) tract before its absorption in the circulation, thus it is totally ineffective when administered by oral route. However, considering patient's resistance to accept injectable insulin, several groups are attempting to develop a system of an envelope or a coating which would prevent digestion of insulin in upper GI tract and facilitate its absorption in an intact form. An Indian group working for Biocon, a biotechnology and pharmaceutical concern based in Bengaluru, is in forefront of the development of oral insulin. They have used polymer technology and their oral insulin (IN 105) is in phase 3 clinical trial. Both rapid and long-acting oral insulin preparations are being developed. Research has been ongoing for years but it still has a long way to come to the market.

## Miscellaneous Noninjectable Insulin Preparations

Looking at the large potential for insulin administration through noninjection route due to severe aversion to lifelong injection of insulin, several groups are working to find out the solution. Subcutaneous patches, orally ingested unfolding microneedle devices and indigestible microapplicator devices that adhere to the GI wall and deliver calibrated dose of insulin, are some of the ongoing projects.

## IMMUNOSUPPRESSION IN THE MANAGEMENT OF TYPE 1 DIABETES MELLITUS

Type 1 diabetes mellitus is due to autoimmune destruction of insulin producing beta cells of the pancreas. Autoantibodies against insulin and beta cell are often present in patients with newly diagnosed T1DM. Thus, therapeutic efforts have been directed toward intervention with various immunosuppressive agents, soon after the diagnosis. Results of initial attempts using steroids, antilymphocytic serum, azathioprine and plasmapheresis have been inconclusive; however, work on agents such as cyclosporine, mycophenolate mofetil, anti-TNF, anti-CD3 and other agents has produced some encouraging results. In a trial on 40 T1DM patients on cyclosporine, it was demonstrated that early treatment with cyclosporine can induce remission from insulin dependence, with half the patients not requiring insulin after a full year. Work in this direction is ongoing.

## EMERGING ANTIDIABETIC AGENTS (OTHER THAN INSULIN)

### Tirzepatide

Tirzepatide is a novel once weekly injectable dual glucose-dependent insulinotropic polypeptide (GIP) and glucagon-like peptide-1 receptor agonist ($GLP_1RA$) agent recently approved in USA for use as an adjutant to diet and exercise to improve glycemic control in T2DM. In addition, it is being developed for use in obesity and nonalcoholic fatty liver disease. In phase III trials, its efficacy has been proved in several comparative clinical trials against anti-diabetic agents including $GLP_1RAs$ (once-a-week semaglutide and dulaglutide), and insulin (glargine and degludec). Its indications are broadly the same as those of $GLP_1RAs$ and needs same precautions while initiating therapy. In order to minimize GI intolerance, it is started in the dose of 2.5 mg SC once a week and every 4 weeks the dose is increased by 2.5 mg. The therapeutic dose is 5-15 mg once a week. In phase III trials, average glycated hemoglobin (HbA1c) reduction of 1.8-2.1% for 5 mg dose, and 1.7-2.5% for 10 and 15 mg dose was observed at the end of 40 weeks. The average weight reduction during the same period was 5.4 kg and 11.3 kg for 5 mg and 15 mg dose, respectively. Thus, the results obtained were superior to the comparator antidiabetic medications for glycemic efficacy as well as weight reduction. Tirzepatide use was not associated with hypoglycemia.

At present, tirzepatide is approved for improving glycemic control in T2DM as monotherapy or in combination with a wide range of antidiabetic medications (excluding other incretin-based agents such as $DPP_4I$ and $GLP_1RAs$). It has a great potential for use as antiobesity agent and for remission in T2DM. In future, it may reduce the need for bariatric surgery.

## Colesevelam Hydrochloride

This new bile acid sequestrant is primarily used for treatment of hypercholesterolemia. In recent clinical trials, it was noted that this compound also has significant blood glucose reducing effect. In a study on T2DM patients on oral antidiabetic agents, 12 weeks treatment with colesevelam, given primarily for hypercholesterolemia, resulted in reduction of HbA1c by 0.5%. The promising effect on glycemic control needs verification in large long-term studies. This agent is already available in the US market as an antidiabetic agent for the last few years.

## Pramlintide

While insulin has been the mainstay of therapy in diabetes, the quest for better control with fewer unwanted effects such as weight gain and hypoglycemia, and the need for constant dosage adjustment has led to search for newer and newer agents and antidiabetic therapy is in continuous state of evolution. Diabetes is a disease with multihormonal defects. Besides insulin deficiency, there is also a deficiency of amylin which is cosecreted along with insulin by the beta cells. The physiological actions of amylin are complementary to those of insulin. Amylin reduces appetite, delays gastric emptying, and suppresses inappropriate postprandial rise of glucagon thus suppressing hepatic glucose production. Amylin deficiency is seen in both T1DM and T2DM. Amylin has a short biological half-life thus has no therapeutic value for day-to-day practice. Pramlintide is a synthetic analog of amylin with a long half-life, making it suitable for twice a day SC injections. It is available in the USA and is indicated as an adjuvant to insulin in those failing to reach glycemic target in T1DM and T2DM. The usual dose is 60 μg twice a day subcutaneously just before meals. Its use leads to significant improvement in metabolic control as judged by HbA1c reduction. Its effect on postprandial blood glucose is more pronounced than that on fasting blood glucose. The plus points of pramlintide are weight reduction, relative freedom from hypoglycemia and simple dosage schedule, which obviates dosage titration. The side effects include nausea, occasional vomiting, and hypoglycemia, induced through insulin which is coadministered. While GI side effects reduce as the therapy is continued, hypoglycemia is tackled by reducing dose of insulin. Pramlintide is also used in dual hormone pumps along with insulin to reduce incidence and severity of hypoglycemia. A dual hormone artificial pancreas is still considered experimental and is not yet in the market.

## Glucokinase Activators

There are four hexokinase enzymes, namely HK1, HK2, HK3 and glucokinase (HK4). The main sites of action of glucokinase are liver and beta cells. Glucose is transported inside these cells by glucose transporter (GLUT). Subsequently, glucokinase converts it to glucose-6-phosphate, which is taken up and further metabolized by the mitochondria in beta cells. ATP formed as a result helps in closure of potassium channels, which leads to depolarization of cell membrane which in turn opens calcium channels, leading to release of insulin. In the hepatic cells, glucose-6-phosphate is converted to glycogen or broken down (glycogenesis and glycolysis). In T2DM, hepatic glucose uptake is reduced. Glucokinase activators are being studied in animals at present. These agents increase hepatic glucose uptake and release of insulin from the beta cells. Potential side effects include hypoglycemia and hepatic steatosis.

## Glucagon Antagonists

One of the pathogenic features of T2DM is increased hepatic glucose production mainly through gluconeogenesis, resulting from excessive postprandial hyperglucagonemia. Metformin blocks about 25% of excessive hepatic glucose production. Administration of glucagon antagonists in experimental diabetic mice has led to reduction of blood glucose by blocking glucagon-induced hepatic gluconeogenesis. Work on human volunteers is in preliminary stage.

## Sirtuins

There are seven sirtuin deacetylases in human body. These enzymes have widespread distribution and perform varied functions. Resveratrol, which is extracted from grapes and which is present in red wine, has a property to activate sirtuin-1 deacetylase. In animals, it has been shown to have multiple beneficial effects including reduction in blood glucose, antiaging activity, prevention of osteoporosis and beneficial effects on cardiovascular system.

## Once-a-week $DPP_4Is$

*Omarigliptin* and *trelagliptin* are long-acting oral $DPP_4I$ available in Japan for once-a-week administration. Clinical efficacy is equivalent to sitagliptin. Cardiovascular Outcomes Trials (CVOTs) have not been performed since companies marketing these molecules are not interested in making them available in USA, the only country where premarketing CVOTs are mandatory to prove cardiovascular safety of antidiabetic agent.

## Emerging Antiobesity Formulations

### Liraglutide

Liraglutide is $GLP_1RA$. It is routinely used in the dosage of 1.2 mg or 1.8 mg subcutaneously once a day in the management of T2DM for more than a decade. Recently, it completed successful clinical trials in obesity.

It was administered in the dose of 3.0 mg once a day subcutaneously in nondiabetic as well as in diabetic patients.

Its use led to significant weight reduction and has received USA FDA marketing approval recently.

## Semaglutide

Injectable semaglutide has established its role as once-a-week agent for management of T2DM. In June 2022, USA FDA gave nod for its use in the dosage of 2.4 mg subcutaneously once a week as an antiobesity agent in those with obesity plus one risk factor.

# DIABETES IN THE 21ST CENTURY

There have been considerable advances in the field of diabetology in the first two decades of 21st century and the future prospects for a diabetic patient are brightening. In the near future, immunosuppression therapy would be perfected. Similarly, islet cell transplantation would be much more successful and progress will be made in fully automating artificial pancreas, embryonic stem cell therapy and insulin gene therapy.

# CHAPTER 27

# Prevention of Diabetes

## INTRODUCTION

Prevention of diabetes like many other diseases can be planned at four levels depending upon the point of time at which preventive measures are initiated. These are as follows:
- *Primordial prevention:* To prevent onset of prediabetes
- *Primary prevention*: To prevent onset of diabetes
- *Secondary prevention*: To prevent onset of complications of diabetes by persistent tight control of blood glucose
- *Tertiary prevention*: To prevent progression of complications which have already set in.

In India, it is estimated that there is at least one prediabetic [impaired glucose tolerance (IGT) and impaired fasting glucose (IFG)] for every diabetic. Every year 18% of Indian prediabetics pass the upper limit of their prediabetic blood glucose levels and become diabetic (the conversion rate is only 5–10% for Western population). "Once a diabetic, always a diabetic". Diabetes, particularly type 2 diabetes mellitus (T2DM) is as much a vascular disease as it is a metabolic disease. Two-thirds of type 2 diabetic patients die of macrovascular disease; among them, three-fourths mortality is due to coronary artery disease. At the time of diagnosis of diabetes, which could be as late as 5 years after the onset in some patients, around half will show some evidence of cardiac involvement, if subjected to investigations with sophisticated diagnostic tools. In advanced countries, where mortality from coronary artery disease is decreasing in general population, it has not decreased to the same extent in diabetic subset. Life expectancy of type 2 diabetic patients is 5-10 years shorter. Thus, if one has to prevent mortality and morbidity from macrovascular diseases in general and coronary artery disease in particular in diabetic patients, it is too late if he starts preventive measures after the diagnosis of diabetes with the intention of primary prevention of coronary artery disease. *The best means of primary prevention of coronary artery disease* is primary *prevention of diabetes*. Considering all these factors, it is prudent to prevent the disease which has no cure but many long-term potentially lethal complications. While it will not be cost-effective and impossible to prevent diabetes in every nondiabetic person, a selective approach of prevention or postponement of T2DM (96% of diabetic patients in our country belong to this subclass) in those who are prediabetic will yield gratifying results. Several large studies on primary prevention of T2DM with lifestyle modifications as well as with oral antidiabetic agents have been done. Some selected studies are summarized below.

## IMPORTANT DIABETES PRIMARY PREVENTION STUDIES

### The Finnish Diabetes Prevention Study

In this study, 522 middle-aged overweight people with IGT were randomized to intensive lifestyle intervention and control groups. Those in intervention group received individualized counseling aimed at reducing weight, total intake of fat, saturated fat and increasing intake of fiber and physical activity. The mean follow-up period was 3.2 years. The cumulative incidence of diabetes at the end of trial was 11% and 23%, respectively, in intervention and control group. Thus, the risk of diabetes was reduced by 58% in the intervention group.

### Diabetes Prevention Program

The 3,234 mostly obese American participants of this study consisted of those having IGT or IFG, those with strong family history or associated risk factors, overweight, and those with history of gestational diabetes. The study period was of 3.5 years. The participants were divided in four groups—(1) intensive lifestyle modifications (150 minutes of exercise per week and aim of reducing at least 7% of the baseline weight), (2) metformin, (3) troglitazone, and (4) placebo. Compared to placebo group, intensive lifestyle management group and metformin group had 58% and 31% reduction in the risk for development of diabetes, respectively. Within 10 months after initiation of study, troglitazone was withdrawn from the market and thus this arm was suspended.

## Study to Prevent Noninsulin-dependent Diabetes Mellitus

This was a 3-year study in which people having IGT were randomized to receive 100 mg of acarbose three times a day or placebo. At the end of study period, there was 25% risk reduction for development of diabetes in acarbose group as compared to placebo group. In addition, there was reduction in cardiovascular risk in acarbose group in respect of development of hypertension and acute myocardial infarction.

## Diabetes Reduction Assessment with Ramipril and Rosiglitazone Medication

In this study 5,269 people with IGT, IFG, or both, and no previous history of cardiovascular disease participated. They were randomized to receive 15 mg of ramipril/day or placebo, or 8 mg of rosiglitazone/day or placebo, by using 2 × 2 factorial design and followed up for 3 years. Use of rosiglitazone led to impressive 62% risk reduction for development of diabetes as compared to only 9% risk reduction in those on ramipril. However, subsequently, due to its cardiovascular side effects, rosiglitazone was banned in many countries including the USA, Western Europe, and India.

## Indian Diabetes Prevention Programme

In this study by A Ramachandran's group, 531 subjects with IGT were randomized into four groups [controls, lifestyle modifications (LSM), metformin, and LSM plus metformin]. The mean follow-up period was 30 months. As compared to controls, the relative risk reduction was 28.5% with LSM, 26.4% with metformin, and 28.2% with LSM plus metformin.

## Troglitazone in the Prevention of Diabetes

This study was conducted on 266 Hispanic women who had gestational diabetes in the past. It was 1:1 double-blind study in which role of troglitazone in prevention of diabetes was compared with placebo. Risk of development of diabetes was reduced by 56% in troglitazone group as compared to control group. During the course of the study, troglitazone had to be discontinued due to its potential hepatotoxicity. Eight months after the discontinuation of troglitazone, the protective effects had continued. Thus, troglitazone was successful in true prevention of diabetes and not only in reduction of blood glucose.

## Xenical in the Prevention of Diabetes in Obese Subjects

In this 4-year double-blind prospective study, 3,305 obese patients were randomized to LSM plus orlistat 120 mg three times a day or LSM only (79% had normal glucose tolerance and 21% had IGT). Orlistat group had 37.7% relative risk reduction for development of diabetes as compared to control group at the end of 4 years.

## ACT NOW Study with Pioglitazone

In a study published in 2011, 45 mg of pioglitazone was compared with placebo in people with IGT. 602 people participated in a trial lasting over 2.4 years. There was 72% risk reduction as regards development of diabetes in pioglitazone subgroup as compared to placebo subgroup. However, weight gain and edema developed in significant number of patients in pioglitazone group **(Table 1)**.

## Prevention of Type 2 Diabetes Mellitus in those with Prediabetes and/or Metabolic Syndrome with Phentermine plus Topiramate Extended Release Tablets

In this study, overweight patients with prediabetes and/or metabolic syndrome were included and divided in three groups: (1) placebo, (2) 7.5/46 mg phentermine-topiramate combination, and (3) 15/92 mg phentermine-topiramate combination. At the end

**TABLE 1: Reduction of diabetes risk in various studies.**

| Study | Intervention | Number of subjects | Diabetes risk reduction in % | Duration |
|---|---|---|---|---|
| FDPS | Lifestyle changes | 522 | 58 | 3.2 years |
| DPP | Lifestyle changes<br>Metformin | 3,234 | 58<br>31 | 2.8 years |
| STOP-NIDDM | Acarbose | 1,148 | 25 | 3.3 years |
| DREAM | Rosiglitazone/<br>Ramipril | 5,629 | 62<br>9 | 3 years |
| Da Quing | Lifestyle changes | 577 | 31–46 | 6 years |
| IDPP | Lifestyle changes<br>metformin LSM +<br>metformin | 531 | 28.5<br>26.7<br>28.2 | 2.5 years |
| Swedish Malmo study | Lifestyle changes | 222 | >50 | 6 years |
| TRIPOD | Troglitazone | 266 women with previous gestational diabetes | 56 | 2.5 years |
| XENDOS | Orlistat | 3,305 | 37.7 | 4 years |
| ACT NOW | Pioglitazone | 602 | 72 | 2.4 years |
| Prevention of T2DM | Phenteramide + topiramate | 475 | 78.7 | 108 weeks |
| CAMELLIA | Lorcaserin* | 12,000 | 19–23 | 3.3 years |

*Lorcaserin was recently banned in USA and many other countries including India.

(ACT NOW: Actos Now for Prevention of Diabetes; CAMELLIA: Cardiovascular and Metabolic Effects of Lorcaserin in Overweight and Obese Patients; DREAM: Diabetes Reduction Assessment with Ramipril and Rosiglitazone Medication; DPP: Diabetes Prevention Program; FDPS: Finnish Diabetes Prevention Study; IDPP: Indian Diabetes Prevention Programme; STOP-NIDDM: Study to Prevent Non-Insulin-Dependent Diabetes Mellitus; TRIPOD: Transparent Reporting of a multivariable prediction model for Individual Prognosis or Diagnosis; T2DM: type 2 diabetes mellitus; XENDOS: XENical in the prevention of diabetes in obese subjects)

of 108 weeks, those in group 2 and 3 had 70.5% and 78.7% reduction in annualized incidence of T2DM as compared to those in group 1 (placebo). The weight reduction noticed over same period was 2.5% in placebo group versus 10.9–12.1% in low- and high-dose phentermine-topiramate group respectively.

## Camellia Study

Camellia study was performed in 12,000 overweight or obese patients with atherosclerotic cardiovascular disease or risk factors for the same. In this study, 10 mg of lorcaserin twice a day was compared with placebo. At the end of 1 year in those who were prediabetic at the beginning of the study, there was 2.8 kg weight reduction and 23% risk reduction for development of diabetes as compared to placebo.

## SUMMARY

Primary prevention or postponement of T2DM is vital and possible with the correct approach at right time. Nonpharmacological measures have given excellent results in Diabetes Prevention Program (DPP) study. However, in a day-to-day clinical setting, it is difficult to sustain intensive nonpharmacological measures over a long-term period. Among the medications, glitazones have given best results while metformin and acarbose have been found to be fairly effective. Though, long-term safety and efficiency of pharmacological agents need to be further verified before they can be widely recommended in day-to-day practice, they offer a great promise to reduce the burden of diabetes on the community. Pharmacoeconomic studies on the role of pharmacological agents in prevention of diabetes are also needed.

In order to detect prediabetic state as early as possible, following measures are recommended.

- Every person should undergo fasting and post-75 g glucose load blood glucose levels at 30 years. These tests should be repeated every 2 years as long as the values are well within normal range.
- Those with family history of diabetes, and those with other cardiovascular risk factors and, those with history of gestational diabetes, or delivering large-sized baby should be screened earlier depending upon individual situation (if a person is diagnosed to have coronary artery disease at 25, he should be immediately screened for diabetes). In those with blood glucose values in IGT or IFG range, nonpharmacological measures to prevent diabetes should be immediately started. Depending on an individual case, if required, one of the pharmacological agents should be added to lifestyle measures. **Table 1** summarizes the designs and outcomes of major diabetes outcome studies.

## OTHER MEASURES TO PREVENT TYPE 2 DIABETES MELLITUS

The usual guidelines for screening for diabetes state that people above 40 (above 30 in India because we are more prone to develop diabetes at younger age), overweight, women with complicated pregnancies, those with family history of diabetes, etc., should be screened. The younger people having minimal probability of diabetes are excluded. The idea is to be cost-effective. But this strategy fails to pick up people before they become prediabetic. Thus, at a personal level, one should not wait to cross 30 or become overweight or have complicated pregnancy to get blood sugar testing. Preventive strategies should start before birth. Those born off women having malnourishment during pregnancy and during breastfeeding are more likely to become diabetic later. Thus malnourishment of women, particularly during child-bearing age should be prevented to prevent prediabetes and eventually diabetes in their offsprings. Chubby, overfed infants and children are more prone to develop diabetes later in life, thus excessive pampering in the form of overfeeding is to be avoided. The idea is to pick up prospective candidates for prediabetes before they become prediabetic, at a stage when their blood glucose is approaching higher limit of normal, before it crosses over to prediabetes range. For example, if somebody has a fasting blood glucose of 97 mg% and/or postprandial blood glucose of 134 mg% at young age of 27 years, he is the candidate to start strategies for prevention of prediabetes. Such approach to prevent diabetes by preventing prediabetes is known as primordial prevention.

## PREVENTION OF TYPE 1 DIABETES MELLITUS

As regards prevention of type 1 diabetes mellitus (T1DM), some preliminary progress has been made. It is now possible to identify potential patients by looking for certain specific markers of disease. Siblings of patients who have been recently diagnosed to have T1DM have increased chances of developing T1DM in future, if they have glutamate decarboxylase (GAD) antibodies or islet cell antibodies in their blood. Hence, in order to prevent development of T1DM, the siblings of recently diagnosed patients with T1DM could be screened for these antibodies and those who are positive could be treated for prevention of diabetes. Among the various drugs, nicotinamide, certain vaccines, low-dose injectable insulin, and oral insulin in capsule had shown some initial promise. However, further studies involving nicotinamide, low-dose injectable insulin as well as oral insulin in high-risk individuals failed to provide beneficial effects. Avoiding exposure to cow's milk in infancy is associated with lesser chances of developing T1DM in future. Recently, a drug called teplizumab, a CD3 antimonoclonal antibody, has shown promise. When administered to siblings of T1DM patients, who were positive for two or more types of antibodies, teplizumab was able to postpone the onset of full-blown T1DM for >2 years in significant number of participants as compared to those who received placebo. Though diabetes could not be prevented, the onset was more gradual and postponement by at least 2 years will help to improve quality of life due to postponement of complications. Teplizumab is already in the market for other indications and has received clearance from USA FDA for use in postponement of onset of T1DM in children aged 8 and above and in adults, on 17th November 2022. As regards inducing remission in those already detected to have T1DM, encouraging progress has been made. In short, even though the prospects of preventing T1DM are considerably more hopeful than a decade ago, formidable problems remain and another decade may pass before we have an acceptable, safe and inexpensive preventive treatment. However, rays of hope are definitely there.

# CHAPTER 28

# Instructions on Selfcare

## FOOT CARE IN DIABETES

Diabetics, particularly those who are long-standing and poorly controlled, are at increased risk to develop various foot complications such as infection, non-healing ulcers, and gangrene, as compared to the general population.

Atherosclerotic peripheral vascular disease leading to poor blood supply in the lower limbs, diabetic peripheral neuropathy leading to impaired sensation and increased susceptibility to infection are the main underlying factors, often operating together and responsible for increased prevalence of the abovementioned complications. In order to avoid these complications, diabetic patients should take meticulous care of their feet (like how a singer would take care of his/her throat, a young actor would take care of his face or a jeweler would take care of an expensive diamond). Of course, energetic and correct management of diabetes, the underlying disease, is equally important.

If a diabetic patient neglects his/her feet, complications gradually set in which could ultimately result in gangrene, requiring amputation. Prevalence of gangrene in the lower limbs is 17 times more common in diabetic patients as compared to nondiabetic patients.

In order to avoid these complications, a diabetic patient should implement the following advice:
- Wash the feet twice a day with mild soap and lukewarm (never hot) water.
- Dry the feet gently with a soft towel especially between the toes.

- If the skin is dry, apply a mild lubricant such as coconut oil, petroleum jelly (vaseline), or cold cream to feet, daily before retiring.
- Keep toenails neatly cut. Always cut straight across, do not cut close to the skin.
- Inspect the feet daily for cuts, blisters, boils, etc. Consult a doctor if required.
- Never walk barefoot.
- Never use a hot water bottle as local sensation might be impaired.
- In order to protect the toes, broad, soft canvas, or leather shoes should be used (avoid *chappals* or *sandals*).
- Gradually break into new shoes by wearing them for a short time to start with. Always buy new shoes in the evening when the foot size is the biggest. Avoid high-heel footwear.
- Use cotton socks only. Do not use socks having tight elastic on it as it will hamper circulation in the legs.
- Inspect the shoes for things like stones, nails, etc.
- Do not cut corns and calluses yourself. Consult your doctor.
- Do not apply strong chemicals to your feet.
- Take regular exercise, it improves blood circulation. Put your feet up when you are sitting. Move your toes up and down for 5 minutes 2–3 times a day. Also move your feet up, down, and inside-outside at ankle joint in similar manner.
- Avoid tobacco in any form.

## MIXING INSULIN

- Thoroughly wash your hands, cleanliness is important and helps prevent infections.

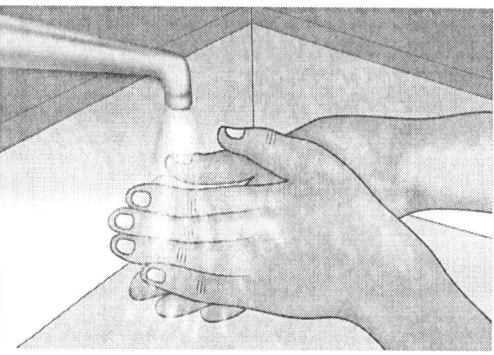

- Slowly roll the bottle of cloudy insulin (Huminsulin N, Mixtard, Insulatard, etc.) between your hands (do not shake). Make sure that the cloudy insulin is mixed completely and that there are no insulin crystals at the bottom of the bottle.

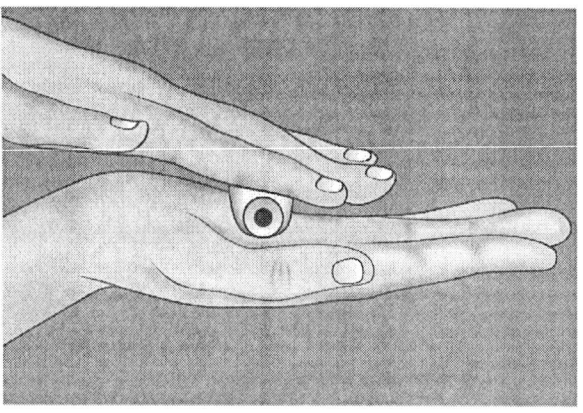

- Clean the rubber stopper of each bottle with spirit swab. For example, we are going to draw a total of 30 units of insulin, 20 units of cloudy insulin, and 10 units of regular (crystalline/plain) insulin (e.g., Huminsulin R, Actrapid).

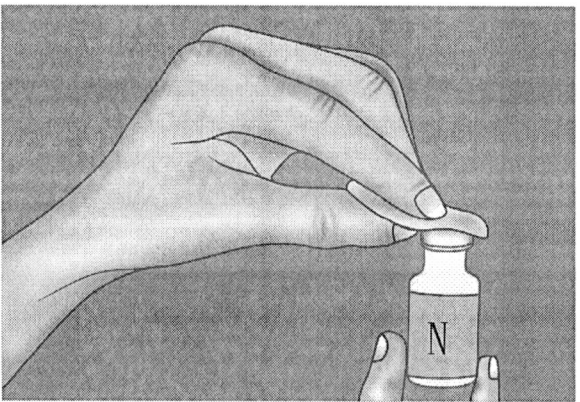

- First, draw air into the syringe to the dose of cloudy insulin. In our example, it is 20 units.

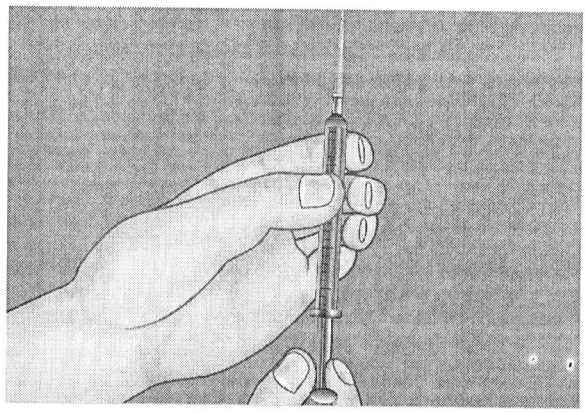

- Insert the needle through the stopper of the bottle of cloudy insulin and push 20 units of air into the bottle. Keep the bottle upright and remove the syringe. Do not draw any of the cloudy insulin yet.

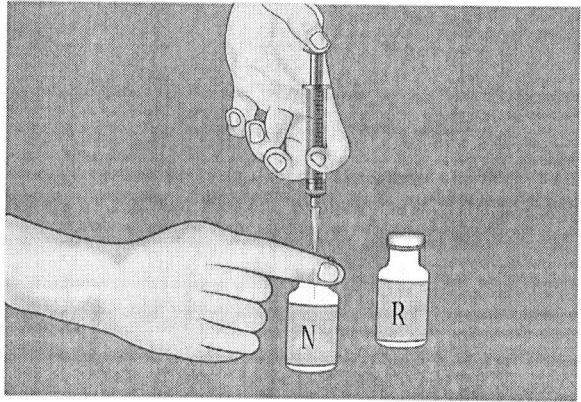

- Now fill the syringe with air equal to the number of units of clear insulin, i.e., 10 units. Insert the needle through the stopper of the regular insulin bottle and push the air into the bottle by pushing on the plunger.

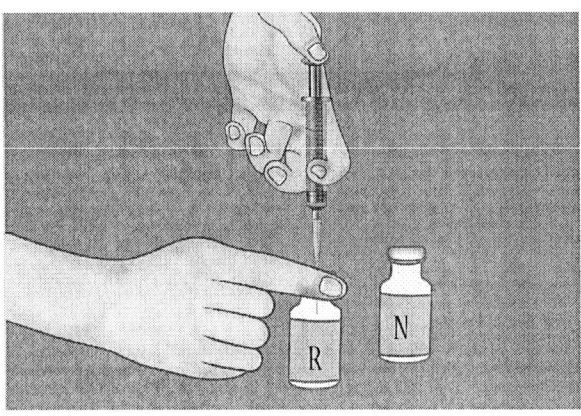

- Leave the needle in the bottle. Turn the bottle upside down. Pull down on the plunger to draw about 15 units of clear insulin, five more units than the 10 units we are using for our example.

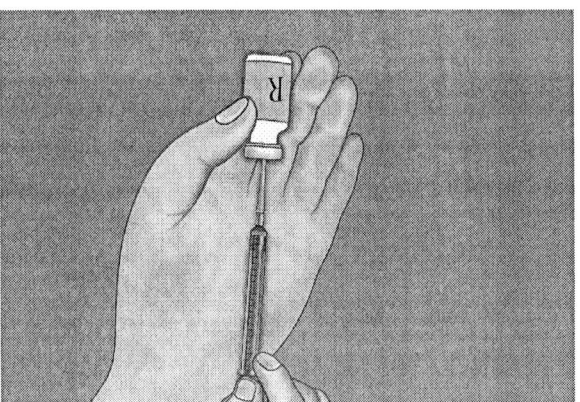

- With the needle still in the bottle, hold it up to the light and check it for air bubbles. If there are no air bubbles in your syringe, push the plunger to the 10-unit mark. Although, this air is not dangerous if injected, you should remove the bubbles from the syringe so that your insulin dose is accurate.

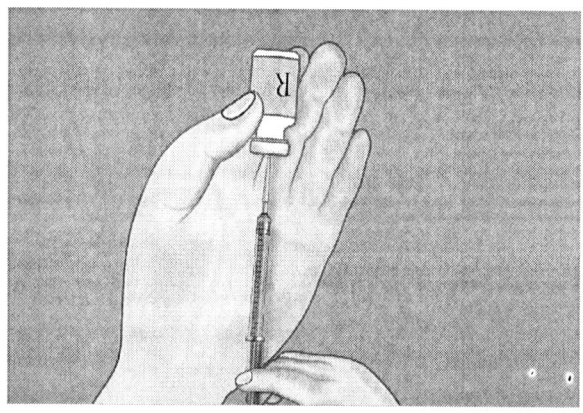

- To remove any air bubbles in the syringe, flick or tap the syringe at the site of the bubbles. This will push the bubbles to the top of the syringe. Push up on the plunger to force the bubbles back into the bottle and pull down on the plunger to draw the 10 units of clear insulin again.

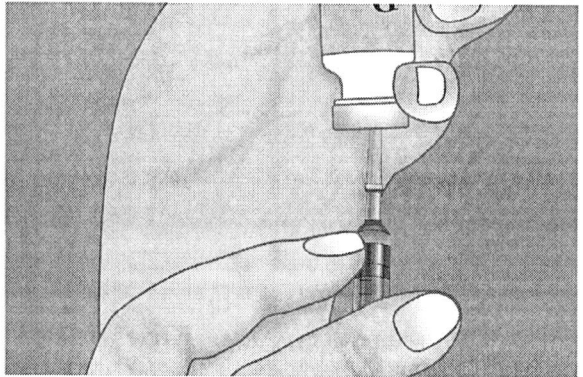

- No air bubbles should appear. If they do, repeat the flicking and pushing step until you draw 10 units of clear insulin without any bubbles. Remove the needle from the bottle, with 10 units of clear insulin in the syringe.

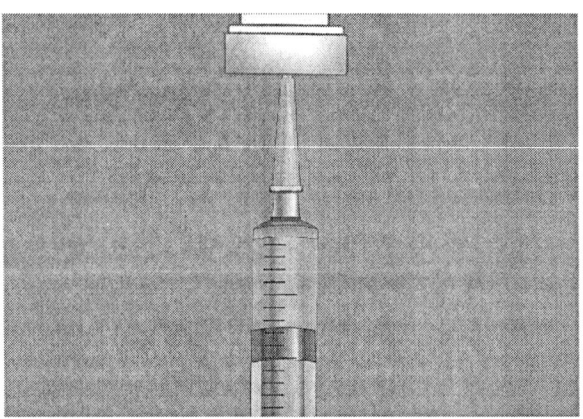

- Holding the bottle upside down put the needle through the stopper of the cloudy insulin. For this example, we are using 20 units of cloudy insulin. Do not push plunger. Since you already have 10 units of clear insulin in the syringe, you will pull the plunger out to the mark showing 30 units, the total of the two types of insulin. Remove the needle with the syringe from the bottle.

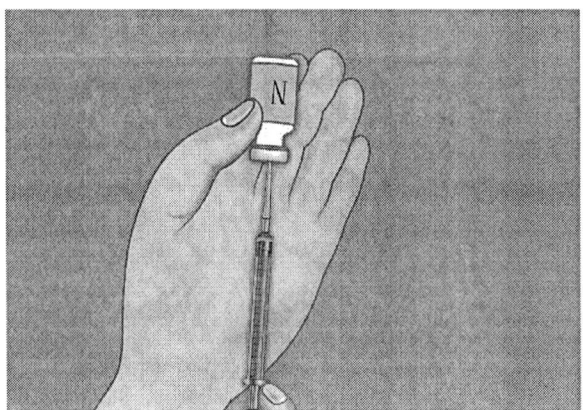

- Check again for bubbles. It is rare to see them at this step, but if you do, discard this syringe and start again at step 1.

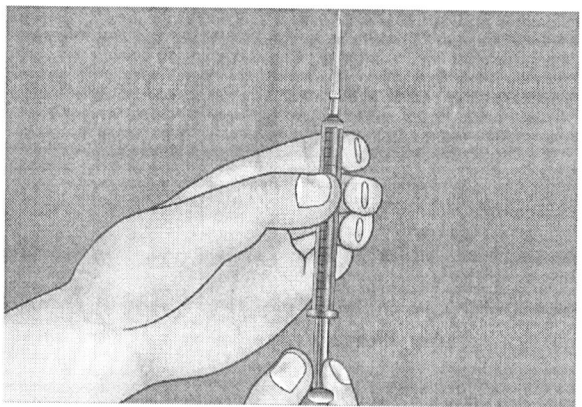

## CORRECT TECHNIQUE FOR SELF-INJECTION

- Wash your hands thoroughly with soap and water and apply spirit or isopropyl alcohol (which is available at the chemist) to the skin at the site of injection. Wait for a minute for the spirit/alcohol to dry up.
- Grip the syringe, and with the other hand pinch up a mound of skin.
- Hold the syringe at an angle of 60° to the skin.

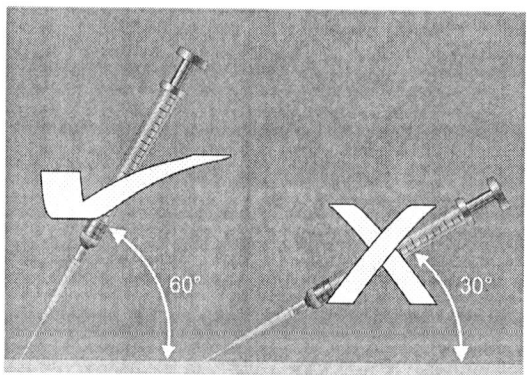

- Press the skin gently with the needle so that it "dimples".

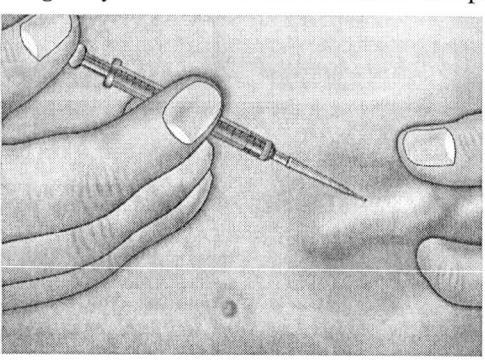

- Insert the needle to its full length.

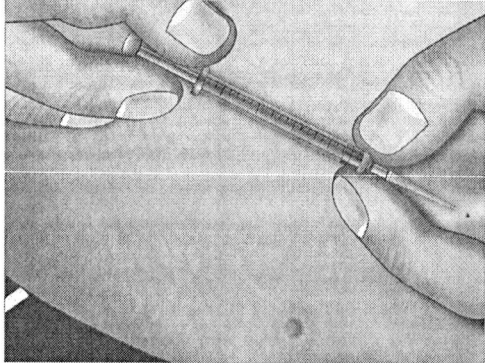

- Let go the skin and grasp the lower end of the syringe.

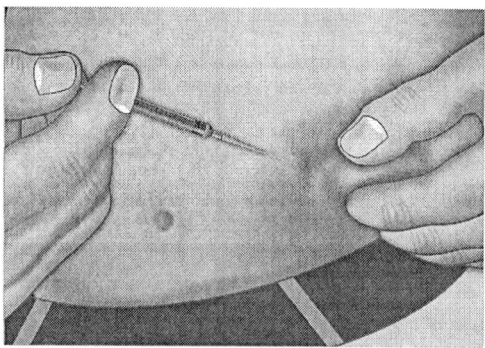

- With the other hand, gently raise the plunger a little way. If blood appears in the syringe, withdraw the needle and start again. If no blood appears, place your thumb on top of the plunger and inject insulin.

- Quickly withdraw the needle and press firmly over the injection site with a clean dry cotton swab for a few seconds. Do not rub.

## STEPWISE PROCEDURE FOR USING REUSABLE INSULIN PEN

1. Pull off the pen cap. Unscrew the pen apart.

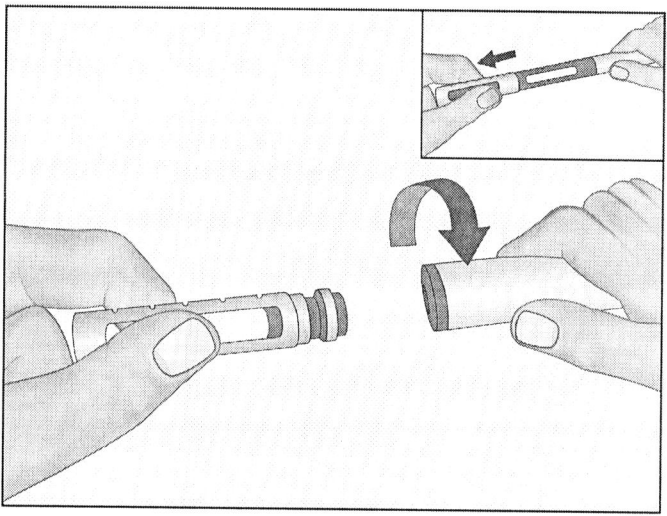

2. Press in the head of piston rod as far as it goes.

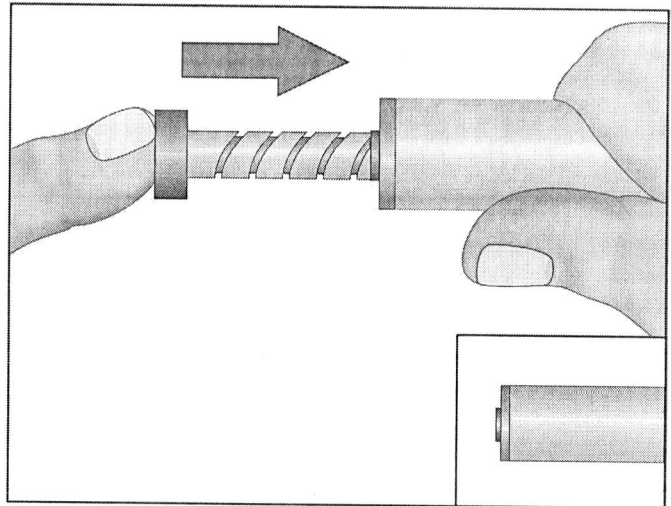

3. Insert insulin cartridge into the cartridge holder. Color-coded cap end goes in first.

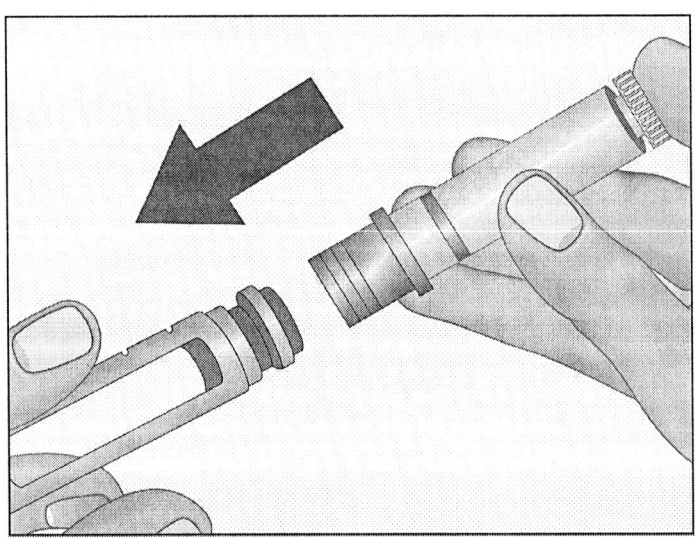

4. Screw together the two parts of insulin pen tightly till the click is heard. Subsequently, screw on insulin needle.

    *Note*: Before inserting cartridge of cloudy insulin (e.g., Mixtard, Novomix), roll it between the palms 20 times.

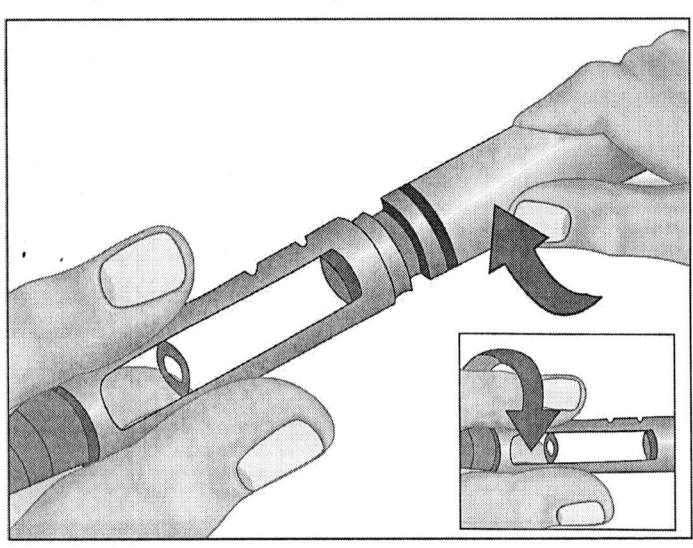

5. Prime the pen by pulling out dose button and turning it in clockwise manner to select 4 (4 units) in case of new cartridge, or 1 (1 unit) in case of cartridge already in use.

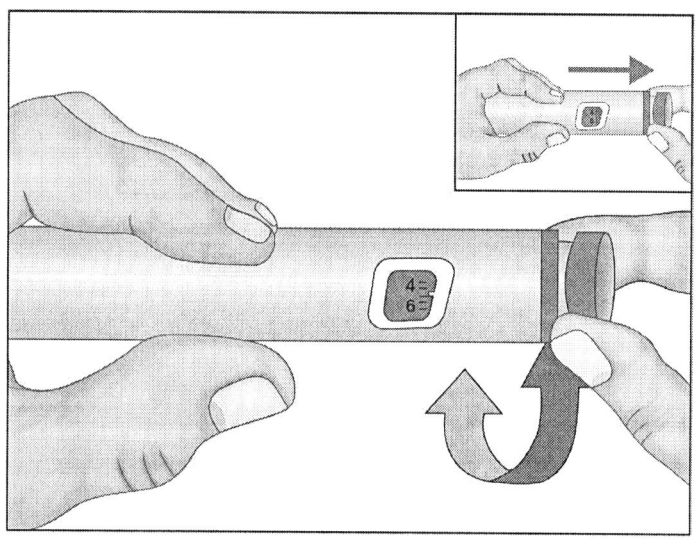

6. Hold the pen with needle facing upward and tap the cartridge holder to raise air bubble if any, to the top of the cartridge.

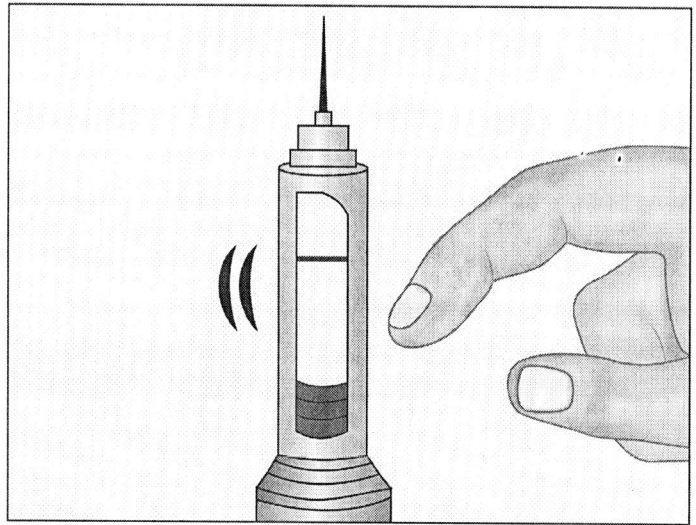

7. Press the dose button completely in until the dose display window shows O. Confirm that a drop of insulin has appeared at the tip of the needle. This confirms that the pen is now primed successfully and is ready for use. If a drop of insulin dose does not appear at the needle tip, repeat steps number 5-7 till a drop of insulin appears at the tip of needle. Now, the pen is ready for use.

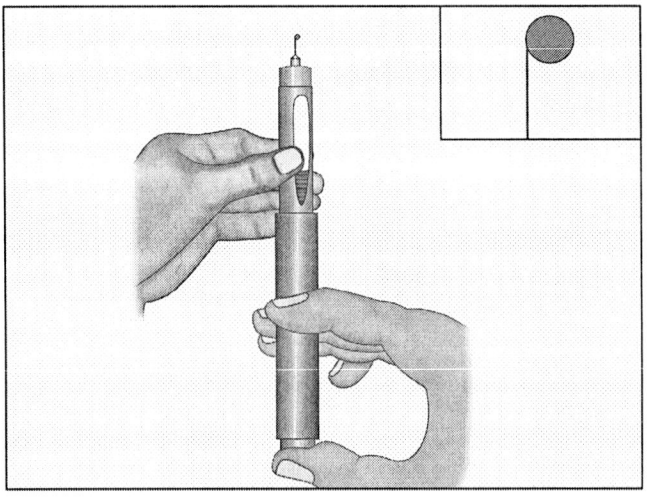

8. *Selecting the dose:* Pull out the dose button and rotate it clockwise till the required dose.

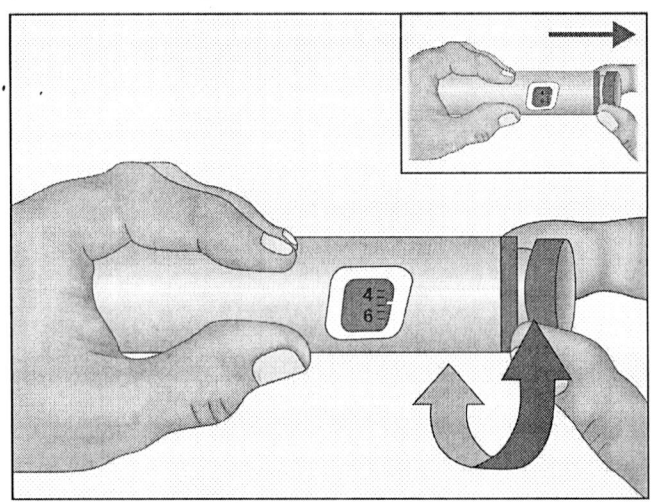

9. *Making the injection:* The actual injecting procedure and the sites of injection are the same for insulin injections through pen and syringes. To inject insulin through pen, press the dose button completely till the display shows 0 and you hear or feel a click. Subsequently, leave the needle under the skin for about 10 seconds. Then, withdraw the needle and replace the needle cap, followed by the pen cap. Please note that as per insulin manufacturer recommendations, the needle needs to be changed after each injection; however, in those who need to economize, the same needle can be used up to 5 times with proper hygienic care.

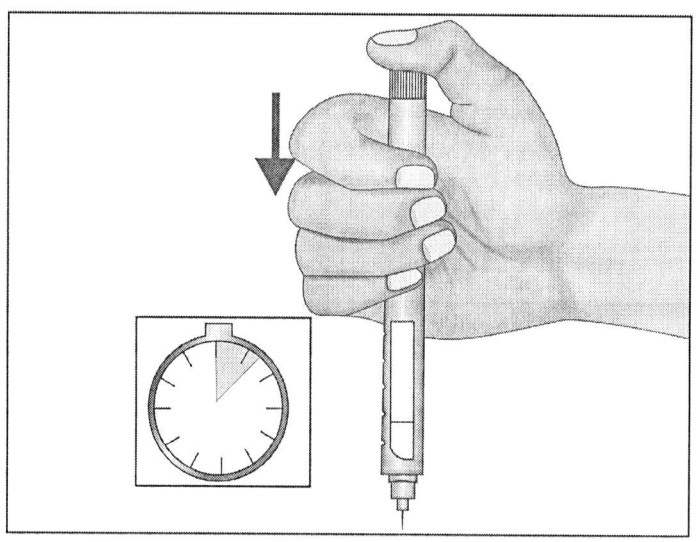

The procedure for injecting insulin from disposable pen is essentially same as that for reusable pen. Since disposable pen is available in ready-to-use form with insulin cartridge inserted at the manufacturer's level, first four steps described above are bypassed. This advantage of disposable insulin pen has to be traded with higher cost of insulin per unit.

*Note*: Today, there are several brands of insulin available in Indian market. Many of these brands are also available in forms suitable for pen devices along with the pens. Some brands are available with both the types of pens (disposable and reusable), while others are available in only one type of pen (disposable or reusable). Thus, there are many pens in market; each brand has its own branded pen. The exact operating procedure for a particular brand of pen may differ from the one described above, even though the basic principles are same. In case of difficulty, one should follow the specific instructions of the manufacturer of pen used by the patient.

## TIPS FOR PAINLESS INSULIN INJECTION

- Remove insulin vial/pen from refrigerator a few minutes before injection so that at the time of injection, temperature of insulin is more or less same as the room temperature.
- Wait for a minute after applying spirit or alcohol. Let alcohol evaporate before injecting.
- Use no. 32 needle for injecting insulin. Better still, use insulin pens for injecting insulin.
- Advance the syringe or pen in swift, linear manner, do not change the direction.

## WHAT ARE THE BEST PARTS OF THE BODY FOR INJECTION?

The best parts of the body for injection are those where a loose fold of flesh can be pinched up **(Fig. 1)**. Absorption speed is fastest from abdomen and slowest from the thigh, while absorption speed from arm is intermediate. Thus, one may prefer thigh for intermediate and long-acting insulin, abdomen for short- and rapid-acting insulin and arm for premixed insulin. Whichever part of body is used, you should vary the injection site each day, moving about 1 inch up or down and across. This is because an unsightly lump due to lipodystrophy will develop if you use the same spot repeatedly and because insulin is absorbed more slowly and unpredictably from such an area. Of course, with gradual shift toward using highly purified porcine insulin and subsequently human insulin, lipodystrophy is very uncommon nowadays.

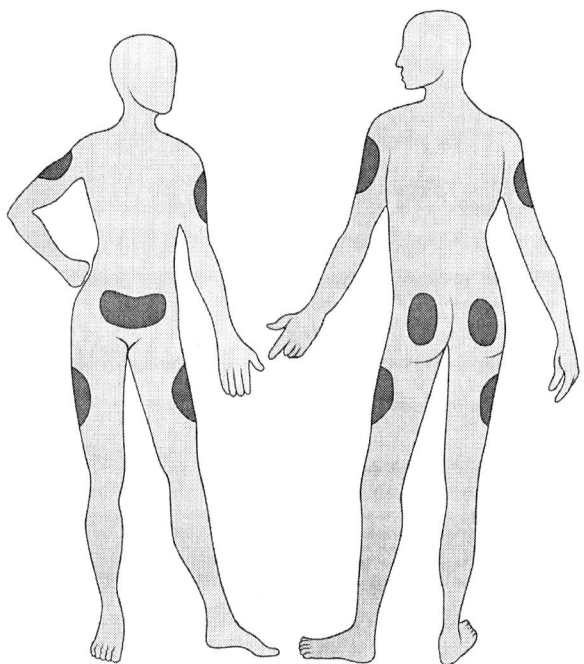

**FIG. 1:** Sites for insulin injection.

The injection site and your hands should be clean. The shaded circled areas **(Fig. 1)** depict best sites for insulin injection.

# Index

Page numbers followed by $b$ refer to box, $f$ refer to figure, $fc$ refer to flowchart, and $t$ refer to table.

## A

Abdominal distention 212
Abscess 242
Acarbose 134, 200
  role of 139
Acidosis 281
  diagnosis of 232
Acidotic breathing 229
Acromegaly 11
Acute coronary syndrome 146, 153
Acute kidney injury 289
Acute metabolic complications 219, 220
Acute respiratory distress syndrome 252, 288
Addison's disease 220
Adenosine triphosphate-sensitive potassium channels 117
Adiponectin 31
Adrenal hypertension 256
Advanced glycated end products 73
Advanced proliferative retinopathy, absence of 87
Adverse intrauterine environment 9
Albiglutide 145
Alcohol 211
  abstinence from 277
  consumption of 230
Aldosterone antagonists 263
Alogliptin 151, 153, 217
Alpha cell 140
  defect 8
Alpha-blockers 263
Alpha-glucosidase inhibitors 63, 115, 138, 139, 197, 212, 216
  combinations of 202

Alpha-methyldopa 264
Alternative insulin
  producing cell resources 310
  regimens 284
Amikacin 56, 235
Amino acid 312
Aminoglycoside antibiotics 56
Aminoglycosides 235
Amputations 78
Android obesity 33
Anemia 240, 252
Anesthesia 281
Anesthetic agents 281
Angina pectoris 262
Angiotensin receptor blocker 236, 260, 265, 266
Angiotensin-converting enzyme 255, 265
  inhibitor 259, 266
Antibiotic sensitivity 251
Antibody, types of 327
Antidiabetic agents 140, 160$f$, 160$t$, 217, 316
  synopsis of actions of 166$t$
Antidiabetic drug 36
  injectable 85
Antidiabetic medications 14, 209, 214, 290
  dosage of 221
  in renal impairment, prescribing 214
Antidiabetic therapy 222
Antidiuretic hormone 121
Antihyperglycemic agents 206
Antihypertensive agents 72, 265$t$
Antihypertensive drug class 261
Anti-insulin antibodies 11

Antiplatelet
  agent 235
  medications 72
Anxiety 221
Arginine 176, 312
Arterial thrombosis 288
Artificial pancreas 307, 319
  future of 309
  limitations of 308
Aspartame 106
Aspirin 211, 235
Atenolol 265
Atherogenic dyslipidemia 268
Atherosclerosis 79
Atherosclerotic cardiovascular
  disease 124, 156, 201, 269, 289
    prevention of 269
    disorders 241
Autoimmune diabetes, severe 15
Autonomic neuropathy 233
Awaiting hospitalization, treatment
  while 227
Azilsartan 260

## B

Back, large carbuncle on 244$f$
Bacterial culture 251
Bacterial infections 242
Balanced food 95
Bariatric surgery 40, 42
  indications for 40
  procedure 42
Basal insulin 176
Basal insulinization 173
Basal metabolic rate 86, 92
Behavioral therapy 36
Bempedoic acid 275
Beta-blockers 165, 262
  selective 262
Beta-cell 9, 117, 140, 147, 200, 219, 317
  defect 200
  failure
    end-stage 172
    progressive 117, 118$f$, 165

  function
    capacity of 175
    genetic defects of 11
Bevacizumab 235
Bicarbonates 231
Biguanide 115, 125, 128, 165, 196
  therapy 128
  use of 231
Biguanide-induced lactic acidosis
  129, 231
    prevention of 232
    symptoms of 231
    treatment of 232
Bile acid 316
  sequestrants 275
Biostator 307
Bisoprolol 263
Blood
  appears 336
  drop for test 68
  ketones 231
  urea nitrogen 282, 283
  vessels, overgrowth of 311
Blood glucose 41, 78, 220, 221, 228, 259, 307, 312
  control 113, 170
    postprandial 173
  data, storing self-monitored 69$t$
  estimating 231, 236
    technique 67
  estimation strip 307
    care of 67
  examination, timing of 65
  fasting 69, 173, 283, 326
  fluctuations 176
  interpretation, normal 57
  level 87
    average 60$t$
    control of 170
  lowering medications,
    combinations of 196
  monitoring of 227, 286
  periodically monitor 122
  postdinner 69
  postlunch 56, 69

predinner 69
prelunch 69
random 50, 62, 181, 220, 227
reduction of 323
self-monitoring of 65
values 48
Blood pressure 46, 71, 75, 80, 87, 254-256, 266
  apparatus 62
  classification of 256*t*
  diastolic 256
  monitoring 255
  systolic 44, 256
Body fat, comparison of 30*t*
Body mass index 14, 29, 32*t*, 33, 40, 46, 99
  category 36
Bon appétit 111
Bone marrow depression 121
Breast, carcinoma of 35
Breathing, rapid 129, 226
Bromocriptine 115, 116, 218
Bronchial asthma 128, 258
Buccal route 314
Bupropion 40

## C

C peptide levels, poststimulation 15
Calcium channel 261
  blocker 261, 265, 266
Calories 101-103, 111, 112
  spent per minute 89*t*
Camellia study 325
Canagliflozin 40, 154, 156, 158, 217, 260
Captopril 260
Carbohydrate 63, 95, 101-103, 108, 109, 140, 209
  counting 108
  insulin ratio 108
Cardiac arrhythmias 286
Cardiac decompensation 227
Cardiac failure 79, 252
Cardiac intervention 233
Cardiogenic shock 230

Cardiovascular disease 30, 275
  clock for 51
Cardiovascular outcome trials 146, 153
Cardiovascular system 252
Carvedilol 262, 263
Cataract extraction 280, 286
Cellulitis 242
Central obesity 33, 45, 46
  waist circumference 46
Centrally acting agents 116, 264
Cereal exchange 101
Cerebrovascular disease 79
Charcot foot 246
Cheiroarthropathy 246*f*
Chemical sympathectomy 281
Chlorides 231
Chlorthalidone 265
Cholecystectomy 280
Cholesterol 259
Chronic kidney disease 146, 153, 156, 290
Chronic obstructive pulmonary disease 231, 255
  severe 128
Cilnidipine 261
Classical acanthosis nigricans 19*f*
Classical neuropathic foot ulcer 250*f*
Clean and dry fingers properly 68
Clofibrate 165
Closed-loop delivery system 307
Cloudy insulin 330
  dose of 331
Cognitive impairments 208
Colesevelam hydrochloride 316
Colon, carcinoma of 35
Coma, ultimately 229
Communicable diseases 21
Complex carbohydrates, digestion of 212
Concentrated glargine 176
Congenital rubella 11
Congestive cardiac failure 258
Connective tissue
  complications 219
  disorders 245

Continuous glucose monitoring 162, 304*f*
  system 301, 305*b*
    applications of 305
  technology 60
Control blood glucose 172
Control cardiovascular risk, action to 81, 83
Conventional glargine 177
Conventional therapy 79
Convulsions 229
Coronary artery bypass graft 287
Coronary artery disease 47, 79, 266, 270, 271, 320, 325
  prevalence of 237
  primary prevention of 321
Coronary heart disease
  primary prevention of 271*f*
  risk of 269
  secondary prevention of 271*f*
Coronary revascularization 275
Coronavirus disease-2019 (COVID-19) 288, 290, 291, 298
  affects people 288
  and diabetes 288, 290
  effect of 292
  first case of 288
  incidence of 289
  infection, active 293
  mortality rate 288
  pandemic 294
  vaccination 293
  vaccine 293
Corticosteroids 11
Cotton swabs 63
Cow's milk 327
C-peptide levels, high 15
Creatine kinase 276
Cushing's
  disease 256
  syndrome 11

## D

Dapagliflozin 40, 154, 156
Deep breathing 129
Deep rapid acidotic breathing 231
Deficient diabetes 15
Degludec 177
Dehydration 226
  profound 229
Dermatitis, exfoliative 121
Detemir insulin 177
Dexamethasone, use of 287
Diabesity 29
  management of 36
Diabetes 40, 170, 219, 237, 254, 319
  action in 82
  and vascular disease, action in 74
  chemical-induced 11
  chronic complications of 233
  classification of 4*b*, 12
  clinic 7
  combination therapy in 196
  complications of 219, 233, 234, 306
  control 78
    and complications trial 50, 70, 73, 79, 83, 170, 234
  cumulative incidence of 321
  cure for 311
  development of 322, 325
  drug-induced 11
  during travel 295*f*
  epidemiology of 21, 83
  foot care in 328
  genetic syndromes with 11
  in clusters 14
  infections in 241
  intensive therapy for 83*t*
  interventions
    and complications, epidemiology of 70, 73
    epidemiology of 83
  long-standing 294
  long-term 295
  management of 84*f*, 170
  meal planning in 94
  mild age-related 15
  mild obesity-related 15
  musculoskeletal complications of 245
  pathophysiology in 171
  populations 163

prevalence of 21, 25, 26f, 213
prevention of 127, 133, 139, 208, 320, 323-325
primary prevention of 208, 320, 321
primordial prevention 320
reduction 324t
  assessment 133, 134, 322, 324
rheumatologic complications of 245
secondary prevention 320
tertiary prevention 320
types of 4, 11, 13, 282
Diabetes mellitus 1, 4, 45, 52, 57, 207, 249, 256
  cardiovascular risk in 268
  diagnosis of 49, 50, 55
  diagnostic test for 57
  epidemiology of
    type 1 23
    type 2 24
  management of 36, 78, 82, 85, 207, 209, 225, 226f, 287, 301, 309, 328
    type 1 315
    type 2 19, 158
  maturity onset 7
  postponement of type 2 321
  prevalence of
    type 1 24
    type 2 26
  prevent noninsulin-dependent 322, 324
  prevent type 2 326
  prevention of
    type 1 326
    type 2 134t, 323
  protein-deficient 13
  risk factors for type 2 9t
  type 1 2, 4, 7, 9, 10-12, 14, 17, 18, 20, 23, 29, 61, 73, 80, 83, 87, 117, 150, 152, 170, 317, 226, 254, 268, 289, 303, 305, 315, 317, 326
  type 2 2, 4, 5, 8, 17, 341f, 49, 71f, 72, 80, 82, 94, 113, 117, 118f, 134, 146, 156, 160t, 161fc, 165, 170, 180, 183, 197, 203, 207, 268, 269, 282, 303, 320, 324
Diabetes Prevention Program 127, 134, 321, 324, 325
Diabetic coma, differential diagnosis of 228t
Diabetic dyslipidemia 268, 272
Diabetic foot 7, 78, 248, 249, 253
  infested 250f
  lesions 253
  management of 251
  problems 209
  treatment of 248
Diabetic hypertensive 259
  treatment of 261
Diabetic ketoacidosis 5, 7, 12, 181, 286, 287
  and coma 171, 226, 229
  development of full-blown 292
  diagnosis of 227
Diabetic ketosis 54
Diabetic kidney 236
Diabetic nephropathy 78, 233, 236, 257
  hypertension without 257
  management of 235
  presence of 267
Diabetic neuropathy 233, 251
  management of 237
Diabetic osteoarthropathy 246
Diabetic patient 214
  surgery in 280
  treatment of 219
Diabetic peripheral neuropathy 328
Diabetic population 254
Diabetic retinopathy 78, 233
  management of 235
  prevention of 235
Diabetic stiff hand syndrome 245
Diabetics and suspected diabetics, investigations in 55
Diabetologist's holter monitor 302
Dialysis intervention 233
Dicumarol 165
Diet 94, 209

Dihydropyridine subclass 261
Diltiazem 261
Dimples 336
Dipeptidyl peptidase-4 inhibitor 114, 140, 146, 148, 153, 197, 212, 216, 217, 290
Disaccharides 140
Disposable insulin syringes 189
Disposable pen 341
Distal stomach 41
Dopamine agonists 115
Down's syndrome 11
Doxazosin 263
Drowsiness 129
Drug
  combinations, fixed-dose 202
  interactions 165, 211
  treatment 210
Dual-acting agents 115
Dual-energy X-ray absorptiometry 34
Dulaglutide 40, 142, 144, 145, 147
  cardiovascular protective effect of 144
Duodenum 41
Dupuytren's contracture 246
Dyslipidemia 40, 45, 269, 273$f$, 279
  management of 268, 269, 272
  type of 268
Dyspnea 129

## E

Edema 137
Efpeglenatide 145
Elastography 240
Electrocardiogram 56, 87
Electrolyte
  disturbances 286
  imbalance, correction of 226
Embryonic stem cell
  research 311
  therapy 319
Emerging antidiabetic agents 315
Emerging antiobesity formulations 318
Empagliflozin 40, 154-156

Enalapril 260
Endocrine disorders 11
Endometrial cancer 36
Enterobacter 249
Eplerenone 263
Erectile dysfunction 263
Ertugliflozin 156
*Escherichia coli* 249
Estimated glomerular filtration rate 128, 210, 215, 217, 218
Evogliptin 151
Exenatide 40, 141, 145, 147
Exercise 85, 210
  benefits of 86
  flexibility 93
  resistance 86, 92, 92$f$
  stretching 93
  type of 88, 89
Eye surgeries 280
Ezetimibe 274

## F

Fasting glucose
  impaired 9, 50, 52, 320
  normal 56
Fasting triglyceride concentration
  HDL concentration 46
Fasting venous plasma glucose 50
  level 50
Fats 34, 96, 101-104
Fatty acid 312
  essential 96
Febrile patient 228
Fenofibrate 278
Fiber 97
  water-insoluble 97
  water-soluble 97
Fibrocalculous pancreatic diabetes 11-13, 13$f$
Finerenone 236
Finnish diabetes prevention study 321, 324
Fluid deficit, correction of 226
Food exchange 101
Foot infections 249

Foot surgeries, types of 280
Fournier's gangrene 242
Frozen shoulder 246
Fructosamine test 60
Fruits 106
Fungal infection 78, 245
Furuncles 242

# G

Galactorrhea 158
Gallbladder disorders 35
Gangrene 78, 244*f*
Gangrenous cholecystitis 242*f*
Gastric banding, adjustable 41
Gastric emptying, delaying 140
Gastrointestinal side effects 38
Gastrointestinal tract 116
Gatifloxacin 211
Gemfibrozil 276, 278
Gene therapy 311
Genetic defects 11
Gentamicin 56, 235
Gestational diabetes mellitus 4, 11, 27, 52
   diagnosis of 51, 52*t*
   epidemiology of 27
   history of 321
   management of 119
   prevalence of 27*t*
Glargine 171, 194, 204, 206, 213, 300
Glibenclamide 116, 118, 120, 135, 208, 215
Gliclazide 116, 118-120, 210, 215
Glimepiride 116-118, 120, 153, 199, 210, 215
Glimepiride-metformin combination 202
Glimins 115, 116, 159
Glinides 123, 223
Glipizide 116, 118, 119, 215
Gliptins 115, 140, 144
Glitazones 115, 124, 130, 132-134
   sensitize tissues 130
Globesity 29

Glomerular filtration rate 215, 235
Glucagon
   antagonists 318
   high secretion of 172
   secretion, postprandial 140
Glucagon-like peptide-1 147
   agonists 1, 291
   levels, reduced 8
   receptor agonist 140, 141, 146, 148, 160, 212, 217
      advantages of 143
Glucokinase 317
   activators 317
   gene mutation 11
Glucometer 62-65
   good 67
   reliability of 64
   use of 62
Glucose 283
   absorption of 116
   blood levels of 259
   concentrations, diagnostic 52*t*
   estimated average 61
   infusion 286
   intolerance 45
   sucrose to 63
   tolerance test 50
      impaired 9, 50, 52, 127, 128
   urine for 227
   value 52
      storage of 304
Glucose-dependent
   enhancement 140
   insulinotropic
      peptide 41
      polypeptide 315
   suppression 140
Glucose-insulin 283
   potassium infusion 284
Glucose-sensitive insulin 313
Glucotoxicity 8
Glutamate decarboxylase 326
Glutamic acid decarboxylase 6, 19, 180
Glyburide 197

Glycated hemoglobin 14, 44, 71, 131, 165, 179, 181, 225*f*, 282, 283, 316
   lowering 234*f*
Glycemic control 82, 226*f*, 254, 292
   maintain 180
   reduces complications 71*t*
Glycemic derangement, management of 240
Glycemic index 107, 109*t*
Glycemic legacy, bad 76*f*
Glycemic threshold 221
Glycogenesis 317
Glycolysis 317
Glycosuria 227
Glycosylated hemoglobin 50, 57, 60*t*, 61
   estimation 56
Gynecoid obesity 33
Gynecomastia 236, 263

## H

HBA1C test, principles of 57
Healthcare professionals 248
Heart failure 160, 262
   congestive 254
   hospitalization for 156
   protection 237
Heart rate, maximal 90
Hemiplegia 229
Hemoglobin, glycation of 57
Hemorrhagic stroke 254
Hemostatic derangements 45
Hepatic failure, severe 180
Hepatic fibrosis 240
Hepatic impairment 123
Hepatic steatosis 317
Hepatocellular carcinoma 241
   development of 240
Hepatocytes 130
Home blood glucose monitoring, equipment required for 63
Human leukocyte antigens 24
Hydrochlorothiazide 265
Hygienic care, proper 341
Hyperaldosteronism, primary 256

Hyperbaric oxygen therapy 252
Hypercholesterolemia 316
Hyperglucagonemia, postprandial 8
Hyperglycemia 10*f*, 57, 66, 158, 223, 263, 281, 302
   control postprandial 173
   fasting 223
   pharmacologic treatment of 161*fc*
   rebound 223
   severe 6, 8, 227, 228, 281
Hyperkalemia develops 236
Hyperketonuria 281
Hyperlipidemia 206
Hyperosmolar nonketotic
   coma 181
   state 286
Hypertension 40, 45, 206, 238, 254, 256, 257, 262, 267, 289
   control of 235
   essential 257
   in diabetes, management of 258, 266*fc*
   meticulous control of 238
   pathogenesis of 254
   prevalence of 254
   renovascular 257
   severe 264
   stepwise management of 264
   supine 258
   surgically curable 256
   treatment of 259
   types of 256
Hypertriglyceridemia 277
   mild isolated 277
Hyperuricemia 45, 122, 286,
Hypoglycemia 62, 63, 66, 120, 122, 125, 140, 148, 175, 184, 205, 206, 208, 211, 214, 220-223, 225, 226*f*, 236, 281, 302, 307, 316, 317
   control 221
   correction of 221, 222
   diagnosis of 209, 220
   episodes of 176
   hormonal response during 221*t*
   management of 223

night-time 212
prevention of 87, 209, 201, 221
severe 220, 225, 225f
symptoms of 184, 190, 222t
treatment of 209
  severe 224
Hypoglycemic action, mild 278
Hypoglycemic coma, differential diagnosis of 228t
Hypotension 226, 230, 281, 286
  postural 264
Hypothyroidism 220, 276, 277

# I

Imeglimin 159
Immune-mediated diabetes 11
Incretin axis, agents acting through 116
Incretin physiology 140
Incretin-based therapy 140
Indapamide 265
Indian Diabetes Prevention Programme 322, 324
Infection 11
  associated 233
  common 242
  in diabetes, management of 245
  mixed 249
  prevalence of 241
  severe 292
Infective tissue complications 219
Inflammation 9
Inflammatory bowel disorders 139
Infusion fluid, selection of 285t
Infusion pump 284
Inhalation route 313
Injection, parts of body for 342
Insulin 1, 73, 88, 170, 180, 204, 205, 212, 216, 254, 292
  adequate 219
  administration of 226
    frequency of 203
  amount of 229
  analog 175, 311, 313
  cartridge 338
  clear 333
  coformulated 179
  dosage of 204, 223, 308
  dose of 285
  exogenous 195
  formulations 182
  gene therapy 319
  glargine 176
  human 342
  initiation 182
  injectable 314
  injecting 341
  intensification of 245
  intermediate-acting 174, 176, 183
  intranasal administration of 314
  large dose of 180, 186, 223
  long-acting 175, 177, 223, 296, 312
  manufacturer 341
  mixing 329
  molecules, novel 313
  newer 311
  peakless 176
  pharmacokinetics 178t
  pharmacology 172
  physiology 171
  prandial 213, 309
  premix 179
  prescribing 187
  pump 299, 306
  purchasing 191
  regimens 183
  release 182
  role of 170
  routes of administration of 313
  secretion 140
  sensitizer 199
  short-acting 172, 174, 184, 216, 285, 342
  strengths of 189
  subcutaneous 227, 285, 305
  synthesis 311
  therapy 282
    intensification of 181f
  treatment, initiation of 182
  twice-daily premixed 297

ultrarapid-acting 174
units of clear 332
vials, use 194
with oral antidiabetic drugs,
 combinations of 203
Insulin deficiency 15
 sever 15
Insulin delivery 305, 306
 systems 306
Insulin infusion 284
 rates 284*t*
Insulin injection 173
 sites for 343, 343*f*
 technique 187
Insulin mixtures 178
 limitation of 179
 ready-made 171
Insulin pen
 reusable 337
 use 194
Insulin plus 205
 alpha-glucosidase inhibitor
 combination 205
 metformin combination 204
 pioglitazone combination 205
 sulfonylurea 204
Insulin requirement
 moderate 175
 variability of 312
Insulin resistance 15, 198, 214, 257
 syndrome 47*f*
 high 15
 syndrome of 45
Insulin secretagogue 115, 116
 therapy 222
Insulin-deficient diabetes, severe 15
Insulin-dependent diabetes mellitus
 4, 5
Insulin-resistant
 diabetes, severe 15
 obese diabetes 15
Intensive glycemic control 71*f*
International Diabetes Federation 46
Interstitial fluid glucose 302
Intestinal mucosa 116
Intraglomerular pressure 258

Irbesartan 260
Iris study 135
Irrational combinations 203
Ischemic heart disease 282
Islet cells transplantation 310
Isopropyl alcohol 335
Itching 7, 18

## J

Jaundice, cholestasis type of 121
Jejunal bypass 41
Joint national committee 255
 guidelines 256*t*
Juvenile diabetes 4

## K

Ketoacidosis 4, 12, 227
Ketones, urine examination for 54
Ketosis 10
Kidney 233
 disease, end-stage 156
 functions, assessment of 282
 transplantation 236
*Klebsiella* 249

## L

Lactic acidosis 128, 230, 231, 283
Latent autoimmune diabetes 6
Left ventricular failure 286
Legacy effect 70, 72
Leprechaunism 11
Leptin deficiency 31
Lethargy 18
Leucocytosis, persistence of 251
Lifestyle modifications 322
Linagliptin 150, 151, 153, 217
Lipid
 levels 71
 profile 55
Lipid-lowering agents 274
Lipoprotein cholesterol
 high-density 15, 44, 46, 48, 86, 277
 levels 15
 levels, low high-density 268

low high-density 238
low-density 44, 75, 86, 136, 238, 268-271
  level of 269*t*
  very-low-density 86
Liraglutide 38, 40, 142, 144, 145, 147
  cardiovascular protective effect of 144
  formulation 39
Lisinopril 260
Liver
  cirrhosis of 240
  concentrate in 313
  fatty infiltration of 239
Lixisenatide 142, 145, 147
Lobeglitazone 130, 137, 138
  indications of 138
Lorcaserin
  cardiovascular effects of 324
  metabolic effects of 324
Lower body obesity 33, 34
Lower limb complications, etiology of 249

## M

Macroalbuminuria 260
Macrovascular complication 170, 233
  progression of 80
Macrovascular disease 71, 79, 206, 237, 259, 320
  management of 238
Major adverse cardiovascular events 146, 153, 156
Masked hypertension 255
Maturity-onset diabetes of young 10, 11
Meal planning 94, 107
  chart 111*t*
Mean blood glucose 60
Meat exchange 102
Medicated spirit 63
Memory deteriorate 209
Metabolic control 220, 234
  criteria for 162*t*
  expressing 61

Metabolic memory 70
  effect 72
  hypothesis 73*t*
  pathogenesis of 73
Metabolic status, deterioration of 251
Metabolic surgery 40
Metabolic syndrome 9, 45-47, 239, 323
  controversy on 48
  diagnosis of 46
  diagnostic criteria for 46*t*
  management of 48
  prevalence of 46
Metabolic tissue complications 219
Metformin 73, 125-128, 134, 136, 160, 198-200, 201, 205, 211, 215, 230, 231, 290, 322
  addition of 204
  mechanism of action of 201
  monotherapy 136
  plus 200, 202
    pioglitazone, combination of 199
  role of 127
  therapy 211
    complication of 290
Metformin-sulfonylurea combination 198
Methyl alcohol 63
Metoprolol 263, 265
Microalbuminuria 45, 259, 260
Microtrauma 247
Microvascular complication 170, 233, 237
  progression of 80
Microvascular disease 233, 234
Mineralocorticoid receptor antagonists 263, 265
Minerals 98
Minor surgical procedures 285
Moderate-intensity statin therapy 274*t*
Monogenic diabetic syndromes 11
Monotherapy 139, 197
Monounsaturated fats 96

Morbid obesity 32
Muscle pains, severe 276
Musculoskeletal complications 233
Myocardial infarction 79, 181, 286
   nonfatal 275

# N

Naltrexone 40
Namaste position 246
Namaste sign 246*f*
   positive 246
Nasal insulin 314
Nasal route 314
Nateglinide 123
National Cholesterol Education
   Program 46
National diabetic associations 107
National Glycohemoglobin
   Standardization Program 50
Nausea 317
Nebivolol 263
Necrotizing fasciitis 242
Neonatal diabetes 11
Nephropathy 71
   advancement of 260
   high prevalence of 15
Nephrotoxic drugs 56
Neuroglycopenic symptoms 222
Neuropathic arthropathy 246
Neuropathy 71, 74
Neutral protamine hagedorn 204
New antiobesity agents 38
Nicotinamide 312
Nitric oxide synthase 74
Nonalcoholic fatty liver disease 131, 233, 239, 276
   diagnosis of 240
   management of 241
Nonalcoholic steatohepatitis 240
   management of 130
Non-antidiabetic agents 241
Nonfetal stroke 275
Noninjectable insulin preparations 315
Noninsulin antidiabetic agents, sites of action of 115*f*
Noninsulin-dependent diabetes mellitus 2, 7
Nonketotic hyperosmolar hyperglycemia
   management of 229
   state 228
Nonpharmacological treatment 272
Nonsteroidal anti-inflammatory drugs 56, 157, 165, 211, 235
Nonsulfonylurea
   insulin secretagogues 123, 216
   secretagogues 203
Normoalbuminuria 260

# O

Obesity 9, 15, 32, 33, 35, 158, 289
   disorders with 35
   mild 32
   onset of epidemic of 29
Obeticholic acid 241
Obstructive disorders 139
Obstructive sleep apnea 36
Olmesartan 260
Omarigliptin 318
Omega-3 fatty acids 96, 241
Omega-6 fatty acids 96
Open-loop delivery system 306
Oral antibiotics 251
Oral anticoagulants 211
Oral antidiabetic agent 113
   therapy 113
Oral antidiabetic drugs 1, 19, 51, 72, 85, 113, 134, 134*t*, 159, 181, 196, 238
   clinical applications of 159
   development of 113
Oral antidiabetic medications, combinations of 196
Oral glucose tolerance-plasma glucose 52
Oral insulin 314, 327
   development of 314
Oral pills 88
Oral semaglutide 40, 113, 145, 147
Orlistat 38

Orthostatic hypotension 258
Osteoarthritis 36
Overweight 9, 32, 33, 100

## P

Painless insulin injection 342
Pancreas 140
Pancreatic diabetes 12
Pancreatic transplantation 309
Pancreatitis 11
Parenteral antibiotics 245
Pathogenic flora 251
PCSK9 inhibitors 275
Pedal edema 261
Pens, types of 341
Periodic lipid profile estimation 279
Peripheral vascular disease 79, 261
Peripherally acting agents 116
Peroxisome proliferator-activated receptor gamma 130
Pharmacological agents 258
Pharmacotherapy 36-38
Phentermine 39
 plus topiramate 323
Phentermine-topiramate 324
 combination 323
Pheochromocytoma 256
Physical activity 100$t$
Physical disabilities, degrees of 208
Physical exercise 210
Physiologically glucose sensors 308
Pioglitazone 114, 130, 131, 134, 199, 200, 205, 212, 216, 291, 323
 acts 199
 combinations 199
Piston rod, head of 337
Placebo 322
Plasma
 lactate 231
 osmolarity, high 229
Plasma glucose 52
 fasting 46, 52, 181
 post-lunch 192
 postprandial 181
Pneumonia 7, 78
 severe 288

Polycystic ovary syndrome 9
Polydipsia 7, 18, 50
Polyethylene tubing 306
Polygenic inheritance 10
Polymorphonuclear leukocytes 241
Polyphagia 7
Polyunsaturated fats 96
Polyuria 7, 18, 50
Poor metabolic control 223
Poorly controlled patients, emergency surgeries in 287
Porcine insulin 171
Postmyocardial infarction 262
Postprandial blood
 glucose 174, 283, 326
  levels 174
Postural hypotension, control of 237
Potassium 259, 263
 channels 317
Potential hepatotoxicity 323
Pramlintide 316
Prazosin 263
Prediabetes 323, 326
 prevalence of 25, 26$f$
Pregnancy
 and lactation 139
 complicated 326
Primary combination therapy 197
Primordial prevention 326
Protein 96, 101-103
 kinase C 73
*Proteus* 249
Pulses and dal exchange 101
Pumps 305

## Q

Quick-release bromocriptine 158
 tablets 158

## R

Ramipril 72, 133, 134, 259, 260, 322, 324
Ranibizumab 235
Rapid-acting insulin 216, 342
 analogs 173, 213

Reaven's syndrome 45
Regimen
   basal-bolus 183
   basal-only 183
   basal-plus 183
Remogliflozin 154, 155
Renal artery angioplasty 257
Renal disease, diet in 218
Renal failure 276, 277, 289
   end-stage 236
   severe 180
Renal impairment 208, 252
   classification of 218$t$
   DPP4IS in 217$t$
   severity of 214
Renal insufficiency 236
Renal protection, degree of 261
Renal transplantation 287
Renin–angiotensin–aldosterone system 237, 260
Repaglinide 123, 203, 204, 222
   combinations of 200
Retinopathy 71, 74
   high prevalence of 15
Rheumatological complications 247
Right foot abscess 244$f$
Roots and tubers 103
Rosiglitazone 114, 130, 133-136, 322, 324
Routine tests 65
Roux-en-Y gastric bypass 41
   surgery 41

## S

Salicylates, large doses of 165
SARS-CoV-2 virus 289
Saturated fat 96
Saxagliptin 114, 150, 153, 217
Scrotum, Fournier's gangrene of 243$f$
Sedentary lifestyle 9
Selfcare, instructions on 328
Self-injection, correct technique for 335
Semaglutide 140, 143, 319
   injection 144, 145

Septicemia 180, 252
Serum
   creatinine 55, 231, 282
   glutamic-oxaloacetic transaminase 132, 276
   glutamic-pyruvic transaminase 132, 239, 276
*SHIP2* gene 311
Shock 230
   septicemic 230
Sirtuin-1 deacetylase 318
Sirtuins 318
Sitagliptin 147, 153, 217
Skin infection 78, 242
Smartphones 307
Smoking, cessation of 273
Sodium 231
   bicarbonate 232
Sodium-glucose cotransporter-2
   enzyme 9
   inhibitor 40, 54, 152, 160, 185, 201, 217, 236, 291
Sodium-glucose transport protein 2
   inhibitor 156
Soft tissue infection 78, 242
SOS tests 66
Spironolactone 235
Statin 11, 72
   indications for 274
Statin therapy 276
   high-intensity 274$t$
   monitoring of 275
Statin–ezetimibe combination, indications of 274
Stethoscope 62
Stevens-Johnson syndrome 121
Stock-keeping units 202
Stop-noninsulin-dependent diabetes mellitus 134
Stress 122, 292
   hyperglycemia, temporary 292
Stroke 79, 286
Sucralose 106
Sucrose 95
Sugar substitutes 106

Sulfonamides 211
Sulfonylurea 40, 73, 116, 122, 123, 160, 185, 198, 203, 205, 210, 211, 215, 222, 223, 291
   long-acting 208
   pharmacokinetics of 118$t$
   therapy 114, 211
   with metformin, combination of 198
Sulfonylurea plus 202
   metformin
     combination 199
     limitations of 199
   pioglitazone combinations 199
Superimposed glucose graphs 304$f$
Suprachiasmatic nuclei, agent acting on 116
Surgery 36
   and anesthesia, metabolic effects of 281
Sweating 221
Switching off metabolic memory 74
Syndrome X 45

## T

Tachycardia 262
Teneligliptin 151, 217
Teplizumab 327
Thiazide 11
   diuretics 259, 260
Thiazolidinediones 114, 115, 130, 131, 160
Thrombocytopenia, severe 293
Thyrotoxicosis 11
Tiredness 18
Tirzepatide 315, 316
Tissue
   glucose concentrations 306
   hypoxia, severe 230
   perfusion, inadequate 281
Topiramate 39
   oral combination 39
Total insulin dose, one-third of 285
Travel and diabetes 294

Trelagliptin 318
Tremors 221
Tricyclic antidepressants 211
Triglyceride 15, 275, 278
Tris-hydroxymethyl aminomethane 232
Troglitazone 322, 323
Troublesome cough 260
Tuberculosis 7, 78, 180, 242
   disseminated 226
Typical butterfly rash 273$f$

## U

Ultrasound 13
Underweight 100
Upper abdominal discomfort 129, 231
Upper body obesity 33, 34
Upper gastrointestinal tract 314
Uric acid levels 259
Urinary albumin 236
   excretion 259
Urinary glucose, sodium salicylate on 113
Urinary ketone 228
Urine 231
   glucose 228
     estimation, limitations of 52
   ketones 228
Ursodeoxycholic acid 241

## V

Valsartan 260
Vascular disease 82
Vascular tissue complications 219
Vegetables
   A group 103
   B group 103
Venous plasma glucose 58
Verapamil 261
Vertical sleeve gastrectomy 42
Veterans Affairs Diabetes Trial 75, 82, 83
Vildagliptin 114, 149, 217

Visceral abdominal fat  31
Vital fatty acids  96
Vitamin  98
  A  241
  E  241
Vitrectomy intervention  233
Vitreoretinal surgeries  280
Vomiting  231
  occasional  317

## W

Waist circumference  46, 99

Waist-hip ratio  46
Water  98
Weakness  7
Weight gain  137, 148
  sulfonylurea-induced  120
Weight loss  7, 18, 50
  goals, setting  36
White-coat hypertension  267
Wound healing  249, 252

## X

X-ray chest  56